# 1 MONTH OF
# FREE
## READING

### at

### www.ForgottenBooks.com

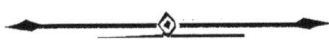

By purchasing this book you are eligible for one month membership to ForgottenBooks.com, giving you unlimited access to our entire collection of over 1,000,000 titles via our web site and mobile apps.

To claim your free month visit:
www.forgottenbooks.com/free795491

ISBN 978-0-483-69030-1
PIBN 10795491

This book is a reproduction of an important historical work. Forgotten Books uses state-of-the-art technology to digitally reconstruct the work, preserving the original format whilst repairing imperfections present in the aged copy. In rare cases, an imperfection in the original, such as a blemish or missing page, may be replicated in our edition. We do, however, repair the vast majority of imperfections successfully; any imperfections that remain are intentionally left to preserve the state of such historical works.

THE

# AMERICAN PRACTITIONER:

A MONTHLY JOURNAL OF

## MEDICINE AND SURGERY.

EDITED BY

### DAVID W. YANDELL, M. D.,

Professor of the Science and Art of Surgery and Clinical Surgery, University
of Louisville.

AND

### THEOPHILUS PARVIN, M. D., LL. D.,

Professor of Obstetrics and Diseases of Women and Children, in the College of
Physicians and Surgeons of Indiana.

LOUISVILLE:

JOHN P. MORTON AND COMPANY,

PUBLISHERS.

# LIST OF CONTRIBUTORS.

RICHARD C. BRANDEIS, M. D.

G. V. BLACK, M. D.

R. F. BLOUNT, M. D.

SAMUEL R. BURROUGHS, M. D.

WILLIAM CARSON, M. D.

W. J. CARTER, M. D.

JAMES R. CHADWICK, M. D.

C. G. COMEGYS, M. D.

JOHN L. COOK, M. D.

A. G. CRAIG, M. D.

E. P. EASLEY, M. D.

E. T. EASLEY, M. D.

C. S. FENNER, M. D.

E. D. FORÉE, M. D.

E. P. GILPIN, M. D.

HON. J. W. GORDON.

HENRY JAMESON, M. D.

W. H. JORDAN, M. D.

G. W. H. KEMPER, M. D.

B. D. KEATOR, M. D.

J. E. LOCKRIDGE, M. D.

T. D. MANNING, M. D.

JAMES D. MAXWELL, M. D.

W. N. McCOY, M. D.

GEORGE N. MONETTE, M. D.

THEOPHILUS PARVIN, M. D.

A. J. SMITH, M. D.

GEORGE SUTTON, M. D.

W. W. VINNEDGE, M. D.

I. C. WALKER, M. D.

DAVID W. YANDELL, M. D.

LUNSFORD P. YANDELL, M. D.

# INDEX.

## Original Communications.

*14690*

## *Reviews.*

## *Clinic.*

## *Notes and Queries.*

# THE AMERICAN PRACTITIONER.

## JULY, 1876.

Certainly it is excellent discipline for an author to feel that he must say all that he has to say in the fewest possible words, or his reader is sure to skip them; and in the plainest possible words, or his reader will certainly misunderstand them. Generally, also, a downright fact may be told in a plain way; and we want downright facts at present more than any thing else.—Ruskin.

## Original Communications.

## NOTES ON THE LIFE AND WRITINGS OF DR. BENJAMIN RUSH.*

### BY LUNSFORD P. YANDELL, M. D.

Dr. Benjamin Rush, at the close of the last century, was not only the most noted medical man in the new world, but was absolutely without a rival to dispute his title to supremacy. He was at once the first writer, the first teacher, and the foremost practitioner of his time in America. During the generation to which he belonged he was more read and oftener quoted, not only than any other American physician, but than all our other medical authors put together. The fame of his writings and teachings, it may be said without exaggeration, filled the land, and his name was upon the lips of the people as well as of physicians. His name, by common consent, has been placed among the worthies of the profession, as one which the world will not willingly let die; but it may well be asked, who now reads his works? There they repose on the shelves of our libraries, gathering cobwebs and dust, beside the works of Sydenham and Cullen, hardly more

* Read before the Louisville Academy of Medicine.

disturbed by readers than the volumes of Boërhaave, Galen, or Hippocrates.

The works of Rush deserve a better fate than this. With text-books, mere manuals, systems of medicine, mutability is the law; they are necessarily short-lived. In a science constantly advancing, like medicine, the system of one age is insufficient for the next, and must yield to others embracing a fuller history of the subject; but the "Inquiries" of our great philosopher abound in original observations, in accounts of epidemics witnessed by himself, in suggestive facts, and bold, ingenious conjectures, which have a lasting interest. I propose to spend an hour, this evening, in a review of some of these, in the hope that I may thereby excite in some of you a curiosity to know more about the labors of this illustrious physician.

Dr. Rush was elected Professor of Chemistry in the Pennsylvania College, now University of Pennsylvania, in August, 1769, when only twenty-three years old, and a little more than a year after taking the degree of M. D. at the University of Edinburgh. And hardly had he entered upon his duties as teacher before he commenced his career as author, for the following year he published a number of "Sermons," as he styled them, written for young men on the subject of temperance and health. But while yet a student he recorded in his diary observations on the yellow fever which desolated Philadelphia in 1762, and these memoranda afford almost the only notices preserved of that epidemic. He loved to write, and urged upon his pupils the great advantage of making notes of all they read or saw, repeating to them often the maxim, *legere sine calamo est somnere.* Though engaged nearly nine years in the study of his profession, we have his own declaration that he never wasted a day in idle or frivolous amusements.

In 1774 he began to prepare those papers which gave him rank at once among the philosophers of his day, and which now are correctly looked upon as the beginning of our medical literature. The first was read as an anniversary oration before the American Philosophical Society, of which Jefferson and Franklin were members. Its subject is the Natural History of Medicine among the Indians of North America. It is a truly remarkable paper, in which every class of readers will find matter to interest and instruct. Its style is fresh, easy, and singularly pleasing. We meet with opinions in which we may not concnr, but the graceful flow of his language must captivate all, as in the following passage: "Some of you may remember the time, and our fathers have told those of us who do not, when the diseases of Pennsylvania were as few and as simple as those of the Indians. The food of the inhabitants was then simple; their only drink was water; their appetites were restrained by labor; religion excluded the influence of sickening passions; private hospitality supplied the want of a public hospital; nature was their only nurse, temperance their principal physician."

In 1780 he wrote an account of a bilious remitting fever as it appeared in Philadelphia that year, and which has since often been described under the term "dengue or break-bone fever." In some cases it was ushered in with coma; in many it was introduced by delirium, and in not a few it was fatal. I may mention, as showing how this disease varies in character, at different periods and places, that I saw it in Memphis, in the autumn of 1860, when out of many thousand persons attacked by it, I believe only a single one died. A distinguishing symptom first noticed by Dr. Rush, which I experienced in my own case and remarked in every instance, was extreme dejection of spirits during the convalescing stage. A young lady, with great feeling, said to Dr. Rush that she thought the complaint "ought to be called break-heart rather than break-bone fever." By giving a gentle vomit of tartar emetic in the forming stage, he says he frequently produced an immediate cure; and in every instance the patient found relief from the pains in the head and limbs by emetics and gentle purgatives. He continues: "I constantly recommended to my patients to lie in bed. Persons who struggled against the fever by sitting up, or who attempted to shake it off by labor or exercise, either sunk under it or had a slow recovery." Sometimes dysenteric symptoms accompanied the fever, when he used opium with good effect; and this leads him to remark that "those physicians enjoy little pleasure in practicing physic who know not how much of the pain and anguish of fevers, of a certain kind, may be lessened by the judicious use of opium."

No remedy is so intimately associated with the name of Rush as blood-letting. His use of the lancet brought great obloquy upon him in his lifetime, and his devotion to the lancet, it was charged by some of his contemporaries, amounted to insanity. And yet, in the fever under consideration, he never resorted to it. "Out of several hundred patients whom I visited," he remarks, "I did not meet with a single case in which the lancet was indicated by the state of the pulse, which was generally full, but never hard;" and he adds that he heard of several cases in which bleeding was followed by fatal results.

Scarlatina, of which he gives an account in the same volume of his Inquiries, appeared to him quite amenable to treatment, "a vomit of ipecacuanha or tartar emetic, mixed with a few grains of calomel, never failing completely to check the disorder in its forming stage," or so far mitigate its violence as to dispose it to a favorable issue in a few days. And he even held that "when the contagion of this disease has been received into the body, a purge has prevented its being excited into action, or rendered the disorder mild throughout a whole family."

His views in regard to cholera infantum were most just. He was fully persuaded that summer fruits had no agency in developing the complaint. His remedies were, first, an emetic, then opiates, the cold bath, and, above all, country air.

Membranous croup, like scarlet fever, he regarded as altogether under the control of medicines. "The bark," he declared, "is scarcely a more certain remedy for intermittents than calomel is in this species of cynanche."

Speaking of intermittent fever, he says he had found that where bark did not succeed after three or four days' trial, the application of blisters to the wrists often rendered it effectual; but that where, from any cause, the disease was protracted into the winter months, he generally cured it by one or two moderate bleedings. He continues: "I have known several instances in which pounds of bark have been taken without effect, in which the loss of ten or twelve ounces of blood has immediately cured the disorder."

On no subject, perhaps, have the therapeutics of Dr. Rush been so grossly misapprehended, not to say misrepresented, as pulmonary consumption. It has been constantly affirmed that he bled his patients in every stage of their disease, shut them up in stove-rooms, and gave them mercury to the point of causing salivation. But so far is this from the truth that he insists, with Sydenham, on horseback exercise as the one great remedy in the disease. He bled for intercurrent inflammations, but says, "If there does exist in nature a remedy that will supply the place of exercise, I believe it will be found in the class of tonics." The prime indication is to "restore the vigor of the constitution." All depends, he taught, upon the tone of the general system. "If consumption be a disease of general debility," as he held, "it becomes us to attempt the cure of it in its first stage; that is, before it produce the symptoms of cough, bloody or purulent discharges from the lungs, and inflammatory or hectic fever." And among his remedies are the cold bath, steel and bark, exercise being put before all.

In dropsy his practice was purely empirical, but, with some good remedies, he gives a number of curious cases; as, for example, that of Dr. Samuel Johnson, who was temporarily relieved by fasting; and that of another patient who was cured by fear; and he concludes the chapter with the following words, in which we have an expression of his singularly hopeful temper: "But let us not despair. It becomes a physician to believe that there is no disease necessarily incurable; and that there exist in the womb of time *certain* remedies for all those disorders which elude the present limits of the healing art."

He has, in the same volume, an interesting chapter on the "influence of the military and political events of the American revolution upon the human body," in which, among others, he mentions the curious fact, that "the population of the United States was more rapid from births during the war than it had ever been in the same number of years since the settlement of the country." This he attributed "chiefly to the quantity of money, and to the facility of procuring the means of subsistence during the war, which favored marriages among the laboring part of the people." Such was the cheapness of living that, he says, beggars of every description disappeared in the year 1776, and were seldom seen till near the close of the war.

Science has been truly said to consist in its facts, and the same may be remarked of the value of Dr. Rush's writings. They constitute a repository of trustworthy observations to which the reader always turns with instruction. I know not where else, in the same compass, so large a number of interesting facts is to be found recorded. He himself felt that his strength was rather in these than in his deductions from them; for, in his paper on consumption, he says: "In relating the *facts* that are contained in this essay, I wish I could have avoided reasoning upon them; especially as I am confident of the certainty of the facts, and somewhat doubtful of the truth of my reasonings." In this the modesty of a true philosopher appears.

His "Account of the state of the body and mind in old age, with observations on its diseases and their remedies," abounds in personal observations, in incidents in biography and history, and in medical facts, and is one of the most charming essays to be found in any literature. Among other means for securing a green old age, he mentions "young company," which, he contends, should be preferred by old people to the company of persons of their own age. And he goes on to say: "I think I have observed old people to enjoy better health and spirits when they have passed the evening of their lives in the families of their children, than when they lived by themselves. Even the solicitude they feel for the welfare of their descendants contributes to invigorate the circulation of the blood, and thereby to add fuel to the lamp of life."

Philadelphia was visited in 1773 by an epidemic of yellow fever more fatal than any that had preceded it, and the year following he published an account of the disease, which forms the third volume of his "Inquiries." He believed, at one time, that the fever was contagious, but had the candor to acknowledge that he was led by the arguments of Webster and of his pupil, Dr. Charles Caldwell, to change his opinion. He thought, for a time, that he was the first to ascribe the pestilence to a domestic origin, but when he learned that Dr. Bond had maintained the doctrine before him he candidly published the fact to the world. No more graphic history of an epidemic is to be found in our language than is here given of yellow fever. He describes with great force the distress of mind with which he saw the scourge advance and his patients sink under it, regardless of his remedies. "Baffled in every attempt to stop the ravages of this fever," he says, "I anticipated all the numerous and complicated distresses in our city which pestilential diseases have so often produced in other countries. The fever had a malignity and an obstinacy which I had never before observed in any disease, and it spread with a rapidity and mortality far beyond what it did in the year 1762. Heaven alone bore witness to the anguish of my soul in this awful situation. But I did not abandon a hope that the disease might yet be cured. I had long believed that good was commensurate with evil, and that there does not exist a disease for which the goodness of Providence has not provided a remedy. Under the impression of this belief, I applied myself with fresh ardor to the investigation of the disease before me. I ransacked my library, and pored over every book that treated of the yellow fever. The result of my researches for a while was fruitless. The account of the symptoms and cure of the disease by the authors I consulted were contradictory, and none of them appeared altogether applicable to the prevailing epidemic. Before I desisted from the inquiry to which I had devoted myself, I recollected that I had among some old papers a manuscript account of the yellow fever as it prevailed in Virginia in the year 1741, which had been put into my hands by Dr. Franklin, a short time before his death. I had read it formerly, and made extracts from it into my lectures upon that disorder. I now read it a second time. I paused upon every sentence; even words in some places arrested my attention. In reading the history of the method of cure, I was struck with the following passages: 'Evacuation by purges is more necessary in this than most other fevers. I have given a purge when the pulse has been so low that it could hardly be felt, and the debility extreme, and yet both one and the other have been restored by it.' Here I paused. A new train of ideas suddenly broke in upon my mind." He at once tried the practice, giving, at first, calomel and jalap in doses of ten grains each, but as this proved to be too slow finally increasing the jalap to fifteen grains; and the effect, he said, far exceeded his expectations. It perfectly cured four out of five of the first patients to whom he gave the purgatives, notwithstanding some of them were advanced several days in the disorder. He imparted the prescription to the College of Physicians, and endeavored to remove the fears of his fellow-citizens by assuring them that the disease was no longer incurable. "I can never forget the transport with which Dr. Pennington ran across the street to inform me, a few days after he began to give strong purges, that the disease yielded to them in every case."

But we must not infer from this strong testimony to the value of purgatives, that he employed no other remedies. With their use he conjoined cool air, cold drinks, cold water bathing, and above all blood-letting. The success of his practice, as has been said, surpassed his fondest hopes, and he exclaims, "Never before did I experience such sublime joy as I now felt in contemplating the success of my new remedies. It repaid me for all the toils and studies of my life. The conquest of this formidable disease was not the effect of accident, nor of the application of a single remedy, but it was the triumph of a principle in medicine." On the 10th of September he wrote in his diary: "Thank God! Out of one hundred patients whom I have visited or prescribed for this day, I have lost none."

The practice, however, was not universally accepted by his brother practitioners; on the contrary, it encountered a storm of opposition. Kuhn, one of his colleagues, as well as Wistar, denounced it as most dangerous; and Currie, a physician and writer of note, went so far as to declare that it "could not fail of being certain death." By many of his brethren he was represented as insane, and some of his fellow-citizens even proposed to "drum him out of the city." "One of my patients," he says, "who had believed it (his insanity) expressed her surprise at perceiving no deviation from my ordinary manner in a sick room." His own health gave way at last under the severe pressure to which it was subjected, and his friends urged him to retire to the country; but to a correspondent he wrote that he "had resolved to stick to his principles, his practice, and his patients, to the last extremity." And he refers to the slanders propagated against him "only for the sake of declaring, in this public manner, that I most heartily forgive them; and that if I discovered at any time an undue sense of the unkindness and cruelty of those slanders, it was not because I felt myself injured by them, but because I was sure they would irreparably injure my fellow-citizens, by lessening their confidence in the only remedies that I believed to be effectual in the reigning epidemic." He adds magnanimously, "I commit them to the dust."

His history of yellow fever is a truly great work. His account is minute, spirited, graphic, and possesses all the interest of a personal narrative. I am sure that no one who begins to read it will be disposed to lay it down without concluding it; and no one can follow the author through his faithful story without a conviction that he was at once a philosopher and a man of true nobleness of soul.

Theory, a hundred years ago, was a leading feature in the teachings of every medical man who claimed to be an instructor. When a student with Dr. Redman, Rush adopted that of Boërhaave respecting fever, that the proximate cause is "a lentor of the blood," together with morbific matters in the vital fluid; but on going to Edinburgh he relinquished this theory and embraced that of Hoffman, which Cullen had accepted and improved, to-wit, that the cause is a spasm of the capillaries of the surface of the body. This he found unsatisfactory when he became a teacher, and so he framed one of his own, according to which fevers of all kinds are preceded by general debility, which gives place, sooner or later, to increased excitability. There is but one cause of fever, and that is a stimulus, which gives rise to irregular or convulsive action in the arteries. And as there is but one cause of fever, so fever itself is a unit, as fire is one and the same whether created by friction, fermentation, electricity, or combustion; pleurisy, dropsy, angina, phthisis, and the rest, being but symptoms of the primary disease in the sanguiferous system. Apoplexy is but an apoplectic form of fever, and so of rheumatism, mania, nephritis, etc. The eruptive state of fever is shown in small pox, measles, and the other exanthemata.

Dr. Rush submitted this theory to his pupils, as a substitute for that of his great master, Cullen, with the lines:

> "We think our fathers fools so wise we grow,
> Our wiser sons, I hope, will think us so."

No professional son of Dr. Rush will ever account him a fool. At the same time it must be admitted that anything more baseless than his theory it would be difficult to find in all the dreams of philosophers. But we are to remember that it was of such stuff that medical speculation had been composed for ages and still consisted in his day, and his hypotheses are as substantial as those that had preceded them. Happily, a change has come over the spirit of medicine, and medical teachers no longer waste much time framing theories of fever.

He had remarked, in the treatment of fever, that convalescence was a pretty sure attendant upon salivation, and naturally but falsely inferred that the specific effect of mercury was curative in such cases; and hence it became a practice with him, which unfortunately obtained long and extensively after his time, to induce ptyalism in acute diseases. I have a most vivid recollection of the appearance of patients in the infirmary at Baltimore, in connection with the University, under the care of his pupil, Dr. Potter, with bowls at their cheeks to catch the saliva as it flowed day after day from their mouths. Long since the barbarous practice has been relinquished, the profession having come to understand that salivation follows convalescence, and is in no sense or degree the cause of it.

The "Inquiries" close with "a defense of blood-letting as a remedy for certain diseases," in which are displayed the boldness, the independence of thought, the earnestness, and the enthusiasm, by which Dr. Rush was distinguished above all his contemporaries. Blood-letting, he taught, was indicated in the inflammatory state of fever; by sudden suppression of natural discharges inducing plethora; by the proximate cause of fever; by the symptoms of its first state; by the rupture of blood vessels; by the relief obtained in fevers; by the immense advantages attending it in inflammatory fevers. Some of these advantages he recites. Thus he says: It frequently strangles a fever; it imparts strength by removing indirect debility; it reduces frequency of pulse when excessive, and increases it when preternaturally slow; it relieves nausea and vomiting; it renders the bowels more soluble by purging physic; it renders the system easier of salivation; it removes or lessens pain in every part of the body, relieves burning heat of the skin, checks sweats, sometimes checks a diarrhœa and tenesmus, after astringents have failed; it removes coma, induces sleep, prevents effusions of serum and blood, and the chronic diseases of cough, consumption, jaundice, abscess in the liver, and all the different states of dropsy, which so often follow autumnal fevers.

The following case affords at once an example of his heroic practice, and some insight into his character as a man. He says:

"My friend, Mrs. Lennox, after having been cured of the yellow fever by seven bleedings, was affected, in consequence of taking a ride, with a slight return of fever, accompanied by an acute pain in the head, which I was afraid would end in a dropsy of the brain. As her pulse was tense and quick, I advised repeated bleedings to remove it. This was not followed. The pain in the meantime became more alarming. In this situation, two physicians were proposed by her friends to consult with me. I objected to them both because I knew their principles and modes of practice to be contrary to mine, and that they were proposed only with a view of wresting the lancet from my hand. From this desire of avoiding a controversy with my brethren, where conviction was impossible on either side, as well as to obviate all cause of complaint by my patient's friends, I offered to take my leave of her, and to resign her wholly to the care of the two gentlemen who were proposed to attend her with me. To this she objected in a decided manner. But that I might not be suspected of an undue reliance upon my own judgment, I proposed to call upon Dr. Griffiths or Dr. Physiek to assist me in my attendance upon her. Both these physicians had renounced the prejudices of the schools in which they had been educated, and had conformed their principles and practice to the present improving state of medical science. My patient preferred Dr. Griffiths, who in his first visit to her, as soon as he felt her pulse, proposed more bleeding. The operation was performed by the doctor himself, and repeated daily for five days afterwards. From an apprehension that the disorder was so fixed as to require some aid to blood-letting, we gave her calomel in such doses as to excite a salivation. By the use of these remedies she recovered slowly, but so perfectly as to enjoy her usual health."

Yet, after all, Dr. Rush was not an indiscriminate bleeder, but points out clearly the state of the pulse and the circumstances in which bleeding is proper or inadmissible; and he alludes to numerous cases in which the lancet, unwisely employed, had seemed to him to have been the cause of death.

An anecdote is related of him, bearing upon his extravagant use of the lancet and calomel, which shows that the idea of insanity which prevailed in relation to him was not altogether unnatural. When the epidemic of 1793 was at its height, he had gone one day over to Kensington, one of the suburbs of Philadelphia, to visit a friend ill with the fever. The fact that he was in the neighborhood soon became generally known, and the friends and relations of the sick collected, according to the story, not by dozens but by fifties and hundreds, near a bridge which it was known he must cross in returning, to consult him. Finding his way blocked up by the great assemblage, and unable to visit all who sought his aid, he directed his carriage to be stopped and requested the multitude to approach him as closely as they could, when he said to them: "I treat my patients successfully by bloodletting, and copious purging with calomel and jalap, ten grains of each for adults, and six for children; and I advise you, my good friends, to use the same remedies." "What!" cried a voice from the crowd, "bleed and purge every one?" "Yes," replied the doctor, "bleed and purge all Kensington;" and then drove on.*

His opposition to nosology is as well known as anything relating to his medical opinions. Rising from his chair as he lectured, it is related by his old pupils, he would exclaim with intense earnestness, in imitation of Cato, "*Delenda, delenda, delenda est nosologia.*" This hostility resulted partly from his peculiar notions about the unity of disease, but was chiefly excited by the routine practice which he saw physicians continually pursuing. Disease he held, and held wisely, is to be treated, not for the name but according to the morbid conditions in each case.

* Caldwell's Autobiography.

An erroneous impression has prevailed that he disregarded the voice of nature in disease, and would "turn the *vis medicatrix naturæ* out of a sick room as he would a noisy cat;" and the idea derives color from his use of the expression quoted. But under what circumstances does he advise such a course? When, in violent diseases or those of feeble reaction, nature is doing nothing but mischief. For example, where there is a burning fever, he would reduce it by cold water; where there are wasting watery discharges, as in cholera, he would check them; where the patient is cold, he would warm him; where he has no appetite, still he would feed him until appetite returns. He would reduce reaction to the level of nature's salutary efforts. Follow nature, he inculcated in his writings and his lectures, but not implicitly or blindly. In many cases there is no guide so trustworthy, but the physician must determine when and how far to follow her. "One of the greatest attainments and frequently the last in the practice of medicine," he said, "is to know when to do nothing." "No medicine," he adds, quoting Hippocrates, "is often the best medicine."

Besides his four volumes of Inquiries, Dr. Rush published a volume of essays, literary, moral and philosophical, the sermons to young men already mentioned, a volume of introductory lectures, and a treatise on diseases of the mind, which appeared only a short time before he died, and may, perhaps, be accounted the ablest of his works. Of all the books pertaining to medicine written in our country, it is the one oftenest quoted by our brethren abroad. In it the author shows that he was abreast with the most enlightened writers of his day on mental diseases. He had caught the spirit of the great Pinel, and recognized the nature of insanity and the true principle in its treatment. To him the new world is indebted for the application of the law of kindness in the management of lunatics, and their condition has been one of steady improvement from his time to the present day. It is a eulogy justly due him that "he opened the prison doors of the maniac, unbarred his noisome dungeon, and knocked the shackles from his limbs, substituting moral treatment for brute force, and love for fear."

Of a most sanguine temperament, he had the utmost faith in the capabilities of medicine, and was persuaded that a beneficent Creator had provided a remedy for every physical as well as every moral evil incident to our present state. One of these he predicted, and in the true spirit of the Baconian philosophy. In the following passage the discovery of anæsthetics in childbirth is clearly foretold: "I have expressed a hope in another place (Med. Repos., Vol. VI.) that a medicine would be discovered that should suspend sensibility altogether, and leave irritability, or the powers of motion, unimpaired, and thereby destroy labor pains altogether. I was encouraged to cherish this hope by having known a delivery to take place, in one instance, during a paroxysm of epilepsy, and having heard of another, during a fit of drunkenness, in a woman attended by Dr. Church, in both of which there was neither consciousness nor recollection of pain."

Not many medical writers have ventured to introduce themselves so often and unreservedly to their readers as Dr. Rush. The act is always one of delicacy and some danger, and if not performed gracefully and with dignity is sure to offend. Dr. Rush is never more interesting than when speaking of himself. Among the many charming features that belong to his writings none are more pleasing than his personal allusions, always unaffected, perfectly devoid of vanity, and in good taste. Nothing that I have read exceeds in beauty or pathos the following passage, for example, in which he refers to himself in connection with his forefathers. He is standing in the cemetery where they sleep. "While considering this repository of the dead," he says, "then holding my kindred dust, my thoughts ran wild, and my ancestors seemed to stand before me in their homespun dresses, and to say, 'What means this gentleman by thus intruding upon our repose?' and I seemed to say, 'Dear and venerable friends, be not disturbed. I am one who inherits your blood and name, and have come here to do homage to your Christian and moral virtues; and truly I have acquired nothing from the world, though raised in fame, which I so highly prize as the religious principles I inherited from you; and I possess nothing that I value so much as the innocence and purity of your character.'"

It is known to you all that Rush was something more than a great medical writer and teacher and philosopher. The storm of revolution, which for a time closed his lecture-room, drove him into politics, and his name appears among those of the great statesmen of his period. A hundred years ago he was subscribing it to our Declaration of Independence, where it will be read by the latest generations of men. Five members of Congress from Pennsylvania had refused to sign the declaration, deeming it premature, and so refusing had retired from the house. Rush was one of those who were elected to fill the vacancies thus created; and so, as has been said, "did not sign the tremendous parchment because he was a member, but became a member that he might sign it."

In the century that has elapsed since that momentous event American medical literature has made very great progress. Many able works have been given to the world by our physicians—works of great research, of true erudition, of immense practical value to the profession—works of which our country is justly proud; but if I were called upon to declare which among them all I would prefer to have written, I should unhesitatingly name the writings of Benjamin Rush.

LOUISVILLE, KY.

A CLINICAL LECTURE ON THE IMMEDIATE APPLI-
CATION OF THE PLASTIC DRESSING IN FRAC-
TURES OF THE LOWER EXTREMITY.*

BY DAVID W. YANDELL, M. D.

*Gentlemen:* The other day, after I had dressed a fractured
leg in your presence, a member of the class asked me, "*What
was the best time to put up such fractures?*" My answer, you
may remember, was, "*The earliest possible moment after the
bone was broken. The sooner the better.*" And now, after
weighing my experience in such cases as carefully as I am
capable of doing, I wish to add this to my reply on that
occasion: *Dress the fracture, if you can, on the spot.* Do not,
if it can be avoided, have the patient moved a single foot
from where he received the injury; for he can undergo no
movement of the limb without augmenting his pain and
increasing his risks.

A little while back a merchant of this city got a simple
fracture of the bones of the leg. He was put in a spring
wagon, and started to his house. On the way the upper end
of the tibia was thrust through the skin, and what, when he
left his store, was a simple subcutaneous wound, had, before
he reached his residence, been made an open wound and
converted into a compound fracture. The second accident
was worse than the first. I saw more than a score of times,
during the late war, soldiers who were started to the rear
with simple fractures of the lower extremity, who, when they
reached the hospitals, had compound fractures. The jolting
inseparable from the best managed transportation on wheels
almost certainly gives rise to pain, which means, in almost
every instance, additional injury to the soft parts, and, as I
have just remarked, it is sometimes even sufficient to change
a simple into a compound fracture. Carrying patients with
broken legs on litters on men's shoulders is safer than on

* Phonographically reported.

wheels, but this can not conveniently be done except for short distances; and no matter how carefully it may be executed, it is nevertheless obnoxious in some degree to the objections I have just named. And this, too, though the surgeon may himself superintend the transfer, and before undertaking it encase the injured limb in a temporary, or what has come to be known as a field dressing; for this dressing, however well applied, is after all but a make-shift— it gives pain and disturbs the fragments of bone while it is being put on, and does the same when it is taken off.

Some years ago, when my lamented colleague, Professor Bayless, was lecturing one day on the subject of fractures, I was called to see a negro man with a broken thigh. I remembered it was the hour for my friend's lecture. The patient, who wished to go to hospital, was only a few blocks from the University. I thought the case would be an agreeable surprise to Dr. Bayless, and would serve better than diagrams or words to illustrate the subject of his lecture, and so after adjusting the fragments and applying a good field dressing to the limb, I placed the patient on a stretcher, and this on the shoulders of four stout men, and putting these under way, I accompanied the cortege to the lecture-room. When we took up our march, I must believe the broken bone was well in place; but when we reached our destination, and removed the dressing, the extremities of the fractured femur were frightfully displaced, and the sufferings of the patient extreme. A part of both these features was due to the motion which is well nigh inseparable from every attempt to transfer persons with broken legs from one spot to another, and a part to the violent spasmodic action of the injured muscles which, primarily lacerated, were still further vexed by being still further disturbed.                    .

So my injunction to you to-day is that if you would encounter a broken leg when the injury done is at the minimum, when in dressing it you would give least pain, and have it most in your power to avert inflammation and all the evils which journey in its train, you must do so on the spot where the accident has occurred, and as soon afterward as you can get to it. , Every inch that a fractured leg is moved is hurtful; every moment lost before putting it up is injurious.

A man in the employ of the gas company here sustained a fracture in the lower third of the leg, within a few feet of my office door. In less than forty minutes after, the plastic dress-ing was drying on the broken limb. Two hours later the patient was removed without the least suffering to his home, a mile away, and had he been accustomed to their use might have walked on crutches the next morning.

It will oftentimes happen, however, that the opportunity to act with the promptness I have advised is not afforded you. You may not see the fracture until after swelling has set in, and the limb has grown painful and red and hot. What then? Why, do just this: Put the fracture up as soon as you can get your dressing ready. Go to work then and there, and encase the limb in some form of fixed apparatus. It may be Paris plaster, or eggs and flour, or glue and zinc, or liquid glass, or shoemaker's paste; only let it be some-thing plastic, and apply it instantly.

Those of you who have been following these lectures long-est can not recall a single instance in which you ever saw me postpone dressing a fractured leg or thigh because of swell-ing in the parts. On the contrary, I have unvaryingly incul-cated that swelling and pain are to be regarded as but so many additional reasons for fixing the limb—for rendering it immovable—for placing the fragments so that neither the movements of the patient nor spasms of the muscles can disturb them. Pain, as Mr. Hilton in his lectures on that subject has so well expressed it, is a monitor—*the* monitor, as he puts it; and here it clearly seems placed to warn the surgeon against further delay in fixing the limb, and so fix-ing it that displacement can by no possibility again occur. Nor is swelling to be regarded as much the inferior of pain itself as a monitor. The two speak the same language. If you are truly wise, you will heed alike the voice of both; their admonitions are the same—they are calls for rest; and

I beg you to believe that the more quickly and the more perfectly you secure this, the more rapidly and the more completely will they quit the broken limb. Oftentimes the injury done to the soft parts by the ends of the bones being suddenly and violently displaced by muscular action, or by change in the position of the patient, gives rise to some of the greatest dangers which occur in fractures. Hence, the sooner you adjust the fragments, and the more securely you provide against their subsequent displacement, the better you will have treated the case. Let neither pain nor swelling deter you from dressing the limb at once. If you see the fracture first at night, I pray you wait not till morning to put it up. Don't trust to sand-bags, or pillows, or splints, or this or that other device, and finally take your leave, saying you will call in the morning. A sight of mischief may occur between midnight and sunrise.

Some years ago a pilot jumped from the hurricane deck of a burning steamboat at the wharf at St. Louis, on to the boiler deck of a boat lying alongside, and sustained a fracture of both bones of the leg. The limb was well put up in splints, and the patient brought by rail to his home in this city. Forty-eight hours after the accident, when I first saw him, the limb was much swollen and very painful. I applied the plastic dressing at once, and had the satisfaction, not only of relieving all suffering immediately, but also of saving a man of very feeble constitution from the long confinement inseparable from any other mode of treatment.

An old gentleman fell, one Tuesday, and broke the two bones of the right leg about their middle. A medical man dressed the parts in the usual way. Thirty-six hours after I found the limb hot, painful, and much swollen. Did I wait for these conditions to abate? Not a bit of it. I ripped up the wrappings in which the leg had been enveloped and put on the final and only dressing which is required in such cases. The next day the patient sat up, and on the following Sunday he went on crutches, with his foot in a sling, two hundred yards to church.

A lady trod on a bit of orange peel, fell and broke her femur ,in its upper fourth. My friend, Professor Bayless, who, though he reposed great trust in the plastic apparatus, preferred waiting the conventional fortnight for the swelling, and so forth, to subside, applied the long splint, and made the orthodox extension and counter-extension enjoined in such cases. The limb swelled enormously, and the pain was extreme. At the end of three days of very great suffering, I saw the case with my colleague, and applied the plastic dressing while the patient was under chloroform. There was no more pain after that, and in a week the lady could, when assisted, get on crutches and move about her room.

From that day, my lamented predecessor became a convert to the immediate application of the fixed apparatus, and among the last services it was my privilege to render him, when his failing health obliged him to abandon such work as called for much physical exertion, was putting up a broken thigh in one of his patients immediately after the accident happened. In that case there was no swelling; none had had time to occur, and the early application of the dressing had most certainly prevented swelling. In proof of this I need only refer you to my own experience in its use, and state that in all the cases in which I have applied it *I have never had occasion to remove it on account of swelling in a single one.* Many times when I have applied it to limbs already swollen, I have been obliged afterward to open it and overlap the edges, or trim them down, in order to adapt the bandage to the shrunken condition of the parts. Nor is this my own observation alone. I may fairly say that it includes the experience of two surgeons very favorably known to you— Professor Cowling and Dr. Roberts, both of whom, former pupils and chiefs of this clinic, are now colleagues, and who, as I believe, have never dressed any fracture of either the leg or thigh by any other than the fixed apparatus. These gentlemen will tell you, as I have done, that when the plastic dressing is applied to a fracture before swelling occurs, none will occur; and that when it is applied after swelling has taken place, the swelling will begin at once to abate and soon disappear altogether.

Nor do these remarks apply alone to simple fractures of the lower extremity. They are equally true of compound fractures in this situation.

A boy, eleven years old, got a compound, comminuted fracture of the left tibia, just below the tubercle. The laceration of the soft parts was considerable. I picked out with my fingers a number of loose fragments of bone, brought the edges of the wound together, and three hours after the accident put the limb in the immovable apparatus. I then cut out a space sufficient to dress and watch the wound. In less than a week the lad went in a wagon, over a rough road, nine miles into the country. In nine weeks he walked into my office with a firm, smart step, and without the slightest shortening.

Three years ago, while Professor Cowling was serving his term at the hospital, Pat Stanton, whom you occasionally see at this clinic, got an extensive compound, comminuted fracture of the right leg. The contusion and laceration of the soft parts were simply frightful. The accident happened in this wise, and I mention it in order that you may the better appreciate the real magnitude of the injury. Stanton and a fellow laborer were engaged in lowering a lot of whisky from the street into a very deep cellar. Stanton's post was in the cellar. By some mismanagement one of the barrels rolled off the ways on which it had been placed, and fell a distance of twelve or eighteen feet on to Stanton's leg. Now, a barrel of whisky, taken at stated periods, is one thing; but taken on a sudden and on one's leg, is another and a very different thing. Stanton was removed to the hospital, where he was soon seen by Dr. Cowling; the internes, in the meantime, having decided that it was clearly a case for amputation. I was sent for, and when, after consultation, it was decided to attempt to save the leg, Stanton drew me near him, and in a feeble voice, for he was still suffering from shock, said: "Doctor, had you told me my leg had to come off, I should

have asked you to put a pistol ball through my head, and let
me go at once." The plastic dressing was used instead of
either the knife or the pistol, and you may now see Stanton
almost any day earning his living on two good legs as a
street cleaner. I hope you will not encounter, indeed it
would be difficult to conceive of, a more unpromising case
than Stanton's, or one which put the fixed apparatus to a
severer test. I am convinced that no other dressing could
have secured the same happy result; and even this would, I
believe, have failed had its application been delayed for the
ten or twelve days advised by some surgeons.

In 1870, when I had six years' less experience than I now
have in the use of the plastic dressing, and when among
surgeons generally there was less positive knowledge of the
inestimable advantages of its immediate application, I stated*
that if the bandages were cut throughout their entire length,
as soon as dry, and their edges subsequently brought together
either by additional strips or by loop-knots, the principal
objection urged against this dressing, namely, that it may
become too tight as the swelling augments, or too loose as
the swelling subsides, would be obviated. This statement
grew out of my respect for the opinions of my seniors rather
than out of the teachings of my own experience; for at that
very time I was unable to recall a single instance where the
dressing once applied, before swelling had occurred, that it
afterward became necessary to remove it because of swelling.
*A limb timely put up in the plastic apparatus will not swell.*
That is my dictum to-day. Hence there will be no occasion
to open the dressing in these cases. Where swelling already
exists it may, on subsiding, leave the limb, as you have seen,
so shrunken as to render it necessary to cut and refit the
bandage; but it is in these cases and these alone.

To conclude: What I wish to impress upon you to-day is,
that the best time to dress these fractures is the first moment
after they have been inflicted. Every moment of delay is

* American Practitioner, July, 1870.

hurtful. The best place is on the spot where they have occurred. Every inch the limb is moved is an injury; and, finally, no dressing is comparable to the fixed dressing.

LOUISVILLE, KY.

---

## FINAL ILLNESS OF DR. JAMES S. ATHON—POST MORTEM EXAMINATION, AND REMARKS UPON THE PREVENTIVE TREATMENT OF APOPLEXY.*

BY I. C. WALKER, M. D.

Since the last meeting of this society, Dr. James S. Athon, one of its old, well known, and most honored members, has passed away. You are familiar with his name, history, and character. He has been the recipient of both medical and political honors; having always discharged the duties with credit to himself and fidelity to his medical and political friends. He had been engaged in the practice of his chosen profession, in this state, for the period of forty years, and consequently was one of the medical pioneers of Indiana. He was self-reliant, possessed of great will power, well developed both mentally and physically, full of personal magnetism, and in point of medical culture far above the average physician of the age in which he lived. He was the first graduate of the Louisville University, at the age of twenty-five years, and was sixty-four at the date of his death. During this long period he was thoroughly identified with our political and medical history, in the capacity of Secretary of State, Superintendent of the Hospital for the Insane, and Vice President of the College of Physicians and Surgeons of Indiana. He also held other positions of honor and trust.

It would seem, in view of the foregoing facts, that a short history of his last illness and death would not be inappropri-

* Read before the Indiana State Medical Society, May, 1876.

ate upon this occasion, and would be of interest to his medical brethren who have so long and favorably known him.

Dr. Athon enjoyed almost uninterrupted health up to the 25th day of September, 1875. Soon after partaking of breakfast, before going to his office, he complained of slight vertigo and pain in the left side, in the region of the spleen and hip. He went to his office at 9 A. M., as was his custom, and commenced examining and prescribing for patients. While looking at a diseased tooth, he had a decided increase of vertigo, with a numbness and loss of voluntary power of the left arm and leg, and would have fallen had he not been assisted to a seat. A death-like pallor was on his face, with an expression of great anxiety. There were no other symptoms worthy of mention; no pain in the head, no loss of consciousness, no paralysis of bladder or bowels, no disturbance of vision, no ptosis, strabismus, nor paralysis of face. The motor paralysis was almost complete for about two days, after which a gradual improvement in the power of the paralyzed limbs was observed up to the 15th day of October, 1875: during all this time he complained of great weakness about the loins and left hip; the arm had improved more than the leg; he commenced walking about his room with the assistance of a cane, but had the characteristic paralytic swing of the limb. In improved condition, while sitting in his chair, drinking a glass of lemonade, his head fell forward, the right arm dropped by his side, and he was heard to utter the word "*paralysis.*" Almost instantly thereafter he became unconscious, with stertorous breathing, slow and full pulse, dilated pupils, and with complete paralysis of the right arm and leg, in which condition he continued for about twenty-four hours, after which there was a partial cessation of the more urgent symptoms. The breathing became less stertorous, with a little evidence of returning consciousness; he would at times appear semi-rational, making indistinct efforts at articulation, and in his better moments seemed to recognize his friends: but no improvement in the paralytic symptoms. Nothing more occurred worthy of note until within thirty-six hours of the close, when the coma again became profound, the breathing stertorous, death-rattle in the throat, pupils widely dilated, sphincters paralyzed, and the surface bathed with a cold perspiration, death ending the scene on the 25th day of October, 1875, just one month from the date of the first attack. During his illness, Drs. Todd and Parvin and the writer were in regular attendance. Drs. Bigelow, Jameson, Woodburn, Thompson, and a number of the other physicians of the city, visited him at irregular intervals.

Dr. Athon's father died of apoplexy at the age of forty-five years. He had three brothers and two sisters, four of whom died of phthisis pulmonalis, and one of acute pneumonia. The cause of his mother's death is unknown.

A post mortem examination was made by Drs. Link and Eastman, twenty-four hours after death, in the presence of about twenty prominent physicians of the city. Weight of brain was nearly fifty-four ounces; a coagulum of blood, about the size of a quail's egg, was found in the anterior portion of the right middle lobe, immediately above the corpus callosum; another clot, three times larger than the first described, was found on the same side, in the posterior lobe, resting in the cornu of the lateral ventricle, pressing upon the corpus striatum. There was some evidence of inflammation, as shown by slight softening of the brain tissue surrounding the first described extravasation. Another clot, about the size of a hen's egg, was found on the left side, in the lateral ventricle, involving the corpus striatum and optic thalamus. The arteries at the base of the brain were generally in a condition of calcification. A branch of the middle cerebral and a branch of the posterior cerebral arteries of the right side were found ruptured, also the middle cerebral artery of the left side. The brain generally presented a healthy appearance.

An interesting question is here presented: Do we know enough of the physiological functions of the various districts of the brain, to enable us to locate the seat of lesion in cases of cerebral hemorrhage? Can it be differentiated from embolism and thrombosis? We are quite sure we can often, from a careful analysis of the symptoms, approximate accuracy, and sometimes determine the question with absolute certainty. How was it with the case just reported? You will remember in the history of the case, in the first attack, there was an instantaneous loss of voluntary power, with slight anæsthesia of the limbs of the left side, without disturbance of mental functions; neither paralysis of face, ptosis, strabismus, derangement of vision, nor serious interruption in the respiratory movements; no paralysis of tongue, nor dysphagia, anæsthesia only transient, no history of heart or lung trouble, nor rheumatic diathesis. Hence we could but conclude the seat of extravasation was within or near the ganglia constituting the motor tract. When the lesion is limited to the corpus striatum of one side, the hemiplegia is on the opposite side. If there be abolition of sensibility, it is but transient. If the optic thalamus is the seat of extravasation, there will be double vision, dilatation or convulsive movements of the pupil, sometimes blindness, anæsthesia, or hyperæsthesia, on the side opposite the brain lesion; hearing and smell may also be disordered. Consequently it was apparent that the lesion did not involve the optic thalamus. Hemorrhage into the crus cerebri causes paralysis of the opposite side with anæsthesia. Ptosis and divergent strabismus would be present on the side of the body corresponding to the seat of lesion, because the third pair of nerves arises from the crus in part, and supplies all the muscles of the eye except the superior oblique and external rectus. Hence it was evident that the crus was free from the influence of the extravasation. When the seat of the hemorrhage is in the pons varolii, the crossed paralysis is still more marked; the limbs are palsied on the opposite side, and the face on the side in which the extravasation is found. If the lesion is in the mesial line, both sides of the body will be paralyzed; consequently we could safely say that there was no trouble in the pons. When the seat of the extravasation is in or near the medulla oblongata, the functions of the glosso-pharyngeal, hypoglossal and pneumogastric, will be impaired or abolished, as shown by the difficulty of swallowing, inability to protrude the tongue, tumultuous action of the heart, and dyspnœa. Hence we know the hemorrhage did not involve the medulla. When the lesion is limited to the cortical gray matter, the symptoms are most varied in their character, differing according to the extent of the injury in different cases. Loss of consciousness may be present, as often incoherence and delirium are manifested. At other times the mental disturbance is marked with merely stupor or obtuseness of intellect. In some cases the paralysis may not be well defined, only great weakness with an unsteady gait; in other instances there is partial and sometimes complete hemiplegia. You will observe there is always more or less mental trouble. This was conclusive evidence the lesion did not occupy the gray substance. We did not suspect meningeal hemorrhage, because cephalalgia was not present, as it usually is to a notable degree, as well as impairment of the mental functions. When the extravasation occupies the cerebellum, there are decided vertigo and pain in the back part of the head; vomiting is much more frequently met than when the cerebrum is the seat of the lesion; loss of voluntary power not so common, and sensibility never disturbed; all of which we accepted as evidence that the extravasation was not in the cerebellum. There was no reason why aphasic symptoms should be present, if the organ of language is located in the third convolution of the left frontal lobe near the island of Reil, as Broca, Dax, Ogle, and others, insist. Extensive hemorrhage may occur in the white substance of the cerebrum, not involving any of the ganglia, and little disturbance of either motion or sensibility result, as was the case with the first described clot found in the white substance above the corpus callosum.'

Then where was the hemorrhage in the first attack?

We could arrive at but one conclusion, that it was in or near the corpus striatum of the right side, causing a loss of voluntary power of left side; and that it was not affecting the cortical gray substance, or there would have been an

instant declaration of unconsciousness or some other manifestation of mental disturbance.

How was it with the second hemorrhage that occurred
twenty days after the first?

You will remember the patient, while taking a glass of
lemonade, was at once profoundly paralyzed in the right side,
with complete unconsciousness; which was evidence to our
minds that a hemorrhage had taken place on the left side in
the great motor tract; and that it was so extensive as to
affect the gray substance of the brain, depriving it of its
normal supply of oxygenated blood.

The heart and lungs were examined and found free from
disease; consequently there was no probability of an embolism. The suddenness of the attack excluded the possibility
of a thrombosis. The post mortem examination fully verified
the correctness of our regional diagnosis.

In the presentation of this case, the causes of arterial degeneration and the preventive treatment should most interest
us. You will doubtless remember nearly all of the arteries,
at the base of the brain, were in a state of calcification. The
father having died of apoplexy, it would be most rational to
conclude that the son had an inherited apoplectic constitution, and should have expected its manifestations at the usual
time of arterial degeneration. With this knowledge, was not
a postponement of the fatal issue possible? Let us examine
the question for a moment.

In speaking of fatty metamorphosis and atheromatous degeneration, Virchow says: "I have, therefore, felt no hesitation in siding with the old view in the matter, and admitting
an inflammation of the inner arterial coat to be the starting
point of the so-called atheromatous degeneration. I have,
moreover, to show that this kind of inflammatory affection of
the arterial coat is, in point of fact, exactly the same as what
is universally termed endocarditis, when it occurs in the parietes of the heart. There is no other difference between the
two processes than that the one more frequently runs an
acute, the other a chronic course."

From the quotation, we are led to infer that the author
believes chronic inflammation of the inner arterial coat to be
due to an acid condition of the blood.    Such is at least a
reasonable hypothesis, as an acid condition is generally admitted in rheumatic endocarditis.    An acid condition of the
blood is undoubtedly more irritating to the internal lining of
the vessels than an alkaline, hence would favor the development of an asthenic grade of inflammation and its consequences, fatty metamorphosis, atheromatous degeneration,
and possibly calcification, with ultimate rupture, when subjected to undue tension.

We have now reached what we conceive to be the most
important part of this paper, and the real object of its production.    What can we do to save our patients from premature death from cerebral hemorrhage?    We see falling, day
by day, the brain-workers and great minds of the country.
Can this appalling mortality be lessened?    Any of us can
write of the symptoms, pathology, causes, and treatment of
apoplexy.    But who knows how to prevent or stay an arterial
degeneration?    In the history furnished us by Sir Thomas
Watson of Dr. Adam Ferguson, the historian, we find an
example from which much may be learned.    He says: "The
doctor experienced several attacks of temporary blindness
before he had an attack of palsy, and he did not take these
hints as readily as he should have done.    He observed that
while he was delivering a lecture, his class and papers before
him would disappear—vanish from his sight—and reappear
again in a few seconds.    He was a man of full habit, at one
time corpulent and very ruddy; though by no means intem-
perate, he lived freely.    I say he did not attend to these admonitions, and at length, in the sixtieth year of his age, he
suffered a decided shock of paralysis.    He recovered, however, and from that period, under the advice of his friend,
Dr. Black, he became a strict Pythagorean in his diet, eating
nothing but vegetables, and drinking only water or milk.
He got rid of any paralytic symptom, became even robust
and muscular for a man of his time of life, and died in full

possession of his mental faculties at the advanced age of ninety-three, upward of thirty years, after his first attack." Sir Walter Scott describes him as having been, "long after his eightieth year, one of the most striking old men it was possible to look at. His firm step and ruddy cheek contrasted agreeably and unexpectedly with his silver locks; and the dress which he usually wore, much resembling that of the Flemish peasant, gave an air of peculiarity to his whole figure. In his conversation, the mixture of original with high moral feeling and extensive learning, his love of country, contempt of luxury, and especially the strong subjection of his passions and feelings to the dominion of his reason, made him, perhaps, the most striking example of the stoic philosopher which could be seen in modern days."

If we learn anything from the above case, it is that cerebral arteries may be so frangible as to rupture under great pressure, and that additional ruptures may be prevented, and possibly the tendency to arterial degeneration stayed, and the already weakened walls strengthened, by the regulation of the nutrition, by abstaining largely from nitrogenous articles of food, and living principally on carbonaceous diet. We also learn that both mental and physical vigor can be maintained to a great age on a diet exclusively of vegetables, water and milk. All this being true, how important is the study of preventing the degeneration of blood vessels, not by medication alone, but chiefly by alimentation. If the doctrine advanced by Virchow be true, that an acid state of the blood favors fatty metamorphosis and atheromatous degeneration, and that the condition of the blood is the same as in endocarditis, it would appear that the way is open to prevent endarteritis and its consequences, by preventing the accumulation of the supposed *materies morbi* in the blood, by the use of agents the tendency of which would be to maintain its normal alkalinity. The object so much desired is to uproot the great underlying cause in the blood. In the selection of means with that view, it should be remembered that almost every particle, however small, that is introduced into the animal economy is decomposed and subjected to chemical changes in the processes of digestion and assimilation. If we have a correct physiological knowledge of these chemico-vital changes, it is logical to conclude that the alkalescence of the blood can be maintained in the selection of a diet with a view to the chemical changes that occur in the stomach without the direct administration of the alkaline salts. It is most certainly true, if we can rely upon the teaching of Dalton, Flint, Marshall, and other physiologists. Dalton says: "The carbonate of soda of the blood is partly introduced as such with the food, but the greater part of it is formed within the body by the decomposition of other salts, introduced with certain fruits and vegetables. These fruits and vegetables, such as apples, cherries, grapes, potatoes, etc., contain malates, tartrates, and citrates of soda and potassa. Now, it has been often noticed, after the use of acescent fruits and vegetables containing the above salts, the urine became alkaline in reaction from the presence of the carbonates." Then in the management of cases in which we have cause to believe there is an inherited predisposition to arterial degeneration, from an acid condition of the blood—and it matters not whether it be uric or lactic—we have but to maintain its alkalinity by interdicting the use of nitrogenous articles of food, and insisting upon the example of the old Pythagorean, "Eat nothing but vegetables, and drink only water or milk." Here let me say water is the most abundant constituent of the animal body, and is a most essential article of food. Its offices are numerous, an important one of which is to dissolve the food, and render it capable of absorption and entrance into the blood. It is abundant in the blood and secretions, and is indispensable in order to give them fluidity, which is necessary to the performance of their functions. It is through them that new substances are introduced into the body, and old ingredients discharged. "The tendency of complex effete matter is to crystallization, in the absence of sufficient water to hold it in solution." Hence effete matter can be conveyed out of the living body only as it is held in solution by the liberal use of water. Then is it not probable, if the fluidity of the blood is well maintained, it will be less irritating to the lining of the cerebral arteries and better suited to the nutrition of the vessels?

Chloride of sodium is found, like water, throughout the different tissues and fluids of the body. It is believed to increase the solubility of the albumen, and perhaps also the earthy phosphates, and is necessary to the proper constitution of the tissues and fluids. The herbivorous animals, when freely supplied with it, are kept in much better condition than when deprived of its use. Thus, we conclude, the moderate use of salt is essential to the proper nutrition of the body, assists in preserving the fluidity of the blood, rendering the vessels less liable to thrombosis and phosphatic deposits.

With the knowledge our patient possessed of his unfortunate inheritance, we think it not irrational to conclude had he kept the blood in an alkaline state by the use of vegetables and fruits, for the last few years, and well maintained its fluidity by the liberal use of chloride of sodium and water, the inherited tendency to arterial degeneration would have been staid, and his life prolonged for a time.

But little need be said as to the treatment of cerebral hemorrhage after the attack. You are supposed to be familiar with the therapeutics of the principal authors upon the subject. I will, however, allude to a few points that may be of interest to the profession. A detailed account of the treatment given the subject of this paper would not be instructive, because the case was necessarily a fatal one, and no form of treatment could have been of the least avail; and more because the second attack, which fatally paralyzed him, came at a time when a part of the treatment of which I desire to speak was about to be instituted—strychnia and electricity. The propriety of blood-letting will arise, and, as Hammond says, "should, in nearly every instance, be decided in the negative." I can conceive of but one condition in which I would expect good results from blood-letting; and then I would much prefer to apply leeches to the inside of the nostrils, the effect of which would be to more directly unload the great venous sinuses of the brain than by any other method. If there was obvious distension of the venous system, indicated by a cyanotic appearance of the face, with impulse of heart strong, its sounds clear, pulse regular, and no signs of commencing œdema of the lungs, I would use leeches as indicated above to remove the venous congestion, the presence of which deprives the ganglion cells and nerve fibers of their normal supply of oxygenated blood.

We must wait, before commencing the use of strychnia, until all symptoms of irritation of the wounded brain have passed away, and the only evidence of ill health is found in the motor paralysis. The extravasated blood must have time to undergo the usual changes of separation and absorption, which changes do not commence before the sixth day. The serum is not absorbed, and the remaining clot encapsulated by a new formation of connective tissue, before the end of the third week. It would not only be useless, but positively unsafe, to attempt to restore the lost voluntary power, with the cause in full force.

I especially desire to speak of the use of strychnia hypodermically. Its effects are much more decided when administered subcutaneously, once a day, in smaller doses, than by the stomach. Hammond says: "In old cases of hemiplegia, the effects of strychnia, thus administered, are often well marked, and are exhibited when administration by the stomach has failed to produce a beneficial result." Dr. Charles Hunter also speaks of the advantages of its use subcutaneously. Dr. R. A. Vance reports several cases in proof of its superior utility when thus used.

Our greatest reliance should be in the use of electricity. No well informed physician, in this age of medical progress, would neglect the use of an agent of such inestimable value in the treatment of motor paralysis and anæsthesia. The same rules prescribed as to time in the use of strychnia, should govern us in the use of this most potent remedy. The improvement is often very decided and satisfactory.

The induced current should be first tried, if the treatment is commenced, soon after the seizure, and will generally produce contractions of the paralyzed muscles. The current should be of sufficient tension to cause slight pain; and if contractions are not produced, it would be better to resort to the galvanic current. In old cases, the loss of electro-contractility is so great that satisfactory results can not be expected from the induced current. The intensity of either current should come short of excessive pain or great fatigue. Friction, kneading the muscles, flexing and extending the paralyzed limbs, should not be neglected. The patient should also be encouraged to move his limbs, from time to time, by his own volition.

INDIANAPOLIS.

---

## SUPPOSED INTUSSUSCEPTION—RECOVERY FROM COPIOUS INJECTIONS, THE BODY BEING INVERTED.

BY M. H. JORDAN, M. D.

The treatment of intussusception by inversion of the body and enemata, has been a most important addition to our therapeutics of this dangerous condition, several successful cases having been reported. I wish to add another to the list, the result being not less prompt than satisfactory.

A child, seven and a half months old, was suddenly taken ill on the night of the twenty-third of March, apparently suffering severe pain accompanied with violent straining to evacuate the bowels, but passing only a little blood and mucus. The physician first in attendance regarding it as a case of dysentery, treated it accordingly. About forty-eight hours after the commencement of the attack, I saw the patient, and found it straining violently, restless, and suffering severely, but without any fecal discharge. Suspecting an intussusception, I passed a gum elastic sound into the rectum; this sound could be introduced some distance, and then met with an obstacle which I believed an intussusception of the large intestine. Having the child inverted, then by means of a Davidson's syringe—the nozzle being wrapped with a napkin external to the anus, and firm pressure being kept up around it to prevent reflux of the water, and this being introduced very slowly, apparently simple points, but of no little importance in such cases—nearly a pint and a half of warm water was thrown into the bowels; at first there was considerable resistance to the introduction of the pipe of the syringe, but by the gradual dilatation of the water it was passed in three and a half or four inches. The injection was retained for a few minutes and then allowed to escape, the infant meanwhile being apparently entirely relieved, and dropping off into a calm sleep. After the escape of the injection, a fecal evacuation—the first since the commencement of the attack—occurred. A repetition of the enema was followed by two more natural discharges. The patient continued to rest well. There were abdominal soreness and tympanites for a few days, but recovery was soon complete.

This case is reported as a contribution to the statistics of this affection, and as a testimony to the value of the treatment employed, and with the hope that it may possibly be of such advantage to some other physician as the reports of similar cases have been to me.

BIRMINGHAM, ALA.

# ℜeviews.

---

Cyclopædia of the Practice of Medicine. Edited by Dr. H. Von Ziemssen, Professor of Clinical Medicine in Munich, Bavaria. Vol. IV. Diseases
of the Respiratory Organs. New York: William Wood & Co. 1876.

These portly volumes continue to appear with a prompti-
tude that bespeaks vigor in all concerned in their production.
This forms the fourth in the series, but is in reality the sixth
published, the fifth and tenth volumes having been issued in
advance of their time. The articles in this volume are by
Drs. Fraenkel, Ziemssen, Steiner, Riegel, and Fraentzel, and
are on a level with those in the preceding volumes, which
have been everywhere accepted as representing the most advanced views of the profession on the matters of which they
treat. Their authors are young but not unknown, having
distinguished themselves as writers, and having enjoyed opportunities which enable them to present their subjects from
a clinical stand-point. We have heretofore alluded to the
biographical sketches prefixed to each volume as a pleasing
feature of this great work, and are glad to see it preserved in
the volume before us.

The first memoir is by Dr. Fraenkel, and relates to diseases
of the nose, pharynx and larynx, their diagnosis and treatment, which are introduced by some excellent instructions in
regard to the inspection of the pharynx. This is done now
in a far more satisfactory way than was possible a few years
ago. In hardly any department of practical medicine has
greater aid been afforded by instruments than in affections of
these parts, and here the reader will find minute directions
how to employ them, made more clear by ample illustrations.
Those instruments may be more complicated than is desirable

for most practitioners, but no one can read this chapter carefully without being better prepared to encounter diseases of
the throat. It may be true that intra-pharyngeal operations
must, as a rule, be left to the specialist; yet it will not be
disputed that every practitioner should be able to use the
laryngoscope so far, at least, as to enable him to arrive at
a diagnosis. Less practice, as is justly remarked by Dr.
Fraenkel, is required to learn laryngoscopy than auscultation
and percussion, without some skill in which no physician
would be content to practice medicine at this day.

Dr. Fraenkel's therapeutics are local; he speaks only of
such as are topically applied to the passages under consideration—solid nitrate of silver, insufflation of powders, the application of fluids by pencilling, the syringe, or the inhalation in
the atomized state.

Von Ziemssen follows in a practical memoir on diseases of
the larynx, connected with anemia, hyperemia and hemorrhage, of which he gives a brief historical sketch, embracing
an allusion to the laryngoscope.

His paper is followed by one on croup by Dr. Steiner. In
looking over the bibliography of this disease, we see that
Dr. Steiner quotes Samuel Bard, but fails to give the name of
Richard Bayley, of New York, who was, perhaps, the first to
detect the true character of membranous croup, and whose
discovery has been recognized by French pathologists. It
was made as early as 1781, and communicated in a letter to
Dr. Hunter. Dr. Rush, too, ought to be noted as a writer on
croup; it is not a little remarkable that his confidence in the
power of remedies in this most intractable affection was so
great. Steiner declares that "we do not at present possess
any which directly influence the morbid process, and upon
which we can rely with confidence."

Dr. Riegel has a much longer memoir on diseases of the
bronchi and trachea. It is a treatise of more than two hundred pages, and is exhaustive. The reader will find in it all
that he desires to learn about these maladies, and we may
remark, in passing, written in a style at once clear and pleas-

ing—a merit for which we have already commended this work.

The concluding paper, by Dr. Fraentzel, is shorter, but makes an essay of a hundred pages. It is directed to diseases of the pleura, and forms a complete monograph on the subject. With the copious index, the volume contains over eight hundred pages, to which our readers are referred as an authoritative and eminently instructive book, which would make a valuable addition to any medical library.

---

**The Medical and Surgical History of the War of the Rebellion.**
Part II, Volume II—Surgical History. Prepared under the direction of Joseph K. Barnes, Surgeon-General U. S. A. By GEORGE A. OTIS, Assistant Surgeon U. S. A. Washington: Government Printing Office. 1876.

The gigantic rebellion has certainly given birth to the most gigantic medical literature ever brought forth by a war. Here we have volume second of two huge quartos devoted to surgery, after two of similar size relating to medicine. These volumes must be studied to be appreciated, but a very cursory glance is sufficient to satisfy the reader that they form a repository of facts such as has hardly its equal in the annals of medicine and surgery. The one before us, like its predecessor, is rendered far more satisfactory by the cuts with which it is profusely illustrated. To the practitioner of surgery it can not fail to be instructive, while to the author it must prove a mine of incalculable value. No one hereafter will think of writing on the subject without a careful reference to its varied contents. Vast as the matter published already is, it is to be followed by a third volume, which has been found necessary to complete the details of the great history. We should fail in duty if we neglected this opportunity to express to the government thanks for having given to the medical profession of the United States a work that reflects so much credit upon our country.

A Manual of the Diseases of the Eye. By C. Macnamara. Philadelphia: Lindsay and Blakiston.

The third edition of this useful book is now before the profession. "The first was published in 1868, and the second in 1872, during my residence in Calcutta. Since my return to Europe I have revised the work, and hope the third edition will be found to sustain the character of those that have gone before it." (Author's preface.)

Those who have either of the former editions need not procure this one, as but few changes have been made, and but little added; and for the best of reasons, viz., but few changes were needed, and but little could have been added while the book remained a manual.

On the first glance over its pages, we find that the author no longer advocates his peculiar views concerning the mechanism of the accommodation of the eye, which are to be found in a former edition.

We then find two very closely written pages on the minute anatomy of the lens, a part of which we quote:

"The lens is made up of layers of these fibers, disposed, as Mr. Bowman observes, like the layers of an onion, one over the other; and in order to carry out the analogy between the lens and voluntary muscle, we have only to suppose the primitive fibers of the latter arranged in layers instead of bundles. I have traced nerves over the capsule of the lens, and there is no reason to suppose that they do not enter its substance, if their presence there is necessary, of which there is no evidence. The germinal matter lining the capsule of the lens is probably sufficient to produce its formed material, and in the growing lens I have found germinal matter scattered throughout its substance, so that there are really no elements in striped muscle not to be found in the lens, except blood-vessels and connective tissue, and these from the nature and functions of the lens could not be admitted into its substance; moreover, they form no part of the essential elements of muscle. If this be the case, and if it has been proved that the lens dilates and contracts, in obedience to a voluntary effort, in exactly the same way that striped muscle does, surely it is far more reasonable to suppose that these changes are effected through an inherent power residing in the lens, analogous to that which exists in voluntary muscle, than to fall back upon the ciliary body as being the active agent in the accommodation of the eye."

After having read the above, we naturally hoped for something further in the same direction; and when the present edition made its appearance, we eagerly turned to the article on the accommodation of the eye, when, to our surprise, we found that the author had "fallen back upon the ciliary body as being the active agent in the accommodation of the eye." His language in the third edition is as follows: "The highest authorities of the day hold that the accommodation of the eye is effected by the action of the ciliary muscle." He quotes Donders in support of this view, and adds: "In support of this idea we can not overlook the fact that in those animals whose range of accommodation is highest, as birds, the ciliary muscle is largely developed; in those, as fishes, in which accommodation is almost *nil*, the ciliary muscle is hardly developed."

Several pages are devoted to the operations known as iridectomy and artificial pupil; and they so concisely and pointedly express the views of all specialists, who have had much experience in eye cases, that we must quote a little from the work:

"*Increasing use of Iridectomy.*—It is remarkable how rapidly the advantages to be derived from the operation of iridectomy have been developed, and its employment extended, since its first introduction at a very recent date into ophthalmic practice. Iridectomy is especially called for in glaucoma, acute choroiditis, irido-choroiditis, rapidly advancing or intractable ulcers of the cornea, in occlusion of the pupil, and in combination with other operative means for the removal of the lens."

Under the head of operations for the removal of cataract, the author first mentions the varied operations as made by others; then he gives his own method, by which he removes the lens with its capsule, through a linear incision made with a peculiarly broad, straight, lance-shaped iridectomy knife at the temporal side of the cornea, without making a section of the iris.

In regard to the propriety of operating on both eyes at the same time, the author says: "It may be laid down as a general rule, that when both eyes are involved, only one should be operated on at a time. I hardly know of any circumstances that would make me perform a double extraction at one sitting, unless in the instance of double traumatic cataract, when we should do well to remove both eyes as soon as possible from the irritation induced by the swollen and opaque lenses."

In the above view the author has a majority on his side, but in spite of it, and the eminence of those who maintain the same, the writer of this believes in a contrary course, and can if required mention a large number of persons from whose eyes he has removed both lenses at the same time, and in whose cases the most remarkably good results have obtained. The age of those persons has ranged respectively from forty-seven to eighty-nine years; some have been in robust health, while others have been bent almost double with decrepitude, and in no instance has a failure resulted when both lenses were extracted at the same time.

Said teaching is, of course, applicable where the operator has not much experience, and such an one would be exceedingly reprehensible did he undertake the operation in both eyes; but it is the belief of the writer that where one has had brilliant results following a certain course, he should continue in the same path. Let us look at the depressing effect which follows the loss of one eye after an operation— how difficult it is for the operator to induce the sufferer to try it on the other eye, when he remembers the pain which followed the loss of the former one; indeed, the fearful apprehension of it is sufficient often to start destructive inflammation in a recently incised eye-ball.

Space will not admit of anything like a complete review of the book, but we can safely and truthfully state, taking all things into consideration, that it is the best manual possible for the busy general practitioner. It has many excellent plates, contains reliable test types, the index is convenient, its marginal references are admirable, and the price is so low that it is within the reach of the most impecunious of our professional brethren. T.

Statistics, Medical and Anthropological, of the Provost-Marshal General's Bureau. By J. K. BAXTER, A. M., M. D. In two volumes. 1875.

We have here two more superb volumes printed at the government printing office in Washington, made up of statistics of the greatest interest to anthropologists as well as physicians, or, in other words, to all classes of readers interested in the study of man. Over a million of recruits, drafted men, substitutes, and enrolled men, are here reported upon, and the data thus recorded afford a fund to the writer on vital statistics more extensive than any ever before collected and published. The volumes may not be much consulted by the busy practitioner, but to students curious in questions that relate to the statistics of disease, and especially to the medical author, they are invaluable.

In addition to many illustrative charts, eleven maps are given, which add largely to the interest of the work. They show, by gradation of color or varying intensity of tint, in an approximative way, the prevalence of diseases of a certain form in the states from which troops were drawn.

We can hardly think of more pleasing volumes than these constitute for a student who has the leisure and the taste to indulge in the researches to which they refer. The author merits and will receive the thanks of his countrymen for his painstaking and most thorough work.

---

**Atlas of Skin Diseases.** By LOUIS A DUHRING, M. D., Professor of Skin Diseases in the Hospital of the University of Pennsylvania, etc. Part I. Eczema (Erythematosum), Psoriasis, Lupus Erythematosus, Siphiloderma (Pustulosum). Philadelphia: J. B. Lippincott & Co.

. We can not speak too highly of this, the first number of Duhring's Atlas of Diseases of the Skin. The form, the text, and above all the chromo-lithographs—of which there are four as indicated in the title above—are all excellent. Without exaggeration, we believe these illustrations vastly better for the practitioner than those of the Sydenham Society. Nor is the price at all exorbitant, as each number will contain four plates, royal quarto, and, with the text, will be furnished at two dollars and a half.

Dr. Duhring's opportunities for the study of cutaneous diseases are ample, and his work on these diseases previously published sufficiently attests his superior abilities. We can recommend these illustrations most heartily to the profession, and even urge upon practitioners the great value they will be in every medical library.

The atlas will be issued in parts, one appearing quarterly, and the work being completed in eight, or at most ten numbers.

# Clinic of the Month.

SULPHATE OF QUININE AS AN EXCITANT OF THE UTERUS.—
In a contribution to *La Presse Médicale Belge* much testimony
is brought forward in support of the power that sulphate of
quinine possesses of awakening and exciting the action of
the uterus. Dr. Paul reports two observations proving its
efficacy for exciting the contractions of the fatigued uterus.
Dr. Voghera says that quinine, given to some women who
during pregnancy were attacked with neuralgia, or for other
causes, provoked abortion; that, given to some women at the
full term of pregnancy, it brought on labor; and that, when
these women experienced slight irregular pains, the sulphate
of quinine rapidly caused the expulsion of the fetus. It likewise facilitates the expulsion of the placenta by exciting uterine contractions; and when in the puerperal state the lochia
are suspended, a dose of quinine is sufficient to reestablish
them. He likewise states that in some rare cases the prolonged use of quinine suppressed the lacteal secretion, and
brought on the menstrual flux. Dr. Ombini Vincent relates
two cases of difficult labor from inertia of the uterus, and
two cases of metrorrhagia, that was overcome by quinine.
Dr. Louis Aporti declares to have found in it a more prompt
and energetic action than in ergot. Dr. Losi Carlo likewise
congratulates himself on having substituted quinine for ergot,
and asserts to have found in it a powerful medicine either to
awaken suspended contractions, or to strengthen them where
they were weakened. Dr. Bouqué recounted a very interesting observation of a case of metrorrhagia, rebellious to every
other treatment than quinine. He admits that quinine is endowed with excito-motor powers over the vaso-motor nerves,
and in this manner explains its hemostatic power in every
case where contraction of the capillaries is insufficient or
wanting. (The Doctor.)

HYPOSULPHITE OF SODA IN DIPHTHERIA.—Dr. Chenery, in the Boston Medical and Surgical Journal, June 8th, speaks highly of the hyposulphite of soda in diphtheria. He also uses the compound tincture of myrrh, made by digesting an ounce each of capsicum, powdered myrrh, and guaiacum, in a pint of alcohol:

"The dose of the hyposulphite is from five to fifteen grains or more in syrup every two to four hours, according to age and circumstances. It can do no harm, but if too much is given it will physic. As much as the patient can bear without physicking is a good rule in the severer cases. The tincture can be used in doses of five drops to a half-drachm in milk. The amount for thorough stimulation is greater than can be taken in water. I usually give it in such doses as can be easily taken in milk, using the milk as food for small children. One fact, however, needs to be borne in mind, namely, the hyposulphite prevents the digestion of milk and should not be given in less than an hour from it. They may be used alternately, however, without interference, in sufficiently frequent doses. Judging in this disease as I judge in others, I am fully persuaded that the treatment I have so long used, and which has not failed me yet, will save nearly every case of diphtheria if seasonably and vigorously employed; and there is no reason why it should not do as well in the hands of others as in my own. In none of my cases have I used any alcohol."

HYDRATE OF CHLORAL AS A LOCAL APPLICATION IN DIPHTHERIA.—In the last number of the *Gazzetta Medico di Roma,* Dr. Cesare Ciattaglia gives an instructive communication on the cure of diphtheria. For some little time he has been wholly successful in treating that ordinarily stubborn malady, his remedies being the chlorate of potash internally, and the application of the hydrate of chloral to the false membranes. With these he has combined a tonic and restorative diet. To children of three to six years of age he has administered the chlorate of potash in doses varying from ten to fifteen grammes a day, dissolved in one hundred and forty of water; while the hydrate of chloral, in the proportion of four grammes of the hydrate dissolved in twenty grammes of glycerine, is painted over the diphtheritic patches three or four times a day. For adults the dose of chlorate of potash is twenty grammes. The *catena* of evidence by which he illustrates this treatment is very convincing—one gratifying observation being the certainty with which the hydrate of chloral and glycerine, from the moment of being smeared on the false membranes or diphtheritic patches, arrested their formation, and removed entirely on the first, or at latest the second day, the offensive and characteristic fetor. Dr. Cesare Ciattaglia, of course, disclaims all pretensions to originality in this treatment. It is to Vogel that we are indebted for the use of the chlorate of potash—a remedy which that distinguished German physician employed for the first time in 1860; while the Italian practitioner, Ferrini, suggested and prescribed the painting of the false membranes with hydrate of chloral and glycerine in the diphtheritic epidemic that ravaged Tunis last year. (Lancet.)

APPLICATIONS OF CAOUTCHOUC IN SURGERY.—Prof. Courty, in reviewing the numerous advantages possessed by caoutchouc in surgery, at one of the meetings of the Association for the Progress of Science in France, showed that the treatment of chronic ulcers of the legs by this means presents numerous advantages. It is carried out in this manner by him: After having washed the ulcer he applies a mild stimulant; he then covers it with a bandage, over which he rolls an elastic band, which in its turn is surrounded with another bandage. When the wound is considerably closed in he abandons this medication and applies ointment on lint to the ulcer, the cicatrization of which is completed at the end of from two to three weeks. Professor Courty has amputated uterine polypi, hypertrophied cervices uteri, tumors of the rectum and anus, etc., by elastic ligatures. M. Gayet reported having divided the pedicle of an ovarian tumor, by the same method, in twenty-two days, without any inconvenience. M. Letenneur removed an epithelioma of the tongue with elastic ligatures, applied in segments, in eight days. M. Laroyenne, of Lyons, remarked that cauterization of tissues rendered anemic by means of Esmarch's elastic bandage gives better results than when it is practiced on parts in which the circulation has not been suspended. Although it is not apparent at the moment of operation, the hot iron produces its effects more deeply. The surface for cauterization contains no liquid, it does not produce vapor, and the operator can watch the exact points to be attacked better. The integuments do not redden under the influence of the radiating caloric, they preserve their color or become slightly pale; the extent and depth of the cauterization are only shown when the elastic bandage is removed. These effects can be explained by the diminished loss of heat that the iron undergoes when it is not in contact with liquids which, as a result of the high temperature, are converted into vapor. When it is necessary to act on fungoid tissues, in osseous parts deeply situated, this means ought to be preferred to all others. (The Doctor.)

WADDING VERSUS SPONGES. — M. Kirmisson publishes a work, in the *Journal de Thérapeutique*, on the employment of prepared wadding instead of sponges and charpie for the dressing and cleaning of wounds, at the instigation of M. Guyon, who has made use of this mode of dressing for a considerable time. Its slow powers of imbibition render wadding not so convenient as the sponge, but this can be overcome by preparing it in the following manner, as recommended by M. Guyon: Cut up the wadding into pieces as large as the hand, and plunge them in a basin of carbolic water—one in fifty—taking care to turn and press them so as to facilitate imbibition. When thoroughly impregnated (which they will be in five or six minutes) press the water out of them, roll them into balls, and place them in a well-stoppered wide-necked bottle. When required for use they have only to be resoaked at the moment of dressing.

# 𝔑otes and 𝔔ueries.

---

AMERICAN MEDICAL ASSOCIATION.—The annual meeting of the American Medical Association, held in Philadelphia June 5th, 6th, 7th and 8th, was a remarkable success as to numbers, more than seven hundred and fifty members being enrolled, and enough outside doctors in attendance to swell the entire number to ten or twelve hundred.

Dr. Pepper, of Philadelphia, delivered an address of welcome with becoming dignity and grace, but apparently with no great enthusiasm and heartiness.

The inaugural address of the President, Dr. Sims, was admirably delivered—indeed the doctor proved himself a real orator in the utterance of more than one eloquent passage—but many of its sentiments met with no little private condemnation. The chief points in it were a criticism of the code of ethics, and a plan for lessening the ravages of syphilis.

The address delivered, Dr. Brodie sprang to his feet with a motion for a vote of thanks to Dr. Sims, and this motion was carried unanimously; had the members had time for reflection, and had they voted as many talked, censure would have been substituted for thanks, or at least the latter negatived. However, when the address is published, there will be time enough for a deliberate opinion upon that which was deliberately determined and uttered; for Dr. Sims knew right well that his views would not be unchallenged, and had fully considered the matter, counted the cost, and said what he conscientiously regarded as wisest and best.

Sarah Hackett Stevenson was admitted a delegate from the Illinois State Medical Society, and when a motion was made to refer the credentials of all female delegates to the judicial council, it was tabled with wonderful promptness. This action of the association was in remarkable contrast with its course a few years before, when Dr. Atlee was almost the only prominent champion of the doctresses, and his arguments were ably met by Dr. N. S. Davis, whose absence was so notable a fact at this meeting, and whose wise counsels were so much needed, and the venerable Dr. Condie, who has gone where all good doctors go, and where there is no dispute as to female representation. Then a large majority was against the commingling of medical petticoats and pantaloons; but now the majority was overwhelmingly reversed. Is this progress, or is it simply an illustration of the uncertain action of popular assemblages!

The McDowell monument fund occupied the attention of the association a little while, a proposition being made to tax the members for an indefinite time one dollar annually—a plan that met with no general approval, but which was surpassed in wisdom and practicability by a proposition to pass around the hat, take up a collection on the spot. The fact is that the whole movement might as well be set down as a brilliant failure, and the less time spent in the association in talking about it—making fine speeches and hatching foolish schemes—the better.

The ethical part of Dr. Sims's address was referred to the judicial council for report thereon at the next meeting of the association, the syphilitic portion was directed to be printed separately for general distribution, and charges were presented against the Illinois State Medical Society for sending a female representative; so the Chicago meeting—for the next session will be held at the Lake City—promises to be one of no little controversy; the dragon's teeth have been sown, and who will doubt a crop of armed men!

Dr. Busey delivered the address on Obstetrics, and it was, of course, an able effort, and elicited marked attention and much praise.

Dr. Garcelon gave the address in Surgery, but the other

addresses were not, because of absence or illness of the parties charged with their delivery.

The following officers were elected:

President—H. I. Bowditch, of Massachusetts.

Vice Presidents—N. J. Pittman, of North Carolina; Franklin Staples, of Minnesota; Joseph R. Smith, of U. S. Army; Samuel C. Busey, of District of Columbia.

Treasurer—Dr. Casper Wistar, of Pennsylvania.

Librarian—Dr. William Lee, of District of Columbia.

Committee on Library—Dr. Johnson Eliot, of District of Columbia.

Assistant Secretary—J. H. Hollister, of Illinois.

Committee of Arrangements—Drs. N. S. Davis, I. W. Freer, H. A. Johnson, T. D. Fitch, H. W. Jones, J. P. Ross, and Lester Curtis.

Committee of Publication—Dr. W. B. Atkinson, Chairman; Drs. T. M. Drysdale, Albert Fricke, Samuel D. Gross, Casper Wistar, Richard J. Dunglison, all of Pennsylvania, and William Lee, of District of Columbia.

And the following are the officers of sections:

Practice of Medicine, Materia Medica and Physiology—Dr. P. G. Robinson, of Missouri, Chairman, and B. A. Vaughan, of Mississippi, Secretary.

Obstetrics and Diseases of Women and Children—Dr. Jas. P. White, of New York, Chairman, and Robert Battey, of Georgia, Secretary.

Surgery and Anatomy—Dr. D. Hayes Agnew, of Pennsylvania, Chairman, and Dr. Moses Gunn, of Illinois, Secretary.

Medical Jurisprudence, Chemistry and Psychology—Dr. Eugene Grissom, of North Carolina, Chairman, and Dr. E. A. Hildreth, of West Virginia, Secretary.

Delegates to the International Medical Congress, to be held September 4, 1875—Dr. H. I. Bowditch, of Massachusetts; E. Seguin, of New York; Thomas L. Madden, of Tennessee; J. S. Welford, of Virginia; A. Dunlap, of Ohio; John T. Hodgen, of Missouri; Joseph Carson, of Pennsylvania; John C. Dalton, of New York; W. O. Baldwin, of Alabama;

D. W. Yandell, of Kentucky; N. S. Davis, of Illinois; Austin Flint, Sr., of New York; T. G. Richardson, of Louisiana; W. F. Westmoreland, of Georgia; A. M. Pollock, of Pennsylvania; Frank Hastings, Hamilton, New York; G. M. Bemiss, of Louisiana; L. A. Dugas, of Georgia; Francis Bacon, of Connecticut; Hunter McGuire, of Virginia; A. J. Shurtleff, of California; E. M. Moore, of New York; O. W. Holmes, of Massachusetts; G. A. Otis, United States Army; F. E. Gunnell, United States Navy.

Just before the close of the last session, Friday morning, a motion was made and carried to invite Dr. Bowditch, the president so wisely chosen for the next year, on the stage, and we immediately supposed he was needed for some oratorical demonstration. Sure enough, in the course of Dr. Sims's eloquent valedictory, Massachusetts shook hands with South Carolina, action corresponding with word; and so the old and new president clasped hands—Dr. Bowditch, in his frank innocence and in the simplicity of a really great soul, thinking that this manual exercise was the custom—the applause thus evoked was hearty and tumultuous. Indeed we could not help thinking that if Dr. Sims had devoted himself to histrionic art, he would have made himself a greater name even than he has in medicine.

During the meeting of the association, Dr. Toner introduced a resolution declaring that those who aid or abet the graduation of medical students in irregular or exclusive systems of medicine, violate the spirit of the ethics of the American Medical Association; and it was passed. This was a blow, right between the eyes, at Michigan University Medical School; how severe the blow, remains to be seen.

Dr. Culbertson, of Zanesville, worthily received a prize for a wonderfully elaborate and exhaustive essay upon *resections,* the printing of which, with its illustrations, we apprehend will cost a few thousand dollars.

A resolution was offered declaring the office of Permanent Secretary vacant, but it was voted down with a storm of indignant noes and hisses. Yet there was considerable dissatisfaction with Dr. Atkinson, and a strong opinion expressed by several in private that it would be for the interest of the association to put in some new man, like Dr. Hutchinson; many Philadelphians themselves were desirous of this change. Dr. Atkinson has worked so hard and so long, that no trivial causes ought to be permitted to even suggest putting him on the retired list.

Undoubtedly there was considerable dissatisfaction with many things; the hall in which the meetings were held was not suitable in form, even if it had been in acoustic properties; fit places for the meetings of the Sections were not chosen at the right time, and properly advertised, no room for the Judicial Council provided, etc. But all these blunders were simply the results of the greater blunder the Association made in Louisville by selecting Philadelphia as the place of meeting in 1876. The Centennial Exposition was a great rock against which the stream of doctors and medical interests was broken into little streamlets, and almost lost. The very newspapers of Philadelphia, if they noticed at all the public proceedings of the association, gave meager if not blundering reports. Indeed Bud Maid and Goldsmith Doble—how the former trotted and the latter talked—were a good deal more prominent in their columns than Dr. Sims and all the other doctors with their deliberations; and a convention of beer-dealers happening at the same time, made a wave that almost drowned out all mention of medical concerns.

Of course the Philadelphia doctors were most courteous and hospitable, several of them giving elegant and costly entertainments. But eating and drinking, fashionable elegancies, feasting and social dissipations, are not the means of advancing medicine, and of increasing the light and power of our great national medical council; nay, they interfere with its true work, and we wish they could be materially diminished, if not entirely abolished. However, space prevents our continuing this topic now, but we mean to recur to it at an early day.

THE RELATION OF MEDICAL EDITORS TO THE MEDICAL
PROFESSION IN THE UNITED STATES.—This is the subject of
the admirable address delivered by Dr. A. N. Bell, of the
Sanitarian, before the Association of Medical Editors at their
annual meeting, in Philadelphia, June 5th. We wish we had
space to publish the entire address, but we must content ourselves and readers with some extracts. Dr. Bell refers to the
duties of medical editors in these words:

"Founded as this association is, upon a common allegiance
to the medical profession, and a clear appreciation of the advantages common to combined effort in the cause of science,
its field of labor is obvious: to cultivate and disseminate scientific truth; to boldly expose without fear or favor the abuses
which threaten the well-being of the profession; to rouse the
attention of the public to a sense of the danger of ignorant
and unprincipled persons, who either assume for themselves,
or have conferred upon them, the titles of 'doctor,' 'pharma-
cist' and 'apothecary'—at the imminent hazard of the lives of
all persons who are so unfortunate as to become the subjects
of their care.

"Emancipated alike from the colleges and the enfranchise-
ments of mouldy 'authorities,' on becoming editors, we enter
a field of labor which admits of no middle ground. Embracing modern research and cultivation, as vehicles for truth
and ordeals for what is unsettled, it is expected of us to perceive the truth and reflect the light. Editors can not afford
to be content with any place below the front rank, and their
duty is to maintain its lines with unflinching integrity; to be
constantly on the alert, to scrutinize, to assault or espouse,
as the case may be, the wrong or the right in every cause for
its inherent qualities; but always with care and politeness,
lest sharp criticism be mistaken for prejudice, or favor for
flattery. Nothing but that which one really performs can be
an honor to him, and what he claims or takes from another
more than he ought, deserves exposure.

"In one respect at least the medical practitioner and the
medical editor occupy common ground: neither is safe in his

practice or his reputation who is afraid to face the case in hand in all its bearings; and in both, he is most to be relied on who is best fitted to intelligently comprehend the emergency before him, and to deduce from the signs or evidences present the probable tenor of coming results. 'If false facts,' remarks Lord Bacon, 'be once set on foot, what, through neglect of examination, the countenance of antiquity, and the use made of them in discourse, they are scarce ever retracted.' Wary, however, as we should ever be for the integrity and honor of our calling, it behooves us at all times to be careful of snap judgments. To no class of men in the world is time for examination, reflection and knowledge, more necessary than to editors, and to no editors so much as medical editors; for in no other profession is the field of innovation so broad, or fraught with the necessity of more careful watching, than medicine. To it the spirit of innovation is literally abroad, from within and without, and so it has been from the beginning—more 'doctors' than of any other occupation."

Again, Dr. Bell thus speaks of the purpose of medicine, and the evils of our present system of medical education:

"The mere 'cure of disease' should no longer obtain as a primary object of medicine in either faith or practice. But instead the admirable object, so well comprehended by the elder Bigelow more than twenty years ago, which may be defined: *A knowledge of diseases and their causes, and the art of preventing them, and curing them when curable.** Let this be made the standard of professional competency, by proper restrictions and tests, and one important step, at least, will have been taken toward the acquirements necessary for a sound professional education, and the exclusion of all those who boast the use of a remedy for every symptom, or one remedy for all symptoms, in the face of their daily history, which gives the lie to all such assertions.

"But let it not be for a single moment supposed that we consider that the course of medical instruction, as ordinarily

---

* Nature in Disease, by Jacob Bigelow, M. D., p. 69.

pursued in this country, calculated to sustain this precept or to hinder the progress of quackery. On the contrary, we think it eminently calculated to promote quackery. From about fifty catalogues and announcements of Medical Colleges before me at the time of this writing, the following extract was selected from the one representing the largest number of students, as a fair representation of the requirements for graduation by colleges of the highest standing:

"'Three years' pupilage, after eighteen years of age, with a *regular physician in good standing*, inclusive of the time of attendance upon medical lectures; attendance on two full courses of lectures, the last being in this college; certificates of at least one course of Practical Anatomy or Dissections; proper testimonials of character; an acceptable thesis composed by and in the handwriting of the candidate, and a satisfactory examination in each of the seven departments of instruction, viz., Practice of Medicine, Surgery, Obstetrics, Materia Medica, Physiology, Anatomy and Chemistry. The examinations upon Practice of Medicine and Surgery include Pathological Anatomy, Ophthalmology, and diseases of the skin. Two full courses of lectures are absolutely required, *and no period of practice is taken as an equivalent for one course.* The candidate must be twenty-one years of age. The three years recognized are considered as ending at the close of the Winter Session. In this provision, the three years date from the time of graduation, and practice before graduation is not counted.' The winter session begins first of October and ends about first of March. A 'Matriculating Examination' on preparatory education is advertised, which 'is optional with the student, and will be given by the faculty to all who desire it. . . . . It is necessary for those only who expect to present their tickets or diplomas for recognition in Great Britain.'

"The faculty for the winter course of this college, including professors of special departments, numbers *nineteen*, and *fourteen* assistants. Besides the duty of hearing so many lectures, numerous hospitals and public institutions have to be visited, dissection practiced, and the use of various instruments and mechanical appliances learned. That such a process of cramming can result in the acquirement of practical knowledge, is inconsistent with human intelligence. At best, it conveys but a mere smattering of the subjects gone over—not even laying a good foundation for subsequent study. Impressed with an idea of a 'regular course' merely, such graduates are, as a rule, only competent to rival quackery—more likely to acquire its arts than to overthrow them.

"While this association does well, not to assert itself in any respect a reformatory body, it should nevertheless be more alive to the general interest of medical instruction, and show less confidence than it has hitherto shown in the promised reform of medical colleges by professors and teachers. *Their* reform consists in the progressive disgrace of the profession, by the bestowment of its honors upon all who are competent to pay the college fees.

"Modern medicine has expanded beyond the bounds of any individual comprehension, and subdivision has become no less essential for its cultivation than its practice. The specialties of a few years ago have become departments; and that the attempt, on the part of professors and teachers, to continue to explain the whole of the sciences now embraced in medicine to students within the brief space of time commonly allowed, has resulted in utter failure and the degradation of the profession, is in no respect surprising. And this undertaking is the more to be wondered at, when we consider that many of the professors and teachers themselves make little or no pretension to practical knowledge outside of their special departments, both in and out of college. And yet we find a dozen or more of the learned gentlemen hammering away at the young intellect at the rate of six or eight hours a day and every night, for two sessions of four months each, and then *passing* them as having acquired knowledge enough to practice medicine in *all* its branches. The absurdity of the system is only exceeded by its danger, and the more from the circumstance that with few exceptions no standard of preparatory education is required."

But what are medical editors to do? Dr. Bell, in the conclusion of his address, uses the following language:

"In view of this showing, and the humiliating advertisement of one of our chief colleges—that the standard of qualification for admission to our ranks is below that which will entitle the holder to recognition abroad—we may well be alarmed at the prospective future of medicine in the United States. This is no time to take part in the conflict of sects for ascendancy in certain universities. It is the time for action on the part of the American Medical Association, by which a standard of professional qualification may be fixed independent of the colleges; a standard to which they—the colleges—shall be required to conform, or else denied the privileges of the association. The time for appointing committees 'to report at the next session,' or for longer dependence on the promises of the colleges, is passed. The danger of all such delays is upon us, and the present is the time for action. The vague and indeterminate generalities which have served no good purpose in the past, are not likely to promise any better results for the future; and if the standard of medical education in the United States is to be raised at all, it must be raised by its highest tribunal, the American Medical Association.

" But medical editors have no need to wait for ceremony in this regard. Their liberty and their duty is to expose existing abuses, and if possible render them so odious as to make their reform a necessity. Our medical colleges must be made to feel that their period of unexampled prosperity, under existing regulations, shall no longer continue to be a period of peace. And if I may be permitted, in conclusion, to apply one of the wholesomest axioms of sanitary science to the most important of all subjects which now concerns the medical profession in the United States—the low standard of professional education—my proposition is, from this time forth, until it is reformed, to treat it as an intolerable nuisance. By universal assent, *the fittest time for the removal of a nuisance is the very earliest day practicable after its existence has been made known.* Who ever opposes the removal of it on that day will be sure to oppose it, if he dare, on every other day."

MEDICAL COLLEGE CONVENTION.—The convention of representatives from medical colleges, which was alluded to in our last, was held in Philadelphia on June second and third. Twenty-three medical colleges had delegates present, and great unanimity characterized the proceedings. Upon the subject of beneficiaries, the following preamble and resolutions were adopted:

*Whereas,* the practice of reducing or remitting in individual cases the established fees of a college has the objectionable feature of discriminating between students who may be equally deserving, and opening the door to possible gross abuses; therefore,

*Resolved,* that this convention regards the above privilege as one to be deprecated in general, and, if put into practice at all, to be exercised both rarely and reluctantly, and only in unusual circumstances, and after unsolicited application by proven deserving candidates.

*Resolved,* that anything like a wholesale system of such reduction or remission of established fees, or any open solicitation of recipients of such favors, be regarded as in the highest degree improper; and that any college indulging in such practices deserves to forfeit its place on the *ad eundem* list of medical colleges.

In regard to consecutive courses of lectures in the same year, the decision was, "that it is the opinion of this convention that no two consecutive sets of lecture tickets shall be regarded as fulfilling the usual prerequisites of instruction for graduation, where the time between the beginning of the first course and the end of the second is less than fifteen months."

It will be observed that both this resolution, and the ones preceding it, have appropriate application to the Louisville-Kentucky Medical College, with its two courses in one year, and its shameless begging for students through newspapers, politicians and college janitors, and then charging its deluded beneficiaries just what the other medical schools of the west charge their students—a generosity which seems like a mere sham.

Professor Waterman offered the following resolution, which was adopted:

*Resolved,* that no medical faculty should issue a diploma not bearing the graduate's name.

In reference to a diploma fee, the convention took this action:

*Resolved,* that it is the sense of the convention that the diploma fee should not be abolished.

As to graded study, the following preamble and resolutions were adopted:

*Whereas,* a knowledge of the elementary branches of medicine should precede a study of the practical branches.

*Resolved,* that, in the hope of inducing students to prolong and systematize their studies, this convention recommends to all medical colleges to offer to students the option of three courses of lectures, after a plan similar to the following: Students who have attended two full courses of lectures on anatomy, chemistry, materia medica and physiology, may be examined upon any of these subjects at the end of their second course. During their third course such students may devote themselves to the lectures upon the theory and practice of medicine, surgery, obstetrics and diseases of women and children, upon which subjects only they shall be examined at the final examination for the degree of M. D.; their standing, however, to be determined by the results of both examinations.

The convention decided upon a permanent organization, as indicated by the subjoined resolutions:

*Resolved,* that this convention now proceed to form a Provisional Association of American Medical Colleges, under its present officers.

*Resolved,* that when the association adjourns, it shall adjourn to meet at the call of its president.

*Resolved,* that the various medical colleges be invited to take into consideration the project of forming, at the next meeting of this Provisional Association, a permanent Association of American Medical Colleges.

*Resolved*, that for the furtherance of this object, a committee of three be appointed at this meeting to confer by letter with the various colleges, and invite their views on the proper object and plan of such proposed organization; and upon the receipt of the same, to draft a constitution and by-laws for a permanent association, to be submitted at the next meeting of this association.

*Resolved*, that the advisory resolutions upon matters of college policy, passed by this convention, be printed and forwarded to all regular medical colleges in the United States for their consideration.

The following resolution is a gentle blow at the medical department of Michigan University:

*Resolved*, that in the opinion of this association medical colleges ought not to recognize or hold fellowship with any school or its alumni in which irregular medicine is taught as a part of the curriculum.

The final resolution of this body was,

*Resolved*, that no degree in medicine should be conferred, under any circumstances, except after an examination in person of the candidate upon all the branches of medicine.

ONLY TWO MEDICAL JOURNALS IN CINCINNATI.—Professor Pooley, whose advent to the corps of medical editors we take pleasure in announcing, in the June number of the Ohio Medical and Surgical Journal, states, "There are no medical journals published in the state except two in Cincinnati, and they by no means so fully meet the demand as to preclude the success of another." The Lancet and Observer—which really represents three journals, for originally as the Observer it absorbed the Western Lancet many years ago, and more recently the Indiana Journal of Medicine, is certainly one of the two, to which, by the way, Dr. Pooley does not allude in the most complimentary manner; but the other one—is it the Clinic or News? Only two medical journals in Cincinnati! Dr. Pooley, possibly borrowing from certain railroad companies that pool their earnings, is pooling the journals, and we fear will have to submit to a thorough course of Hamilton on Logic.

THE AMERICAN GYNECOLOGICAL SOCIETY.—A meeting of those interested in the formation of a society devoted to the study of diseases of women and of obstetrics, was held in the hall of the New York Academy of Medicine, on Saturday, June 3d. Dr. Peaslee, of New York, was elected temporary President, and Dr. Chadwick, of Boston, Secretary.

A committee to present a constitution for the society was appointed; the committee being Dr. Thomas of New York, Dr. Byrne of Brooklyn, and Dr. Parvin of Indianapolis. The constitution adopted limits the membership to sixty, provides for an annual meeting, makes the officers a president, two vice presidents, a treasurer, and a secretary: these officers, with four more, shall constitute the council.

A committee on nominations, composed of Dr. Jenks of Detroit, Drs. Lusk and Nœggerath of New York, Dr. Sinclair of Boston, and Dr. Trask of Astoria, was appointed. This committee reported the following officers: President, Dr. B. F. Barker, of New York; Vice Presidents, Dr. Atlee, of Philadelphia, and Dr. Byford, of Chicago; Secretary, Dr. Chadwick; Treasurer, Dr. Paul F. Mundé; Council, those just mentioned, with Drs. Sims, Goodell, Lyman and Parvin.

It was determined to hold a meeting of the society in New York the next week after that in which the International Medical Congress is held, and several papers were promised in addition to the inaugural address of the president.

"A GREAT MISTAKE."—The Medical Record, June 15, remarks, in referring to the last meeting of the Indiana State Medical Society: "In the course of the meeting a resolution was adopted to the effect that no paper be published in any medical journal before its appearance in the transactions, which we believe is a great mistake."

ADVERTISEMENTS OF MEDICAL COLLEGES.—We direct the attention of our readers to the advertisements of the medical department of the University of Pennsylvania, of the medical department of the University of Louisville, and of the College of Physicians and Surgeons of Indiana.

THE SUBJECT OF VIVISECTION BEFORE THE BRITISH MEDI-
CAL COUNCIL—*Remarks of Sir Dominic Corrigan.*—"An Act
to Prevent Cruel Experiments on Animals," known as Lord
Carnarvon's Bill, being under consideration by the Council,
the following is a part of Sir Dominic's speech upon the subject: "The crimping of salmon was one thing which might
be retaliated upon those who were striving to inflict penalties
on medical men only. Immediately on being taken out of
the water, the fisherman seized the fish by the head and drew
his knife across its body at intervals of about two inches from
the head to the tail. This was done to make the fish firm,
and the noble lord who owned the fishery got two pence a
pound more for the salmon when they were crimped than
when they were not crimped. When, therefore, a professional
man was taken before a magistrate for making an experiment
on a conger eel, the proper reply would be to ask the magistrate, 'What do you do in your salmon fishery?' When a
witness was examined before a committee of the House of
Commons as to the details of cutting off a rat's tail, a fair
answer would be, 'What do you do with the fox's tail when
the hunt is over?' In order that the tail might retain its
hairs, it was cut off while the animal was still alive, and then
the fox was left to be torn to pieces by the dogs; and at
hunting balls the lady who could show the greatest number
of fox-tails on her flounces was considered the belle. Ostrich
feathers, which were so commonly worn by ladies, were obtained from ostrich farms, where birds were reared for the
purpose; but in order that the feathers might preserve their
freshness and color, it was necessary that they should be
plucked out while the bird was living. Not long since ladies'
bonnets were commonly ornamented with little stuffed birds,
such as the wren and humming-bird, but it was not always
borne in mind that the skins were taken off those birds before they were dead. In Devonshire, too, ponies were branded
when very young, and branding a pony one month old was as
painful an operation as firing a horse. The cramming of fowls
and turkeys was a cruel thing. The food was thrust every
two hours down the bird's throat, and the result was that it

lost for life the power of voluntary swallowing. At Hurling-
ham he once saw a little pigeon which had been wounded,
after having its tail cut off to make it fly straight, take shelter
on the dress of a lady, and there was a wonderful expression
of sympathy, not for the little bird, whose bowels were hanging out, but for the lady's silk dress. The manufacture of
cocktails to horses inflicted frightful pain, in order that the
fashionable owner might ride a cocktail horse. One gentleman, a colonel, had recently written to the Times to say that
in the stables over which he had control firing had been abolished, but the substitute was an application of red iodide of
mercury, which caused a thousand times more pain than
firing. The pain caused by fire was over in a few minutes,
but three weeks would not see the end of the pain caused by
the red iodide of mercury."

A Curious Document.—Whilst the anti-quackery bill was
pending in the California Legislature, the Hon. Mr. Clarken,
of San Francisco, made an impressive speech in its favor. A
few days afterward he received a communication of which the
following is a copy:

To the Hon. Sir Clarken, of the Assembly of Law makers at Sacramento:

Most Respected Sir:—May the blessings of all the sick
overshadow you. The men from the flowery kingdom who
heal the sick in California beg you no more to say so good
words for the law which will take away from them their
bread. There are many in California (China doctors) we
guess fifty and we guess one hundred. They cure white
people many. Fine ladies ask us for cure when the white
doctors can not. They would die many good wives of rich
and noble white man if the law do command us to give them
no medicine. Some of us have lived here twenty-five years
and made well the sick by much skill all that time. Then
would be cruel to drive us away. We ask you very loud to
keep close your lips and no more praise that bad law. We
ask you to read this writing to the great assembly of law-
makers. Read it with much voice that all shall hear. Written by command of the Company of Chinese Doctors in San
Francisco the 18 day of March, 1876.

　　　　　　　　　　　Doctor Lang Fo Chung,
(San Francisco Med. Jour.)　　　　　　Obedient writer.

Dr. Haughton.—We have been desired to state that Dr.
R. E. Haughton, formerly of Richmond, is now permanently

# THE AMERICAN PRACTITIONER.

## AUGUST, 1876.

Certainly it is excellent discipline for an author to feel that he must say all that he has to say in the fewest possible words, or his reader is sure to skip them; and in the plainest possible words, or his reader will certainly misunderstand them. Generally, also, a downright fact may be told in a plain way; and we want downright facts at present more than any thing else.—RUSKIN.

## Original Communications.

## STRUMOUS OPHTHALMIA.

### BY C. S. FENNER, M. D.

Strumous ophthalmia, called by McKenzie phlyctenular ophthalmia, and known in the modern text-books as herpes corneæ, herpes conjunctivæ, according as the eruption appears on the cornea or on the conjunctiva, is one of the most troublesome affections the physician is called upon to treat, and one in which both he and the patient, or the friends of the patient, often become heartily tired of each other.

I do not propose, in this paper, to write an exhaustive account of the symptoms and pathology of strumous ophthalmia, but rather to give to the general practitioner some points in regard to its causes and of the treatment which I have found to give the most satisfactory results.

On the first appearance of the affection, minute white elevations or eruptions are noticed on the cornea or conjunctiva, covered by epithelium. There may be but one or two of these phlyctenulæ, which may be either on the cornea or on the conjunctiva; or they may be more numerous and found

VOL. XIV.—5

both on the cornea and conjunctiva, and also on the surrounding external skin.   One or more is often seen at the sclero-
corneal junction.   The epithelial covering of the elevations is
soon absorbed, allowing the contents of the vesicle to escape,
leaving small superficial ulcers.   On the cornea, however, the
ulcers may extend more deeply and be covered with a yellowish opaque matter.   The ulcerated surfaces soon heal, and
are, when on the cornea—unless, indeed, the ulceration has
penetrated to a considerable depth—again covered with trans-
parent epithelium.   Another crop of eruptions soon follows,
and these are in turn succeeded by others.

The appearance of the pustules is accompanied by great
irritability of the eyes, slight conjunctival redness, and by a
most painful sensitiveness on exposure to light (*photophobia*).
There is a sensation of smarting beneath the lids, with a
copious flow of scalding tears, that excoriate the skin of the
face over which they pass.   These tears, entering the nose
through the nasal duct, irritate the schneiderian membrane,
causing an acrid discharge, which often excoriates the alæ
nasi and skin of the upper lip.   The extreme pain and irritation induced by light, cause, through reflex action, a spasmodic contraction of the orbicularis, which presses strongly
on the eye; but when the light is excluded the spasm ceases,
and the lids can be freely opened.   The child will for hours
bury its face in its mother's lap, or seek some dark place, as
behind the bed or a darkened corner of the room, instinctively
avoiding the light; but as soon as the sun goes down, opens
the eyes, runs about, and becomes lively and cheerful.

The above mentioned local symptoms are the most prominent ones of this troublesome affection, which is rarely seen
except in children and young persons having a decidedly
marked strumous constitution; hence, the very expressive
name of scrofulous or strumous ophthalmia, which of itself
indicates the underlying cause of the disease, and plainly
points out the course of treatment which should be pursued.
The tongue is furred, the breath fetid, the upper lip and alæ
nasi swollen, the abdomen tumid, the bowels torpid, appetite

morbid, and often redness and excoriation of the external ear. Usually both eyes are affected, but one is much worse, and they alternate in this respect. As stated by Mr. Lawrence, "The inflammation may suddenly get better, and will return as suddenly. There are often repeated attacks at longer or shorter intervals, and slight exciting causes will renew the disorder when the disposition is strong. In this way the affection lasts for many months or years, and it is difficult to say when the patient is permanently recovered. The affection of the eye often alternates with other symptoms; the ears get worse, and the eyes get better, or *vice versa.*"

The strumous constitution is so graphically described by Mr. Lawrence, in his able treatise on the diseases of the eye, that I give it place here, believing that it will be appreciated by the readers of the Practitioner as highly as it has been by the writer of this article:

"*Scrofulous Constitution.*—All mankind are not formed after one pattern; if it had been so, the business of the physician and surgeon would have been much more simple than it is. There are diversities of natural organization, and analogous varieties in the forms of disease. Each individual has something peculiar in constitution, as well as in form and features. But the peculiarities with which it is more important that we should become acquainted, medically, are those which distinguish classes more or less numerous; and of these none is more common than the scrofulous. The word *scrofula* is used in two senses; either to designate that assemblage of characters which marks a particular disease, or to denote the peculiarity of constitution, generally original or connate, from which such distinctive characters are derived. In the former sense, *scrofula* is equivalent to *scrofulous disease;* in the latter, to *scrofulous constitution.* We can point out certain external marks of scrofula; but we have not yet discovered the differences in the elementary composition of the frame on which the characteristic of scrofulous disease depend. The morbid disposition, however, is strongly marked; certain forms of disease are so easily excited, and return so readily, that it is almost impossible to keep them off. The absorbent glands, and some other organs of glandular structure, the mucous membranes and skin, the lungs, bones, and joints, are the parts most liable to scrofula. Of the membranes, such as are exposed to the external air suffer most; for instance, those of the eyes, nose, and lungs. Two kinds of constitution, differing considerably in some respects, are observed in persons called scrofulous. In one there is a pale and bloated countenance, a swelling of the upper lip and septum of the nose, and tumid abdomen. The mucous membrane of the stomach and bowels is easily disordered by errors of diet, or by trifling causes, which have but little or no effect on other persons. When these important organs are disturbed, the nutrition of the entire body is more or less impaired. There is a languid state of the circulation, so that the skin is pale and rough, and the extremities are cold; the muscular flesh is loose and flabby; and there is a kind of torpor in all the functions, bodily and mental. In the other set of subjects the integuments are thin, and the ramifications of the cutaneous veins are distinctly seen; there is an almost unnatural color in the cheeks. The circulation is rapid, the nervous system irritable, and both are easily excited. The various functions of the body and mind are performed quickly. A premature development of intellect is often observed in such children, and they are affected powerfully by all external influences."

Mr. Lawrence adds: "The liability to scrofula does not extend equally through the whole of life. Disease of this character generally, and strumous ophthalmia in particular, are not seen in infants at the breast, which, being kept warm, and having a supply of wholesome food prepared by nature, escape the two great exciting causes. They prevail, however, extensively from the end of suckling to the age of puberty, in which period the processes of nutrition and growth are going on actively, and easily disturbed by the circumstances already alluded to. Strumous ophthalmia is seldom seen after puberty; but other forms of ophthalmic inflammation are often found more obstinate in persons of scrofulous constitution."

The phlyctenulæ or pustules may occur in children free from struma, and strumous ophthalmia may exist without the eruptions; but these exceptions are rarely met with.

In this, as in other affections, the symptoms often vary in different cases; and, in reference to this subject, I must again quote from Mr. Lawrence, who says: "In describing diseases, we find it necessary to select the instances in which the characters are best marked. We do not find them exactly as they are described in books and lectures; and they, who are only acquainted with them from such sources, discover, when they have to examine the sick, that several morbid affections are not so clearly characterized as they expected. We give names to such forms of disease as are clearly marked, but we see many cases which do not come under our descriptions. There is an insensible gradation from one form to another, so that we can not draw an accurate boundary between them. This is the case with strumous and common ophthalmia. If we find the nosologies imperfect, we must recollect that they are not the productions of nature, but the work of man."

*Treatment.*—Since the treatment of eye diseases has largely fallen into the hands of specialists, I am satisfied from extensive observation that those ocular inflammations having their origin in constitutional causes, are not now so successfully treated as in former times, when this branch of medicine fell chiefly in the practice of the general surgeon, who habitually takes a broader and more comprehensive view of the causes of disease than do those whose minds are constantly directed in a single channel and to a single organ. Hence, the tendency of the specialist is to regard the diseases which he treats as of local origin, to be relieved chiefly by local treatment. This is exemplified in the modern text-books on the diseases of the eye, where take, for example, the chapters on phlyctenular ophthalmia, several pages are devoted to local treatment, while the constitutional treatment is disposed of in a very few lines.

*Constitutional Treatment.*—As strumous ophthalmia is but the local development of a constitutional affection, it follows that the chief object of treatment should be to overcome that defective organization, and the various morbid conditions to which it gives rise, and which are always found accompanying this affection.   As the bowels are torpid, and the stomach distended often with indigestible food, the use of purgatives is strongly indicated, and calomel or blue mass, combined with rhubarb or jalap, given so as to produce a free action of the bowels, will give much relief; frequently several doses are necessary before the tongue becomes clean and the tumidity of the stomach disappears.   As soon as the latter results take place, there is almost invariably a marked improvement of the inflammatory symptoms of the eye; the sensitiveness to light is less or disappears, the redness decreases, and the ulcerations rapidly take on the healing process.   I know of no remedy which has so powerful an influence over the morbid conditions accompanying strumous ophthalmia as mercury, given in minute alterative doses; and when the symptoms are very urgent, calomel or blue mass, with a view to its purgative effect.   The distended stomach, furred tongue, and fetid breath, rapidly disappear under this treatment.

Sir William Wilde says: "There is a peculiar heavy breath belonging to strumous patients, which it is difficult to describe, but which, once perceived, is easily recognized ever after.   I may here mention that I do not remember a single instance in which, for any cause, mercurial action was fully produced in a person possessing naturally what is termed 'bad breath,' that that most unpleasant affection was not removed by it."

I usually prescribe one or two grains of hydrarg. cum creta, with two or three grains of pulverized rhubarb, to be taken every second or third night, or sufficiently often to keep the bowels freely open.   By far the most efficacious form in which mercury can be administered as an alterative to produce permanent effects, is the bichloride or corrosive sublimate.   This medicine exercises a powerfully controlling influence over that defective organization which underlies or gives rise to these morbid conditions usually found in persons having the well marked strumous diathesis.

I again quote from Wilde, who says: "The third and perhaps the most efficacious form in which mercury may be used, is that of the bichloride, still commonly known in this country as the oxymuriate, one of the most valuable medicines in the entire pharmacopœia. A treatise might be written on the virtues of this remedy, and the vast field of disease over which it exercises a sanative influence, combined with Peruvian bark, which the chemists say is incompatible, but the product of the decomposition said to be produced by which may be the very substance which acts more beneficially; it is almost a panacea for most of the strumous inflammations in children and young people, and its power in controlling scrofulous ophthalmia, corneitis, iritis, etc., extends equally to the cure of kindred affections in the ear. . . . It is, moreover, when properly administered, one of the safest as well as the surest preparations of mercury; it leaves no ill effects, it rarely induces ptyalism, and patients improve in health, and absolutely grow fat, while using it."

I am able to confirm all that Mr. Wilde has said in regard to the efficacy of this most potent remedy. I have given it continuously, in hundreds of cases for many months, without producing any unpleasant results, and rarely without either entirely relieving or greatly ameliorating the ophthalmic symptoms, and at the same time improving the general condition of the patient. The following formula I have used for many years: Hydrarg. bichlor., two grains; aquæ dist., half an ounce; ammon. chlor., q. s. Dissolve and add tinc. cincho. comp., four ounces; syrup sarsapar., three ounces and a half. Dose, from one to two teaspoonfuls three times a day, just before eating.

*Tonics* are always indicated in strumous ophthalmia, and the most efficacious I have found to be quinia and iron. Dr. Isaac Hays has strongly recommended the syrup of the ioduret of iron. I have derived more benefit from the phosphate of iron, given in from five to ten grain doses three times a day. This may be combined with quinia given in grain doses, or the iron may be administered during the day and the quinia

taken at bedtime.   Cod liver oil, where it does not disagree
with the stomach, may be of benefit; indeed, all remedies
which give tone to the system are admissible.

The diet should be carefully attended to, both with regard
to quality and quantity of food, the meals regular; and indigestible food, such as cakes and candies, avoided.   Meat may
be allowed at breakfast and dinner, but not for supper.   The
diet should chiefly consist of meat, milk, vegetables, bread,
and other farinaceous articles; ripe fruit is admissible, taken
in moderate quantities.   Exercise in the open air is desirable,
whenever the photophobia will admit of it.

*Local Treatment.*—When the orbicularis muscle, from excessive use, has attained abnormal strength and development,
canthoplasty is advisable in order to weaken the action of the
muscle and diminish the pressure on the eye.   One great objection to the use of local applications arises from the fact
that, owing to great pain and irritation induced by light and
the irritability of the child, the effort to open the lids is powerfully resisted, and force must necessarily be applied sufficient
to overcome the utmost tension of the muscle.   This effort
often produces so much pressure on the eye and is attended
by such an amount of irritation, as to more than counterbalance any benefit that might otherwise result from local
applications.   A solution of the sulphate of atropia, of the
strength of two or three grains to the ounce of distilled water,
dropped in the eye once a day, is a most effectual remedy in
relieving the intolerance of light and in allaying the irritability
of the eye.

After the inflammatory symptoms have partially subsided,
it is a general practice now to dust a small quantity of calomel
beneath the lids.   This substance is supposed to exercise a
chemical effect, so as in some unexplained manner to produce
contraction or obliteration of the terminal branches of the
blood vessels.   If the margin of the lids be inflamed, or the
external skin excoriated, an application of the amorphous
yellow oxide of mercury in the proportion of ten to fifteen
grains to the ounce of simple cerate, or the glycerole of

starch, will be found of benefit. An alum curd in such cases, placed over the eyes and retained by a bandage, is useful and often grateful to the patient. Pledgets of lint soaked in a weak solution of alum, placed over the eyes and confined, by a compress bandage, will be of service, not only by the astringency of the alum relieving the excoriation, but by restraining the motion of the eyes, portions of whose surfaces have lost their epithelial covering, leaving the terminal nerves exposed to the friction of the lining membrane of the lids. For the excoriations of the alæ nasi, septum nasi, and schneiderian membrane, I have derived much benefit from the use of resin (basilicon) ointment.

LOUISVILLE.

---

# A CASE OF CUT-THROAT—MARKED EFFECT OF OPIUM ON THE RESPIRATORY MUCOUS MEMBRANE.

BY E. P. EASLEY, M. D.

Jacob R——, a large, vigorous German, aged fifty-five years, after murdering his wife, set the house on fire, and attempted suicide by cutting his throat with a dull Barlow knife on September 25th, 1875. He severed the anterior jugular veins, superior thyroid artery, sterno-hyoid and sterno-thyroid muscles and trachea. When seen a few hours afterward there had evidently been profuse hemorrhage and great shock. The second ring of the trachea was removed and a part of the first, which was partially detached from the cricoid cartilage, and the ends of the trachea were united with wire sutures, and the external wound brought together with silk. Reaction came on during the evening through the use of stimulants. The parts became greatly swollen, suppurated, and on the fifth day the sutures cutting out the wound reopened, presenting a cavity filled with offensive pus, which running into the windpipe produced intense dyspnœa, which was relieved by placing the patient in the "all fours" position, thus allowing the pus to escape from the trachea.

The curved end of a gum catheter was now introduced through the wound into the trachea. This prevented dyspnœa, but had to be removed occasionally and cleared of the tenacious mucus; so I had constructed a silver tube, four inches long, with a caliber of three-eighths of an inch. He wore this six weeks, and while it remained *in situ*, respiration was carried on solely through it. This larger tube would also become occluded and cause violent dyspnœa, and would have to be removed instantly, cleaned and replaced.

The depressors of the larynx being severed, the elevators drew the larynx close up to the base of the tongue. A mirror introduced into the wound, with its reflecting surface looking upward, reflected a perfect view of the larynx, showing the relation of all the parts to one another. During inspiration and deglutition the vocal chords approached each other, and lay side by side, and in expiration separated. Aphonia was complete, but attempts to articulate contracted, separated, and rendered the chords pale. These movements were abnormal, for laryngoscopical examinations show that the action of these parts in the normal condition is the reverse of what I have described, except during deglutition. Aphonia, it appears, is due to a non-approximation of the vocal chords, let the pathological condition be what it may. Respiration was comparatively easy through the larger tube. The rings of the trachea were reproduced, and the trachea united, with the exception of a small opening in front. The external wound cicatrized, and the patient's general condition improved so that he was soon able to walk around; but in a few days œdema of the feet and ankles appeared, with paroxysms of dyspnœa; his pulse became very weak, and on the 25th of November he fell from his chair and instantly expired.

I made an autopsy, and found the lungs normal. The pericardium contained from five to six ounces of serum. The walls of the right heart were in an advanced state of fatty degeneration, the finger being thrust through with ease. The columnæ carneæ and musculi pectinati were so soft as to be rubbed off with the thumb. The right ventricle was dilated with coagulated blood, and a coagulum composed of several layers extended three inches into the pulmonary artery, from the end of which a piece had been detached and carried into the lungs, thus producing the dyspnœa and instant collapse. All the essential factors for the production of a thrombus in the pulmonary artery were present, viz., a dilated and fatty heart, and an obstructed circulation in the lungs consequent upon violent and prolonged fits of coughing.

The remedies employed externally were water dressing, carbolic and salicylic acid; internally, opium, bromide of potash, muriate of ammonia and tonics. The bromide was given to obtund the sensibility of the mucous membranes of the larynx and trachea, and the ammonia for the bronchitis; but neither had the slightest effect. The opium given had a marked effect in allaying the cough and checking the enormous pulmonary and tracheal secretions. The mucus, which had been thick, tenacious and ropy, and had to be detached from the tube by a pair of forceps, became diminished in quantity and changed in character, so it could be expectorated with ease. If the opium was discontinued the cough returned and the expectoration assumed its original character. After this experience with opium, I would not hesitate to employ it in croupous or catarrhal inflammation of the lungs, and in bronchitis.

It is quite evident that this patient died of pulmonary embolism, and the remarkable effort of the trachea to repair the injury under such unfavorable circumstances proves that tracheotomy is not a very grave operation *per se*, and should be resorted to in the majority of cases where life is in danger from laryngeal stenosis.

NEW ALBANY, IND.

## CHOLERA INFANTUM.

BY A. G. CRAIG, M. D.

*Formerly Resident Physician of Cincinnati Hospital.*

Cholera infantum, or, as it is generally called, summer complaint, is not as supposed by some a disease peculiar to this country. English writers describe the morbid phenomena of this affection under the head of infantile diarrhœa. Trousseau adopts the term infantile cholera. By other French writers it is usually called choleriform diarrhœa. It is an affection that occurs in this country from the month of May to October, its maximum frequency and severity correspond with the degree of heat, the disease increasing or decreasing as the mercury rises or falls in the thermometer. The disease is most prevalent in the months of July and August. It is not a disease confined almost exclusively to large cities, as is generally taught in our text-books. It is frequently met with in the rural districts, under the most favorable hygienic conditions. By some writers the term cholera infantum has been extended so as to include all the diarrhœal maladies of infancy, during the hot season. I shall restrict it to that form of infantile diarrhœa in which the stools are frequent and watery, accompanied by vomiting, great thirst, high temperature, and rapid emaciation.

Cholera infantum occurs commonly under the age of two years, and generally during the period of early dentition. For this reason the malady is associated with teething in the popular mind, and even some practitioners consider dentition a cause. The eruption of the teeth is doubtless often retarded by this affection, and the disease frequently aggravated by irritation of the gums, but dentition will not of itself produce it. During infancy, which extends from birth to the age of two and a half years, there is great functional activity and rapid development of the intestinal follicles, and the disease should be attributed to this cause, rather than to dentition.

But the most obvious cause of this malady is the intense heat of summer, and the anti-hygienic conditions to which it gives rise. In the large cities the heat is greater than in the country, the atmosphere is loaded with noxious vapors, especially gases arising from animal and vegetable decomposition. Children of the poorer classes, in insalubrious locations, living in crowded tenement houses, and in an atmosphere rendered impure by personal and domiciliary uncleanliness, are peculiarly liable to be affected, but the children of those surrounded by the most favorable hygienic circumstances, by no means escape. In many cases another cause coöperates, namely, indigestion induced by the use of improper food, which tends to impair the whole alimentary tract. Bottle-fed infants are especially subject to this affection. In some cases malaria contributes to the intensity of the disease.

Cholera infantum in the great majority of cases is preceded by simple diarrhœa, the dejections being more or less numerous and copious, but not such as to excite much alarm. In other cases the attack commences abruptly. The diarrhœa is profuse, the stools often of a green or yellow color, but more commonly light-colored and watery, and almost always contain particles of food, especially undigested milk. The discharges are generally offensive from the onset, and when the disease is protracted, they are frequently streaked with blood. The diarrhœa rarely continues for any length of time before an extreme irritability of the stomach manifests itself. Vomiting is a prominent and persistent symptom, everything taken into the stomach being immediately rejected, sometimes with great violence. In other cases there is constant retching without vomiting. In many cases the irritability of the stomach continues throughout the attack; in others the vomiting ceases while the purging continues unabated, or even increases in violence, and whatever food or drink is taken passes off rapidly without undergoing much change. In some cases the dejections are so thin and watery, as to soak into the diaper, and scarcely produce more of a stain than does the urine, and occasionally are almost odorless.

Thirst is a prominent and persistent symptom, the little patient craves constantly cold drinks, and ice is taken with great avidity. The appetite is gone, yet the infant seizes the breast eagerly in order to relieve the great thirst. The tongue in the commencement of the attack is covered with a white, slimy mucus; in protracted cases it becomes red and dry. The pulse is usually quick, frequent, small and tense, and the respiration somewhat increased in frequency. The skin is dry and harsh, the head and abdomen are hot. The thermometer indicates a temperature of 103° to 107°, and in one case under my care, which proved fatal, 110¼°. The infant is restless, and fretful, and generally sleeps with its eyelids partially open. The emaciation is more rapid than in any disease, except Asiatic cholera. The eyes are sunken, languid and glassy; the countenance pale and shrunken; the lips thin, dry and shriveled. As death approaches, the infant rolls its head about; utters plaintive, scarcely audible cries; the abdomen becomes tympanitic; the hands and feet of leaden hue, and sometimes œdematous; the skin has a clammy coldness; the discharges from the bowels frequent and very offensive; urine scanty or suppressed; complete coma results, death being in many cases preceded by convulsions. In some cases effusion takes place in the brain, and the patient has all the symptoms of acute hydrocephalus.

Cholera infantum is essentially an inflammatory malady. In inflammation of mucous surfaces the redness is apt to partially disappear in the cadaver. After death an examination reveals turgescence of the intestinal follicles. The mucous membrane is vascular and softened, and the solitary glands, and the patches of Peyer, present an inflammatory hyperæmia; and sometimes ulcerated patches are found throughout the intestinal canal. When the brain is involved there are found softening and injection of the cerebral tissue, and congestion of the cranial sinuses, veins, and capillaries.

*Treatment.* —This remains a *quæstio vexata.* The great variety of treatment instituted for the relief and cure of this affection, is evidence of the difficulty experienced in the man-

agement of it. I am, from no limited experience, a believer
in calomel in the early stages of this disease. Given at once,
so soon as the disease manifests itself, nothing else will so
promptly restore the healthy action of the stomach and bowels. The medicine is best administered dry on the tongue,
for being tasteless it is swallowed without repugnance. It is
one of our best remedies for the relief of sick stomach in this
affection. I have known it to succeed after all other means
had failed. I administer from one-fourth to two grains, two
or three times daily, or every two or three hours in urgent
cases, when the discharges are frequent and exhausting. A
spice poultice, wet with brandy, should be kept over the abdomen so long as the vomiting continues, and should be
renewed frequently, so as to maintain its strength. A sinapism to the epigastrium is often necessary. Pounded ice may
be given to quench the thirst. When the stomach is very
irritable, water should be given sparingly or withheld altogether. In a majority of cases opiates are indispensable. The
paramount object is the arrest of the exhausting discharges,
and to relieve the griping, until the calomel has had time to
effect a change in the secretions. The remedy on which most
dependence is to be placed in effecting this object is opium.
Laudanum is a most eligible preparation. When the stomach
is very irritable, and the discharges frequent and exhausting,
and attended with griping, it should be given by the rectum
in starch-water. Sometimes acetate of lead injections—from
two to four grains, in starch-water—may be farther needed,
for the same intent. So soon as the irritability of the stomach
is sufficiently quieted as to allow of its administration, the
remedy which I have found generally to promptly restrain the
disordered action of the bowels, is a combination of calomel,
prepared chalk, acetate of lead and opium.

   R. Hydrarg. chlor. mit.,  . . .   gr. iv.
     Cretæ præp.,  . . . . .   gr. xxxvj.
     Plumbi acetat.,  . . . . .   gr. xij.
     Opii pulv.,  . . . . . .   gr. j.

 M. ft. ch. No. xii. One powder every two to four hours to
an infant one year old.

I have also used the following formula with the best results in this affection. The dose is for an infant of one year:

R. Tinct. opii, . . . . . . . gtt. xxiv.
Bismuth subnitrat., . . . . ʒij.
Mistur. cretæ, . . . . . . ʒij. Misce.

Shake bottle thoroughly, and give one teaspoonful every three or four hours.

In some cases I have used with gratifying results the subnitrate of bismuth and the compound powder of chalk with opium, combining as it does an astringent, alkali, and opiate. The bismuth is an efficient anti-emetic, and is a valuable remedy, not only in this disease, but in all of the diarrhœal maladies of infancy. Its effects are entirely local, namely, upon the gastro-intestinal surface. It undergoes some chemical change with the secretions, which turns it black, and gives more consistence to the discharges. There is no positive evidence of its absorption.

Creasote is a valuable anti-emetic in this affection, counteracting as it does fermentation in the alimentary mass. It is best given in mucilage. Lime-water and milk, besides being nutritious, are efficient in relieving the irritability of the stomach. There are exceptional cases of cholera infantum in which we are left in no doubt as to their malarious nature. Such cases will require quinia or cinchonidia in conjunction with other remedies. •

In protracted cases the vegetable astringents are of service. A decoction of the root of geranium maculatum, sweetened to the taste, is the best; it checks the discharges, and promotes digestion.

If the head be hot, and stupor or coma be threatened, with other marked cerebral symptoms, the opiate should be omitted. In these cases a few leeches behind the ears, and the application of cold water to the head, may be proper.

In every case the gums should be carefully examined, and if found to be swollen and inflamed, they should be freely lanced.

Attention to diet and regimen is of the greatest importance.

If the milk of the mother, from pregnancy or other causes, is found to disagree with the infant, it must be weaned, and fed upon rich cow's milk, sweetened but not diluted. Pure milk is generally considered by physicians as the most appropriate article of food in this affection; but I have frequently met with cases in which the vomiting and purging were increased by confining the little patient to a milk diet, large masses of caseum being ejected from the stomach, and passed from the bowels. Egg-water, made by dissolving the whites of four eggs in a pint of iced water, to which a teaspoonful of bicarbonate of soda has been added, is, in my opinion, one of the very best articles of diet in cholera infantum. By the use of this drink I have seen patients rescued from imminent danger of collapse. It is taken with avidity by very young children, and is very seldom ejected, is readily digested, the albumen passing into the circulation and replacing that element of the blood exuded in the watery evacuations. In some cases I have administered, with the best results, the white of an egg beaten well with a spoon, to which a lump of ice had been added. Arrow-root, farina, chicken-water, essence of beef, strong broths, and broiled tender beef, have been found to answer best with some. Trousseau and others recommend raw meat made into a kind of *purée* by being reduced to a pulp in a mortar and pressed through a fine sieve, so as to separate the vessels and areolar tissue. I have had no experience in the use of raw meat, but the liability to tænia and trichina, as a result of eating uncooked meat, is not to be overlooked. Vegetables and fruits, and every kind of food which is not readily digested, should be prohibited. Many children will require alcoholic stimulants, preferably with their food, for support. Pure brandy, if it can be obtained, is the best stimulant. Elixir of calisaya bark is an eligible preparation, combining as it does a tonic and stimulant, agreeable to the taste. Pepsin is often beneficial.

The child should be bathed daily. Its apartments should be clean, dry, and freely ventilated, and so arranged as to be darkened during the day. The clothing should be sufficient to protect the child against the sudden changes of the weather, but not so warm as to overheat the body. The custom of dressing the child in flannel and other warm clothing, can not be too much reprehended. During the extreme heat of the day, a thin cotton dress is all that is required. The babe should be carried into the open air in the shade of trees, but should not be exposed to the warm rays of the sun.

In the close built parts of a large city, all treatment may fail in some cases of cholera infantum, but the patients will speedily recover on being carried into the salubrious air of the country. The details of the treatment above indicated, must, of course, be left to the judgment of the medical attendant. Protracted summer complaint affords scope for perseverance and contrivance in finding remedies to control the vomiting, to restrain the exhausting discharges, and to improve the digestive powers of the little sufferer.

GHENT, KY.

---

# CAPILLARY BRONCHITIS.

## SYNONYMS—CATARRHAL PNEUMONIA, BRONCHO-PNEUMONIA.

### BY JOHN L. COOK, M. D.*

After reading Juergensen's article on catarrhal pneumonia, in Ziemssen's Cyclopædia of the Practice of Medicine, Vol. V, I announced before the Henderson Medical Club that the disease described was really capillary bronchitis.

Catarrhal pneumonia, so called, is a secondary affection, generally commences in the external air passages, and travels inwards towards the lungs. It is preceded by a common cold, which passes downwards into the large bronchial tubes, where it is known as ordinary bronchitis. Finally, when the inflam-

* Remarks made before the Kentucky State Medical Society at Hopkinsville.

mation extends to the minute bronchial tubes, we have capillary bronchitis, the disease under present consideration. This is the complication which destroys so many children with hooping-cough, and so many patients with measles. Indeed, it is claimed by high authority that lobular pneumonia in children under five years of age is not inflammation of the lung substance at all, but a form of bronchitis.

Capillary bronchitis is a very grave, and frequently a very rapid disease, death ensuing in from three to five days. The patient may have an ordinary bronchitis, in which he is doing very well; but when the minute tubes are invaded, alarming symptoms at once show themselves. While in this, as in all acute inflammations, fever is usually present, the danger of death is not from excessive temperature, but from asphyxia. The respirations often reach fifty per minute; the pulse beats one hundred and fifty in the same time. The surface of the body is blue, from the want of aeration of the blood. The absence of pain in the chest presents a striking contrast to acute lobar pneumonia. Furthermore, the malady is always bilateral. The product of the inflammation is serous in character, in which there is proliferation of epithelial cells.

But what does physical exploration of the chest reveal? It discloses the subcrepitant râle, as Juergensen says, but when it does so, it is pathognomonic of capillary bronchitis, of which it is the physical sign, when pulmonary tuberculosis, hemoptysis, œdema of the lungs, etc., are excluded; but then the history of the disease under which the patient is laboring should be taken into consideration. As ordinary bronchitis is associated with the malady, the sibilant, sonorous and mucous râles will be observed. There may be no change in the percussion note, but should collapse of the lobules of the lungs occur, as is often the case, there will be dullness on percussion.

In order to make the subject clear and satisfactory, it will be proper to refer briefly to acute lobar pneumonia, its history, and its physical signs. Croupous pneumonia, as it is termed, seizes the lung suddenly and directly, and is generally unilateral. In the midst of the night, perhaps, the patient is attacked with a chill, pain in the side, and difficulty of breathing. Fever soon follows. The pulse is from one hundred to one hundred and twenty per minute; the respiration from twenty-five to forty; the mouth is dry, and the secretions in general scant. A distressing cough, at first dry, annoys the patient, but the characteristic rusty-colored expectoration soon makes its appearance. This is the first stage, or that of congestion. Physical examination discovers the crepitant râle, which is due to a slight exudation of plastic lymph into the air cells, and a closure and separation of their walls during inspiration and expiration. In addition, there will be broncho-vesicular respiration and exaggerated vocal resonance. Distinct dullness on percussion will be readily detected.

Here is presented an opportunity for the physician to accomplish much good. Heroic measures, properly directed, may abort the disease. But if we stand by, with our hands folded, or rely upon expectant treatment, we may have the proud consolation of knowing the patient has "typhoid pneumonia," or the second stage, that of consolidation, has been reached. In that event, the air cells are completely blocked up with the exudation of lymph. The vesicular murmur is entirely suppressed. The broncho-vesicular respiration is supplanted by the bronchial respiration, and the exaggerated vocal resonance gives way to bronchophony and whispering bronchophony, which are the correlative signs.

The physical signs which obtain in the solidification of croupous pneumonia are present also in the solidification of catarrhal pneumonia, when there is dullness from the collapse of the lobules of the lungs. In other words, the pitch, quality and intensity of the broncho-vesicular respiration, bronchial respiration and bronchophony, do not depend on the character of inflammation, whether croupous or catarrhal, but on the degree of consolidation.

One strong point which I wish to urge here, is that in the inflammatory product of catarrhal pneumonia there is no lymph. This being true, there can be no crepitant râle in the disease, for this sign depends upon this glutinous deposit. Juergensen states that his ear is unable to distinguish the crepitant from the subcrepitant râle. Practically the crepitant râle is a dry sound, heard in inspiration only; whereas the subcrepitant râle is a moist, bubbling sound, usually heard both in inspiration and expiration.

It is not my design to say that catarrhal inflammation may not dip down into the air cells; but should it do so, we possess no means which would enable us to make a correct diagnosis.

CARDINAL DIFFERENCES TABULATED.

| *Croupous Pneumonia.* | *Catarrhal Pneumonia.* |
|---|---|
| 1. Seizes the lung directly and suddenly. | 1. Commences in the external air passages and travels inward. |
| 2. Generally unilateral. | 2. Always bilateral. |
| 3. Crepitant râle. | 3. Subcrepitant râle. |
| 4. Plastic lymph. | 4. No plastic lymph. |
| 5. Dullness from exudation. | 5. Dullness from collapse of lobules. |
| 6. Fever high. | 6. Fever not marked. |
| 7. Pain in the side. | 7. No pain in the side, or but little. |
| 8. Death from asthenia. | 8. Death from asphyxia. |
| 9. Pulse 100 to 120. | 9. Pulse 150 or more. |
| 10. Respirations from 25 to 40. | 10. Respirations, 50 or more. |
| 11. Cyanosis late, if at all. | 11. Cyanosis early. |
| 12. Rusty-colored expectoration. | 12. Muco-purulent expectoration. |
| 13. Death rate not more than ten per cent. | 13. Death rate two-thirds or more. |

In my opinion all diseases in which there is generally a rapid and fatal course, should be met with heroic treatment. The attempt should be made to arrest the onward march of the disease, subdue its active forces, and relieve its pathological changes. Nature does her part nobly, but because she is faithful that does not prove that she does not need aid. In most cases she is victorious, but in many instances she is pushed to the wall. In the first stage of capillary bronchitis, I should administer such sedatives as veratrum, ipecac, ergot and quinia, to which ammonia might be added. Thus:

R. Syr. ipecac., . . . . . . ℥vj.
Verat. tinct., . . . . . . gtt. xxiv.
Quiniæ sulphat, . . . . . gr. xxx. Misce.

Dose, a teaspoonful every two hours if necessary. If the pulse become weak, five grains of carbonate of ammonia should be added to each dose.

The danger in this disease is not from exhaustion, but from asphyxia; therefore, we should control the inflammation as much as possible, so that sufficient air can enter the lungs. Active remedies, when properly administered, control inflammation and the morbid processes to which it leads. It should be remembered that exhaustion by excessive action is very dangerous. Sedatives prevent such disturbances, and so restore the patient. Bring the pulse to the normal standard, and there hold it. Then use quinia, ergot, etc., to constringe the blood vessels in the engorged bronchial tubes.

Should exhaustion manifest itself, heroic measures must be suspended, and then rely on whisky, quinia and ammonia, in full and repeated doses. Opium, if used, should be given with great circumspection.

HENDERSON, KY.

—

## AN ORIGINAL SUICIDE.

BY W. W. VINNEDGE, M. D.

On Saturday, the 10th day of June, 1876, James A. Moon, a farmer, thirty-seven years of age, residing on the Wea Plains, nine miles west of Lafayette, left home and came to this city, and made every preparation to make his name notorious. On his arrival in the morning he registered his name at the Lahr House, and told the proprietor "he would like to have a *good* room shown him, as he would probably occupy it three or four days." A number of rooms were then shown to him before one was found suitable, it being No. 41, on the upper floor, immediately over the market space, and not accessible to view from any direction. While selecting the room he remarked to the porter, "that he wanted a room as far away from the noise as possible, as he slept but little except in a quiet room, and not at all if troubled by noise." After selecting his room, he remarked, "Room 41 suits me first-rate." He then locked the door, left the house, and was not seen again until late in the afternoon.

On his second visit he brought a heavy trunk, which he charged the porters to carry right side up and with great care, as its contents would not permit "jostling." To see this order properly executed, he followed the men to his room, showing just where and how to place the trunk. He then again went down on the street, was shaved, visited a short time with two or three old soldier friends, returned to his room between eight and nine in the evening, and was not seen again alive. During the entire time of these preparations he was cheerful, laughing and talking familiarly and freely with his acquaintances, giving especial attention to army reminiscences. When the boy at the foundry, who drilled the holes in the pole of the broad-ax used in his destruction, and through the iron upright bars to which the broad-ax was attached by bolts and screws, asked him what he intended to make, he replied, "An instrument for making fruit-baskets."

The room that he selected at the hotel is twelve by fourteen feet, having but one window which opens towards the west, and two doors, one in the south wall opening into an adjoining room, and one in the east wall opening into the hall. The furniture of the room consisted of a bed, wash-stand, table, and the trunk which contained the instrument of death, and which, on account of its construction and *modus operandi*, has been called "the Moon guillotine." The essential parts of the instrument are a broad-ax and lever screwed at one end to the floor. The ax was secured to this lever, seven feet in length, the lower two-thirds of which consisted of wood, by upright pieces of bar-iron fastened with bolts and screws. The lever was composed of three separate parts, for convenience in transportation, firmly bolted together, the widened end being attached to the floor by means of hinges to prevent any possible lateral motion. At the other end of the lever, the iron bars to which the ax was attached were very heavy, in order to give the machine great effectiveness when put in motion. The ax being elevated, was sustained at the proper angle for falling the greatest distance possible by means of a double cord attached to the free end of the lever, and to a small hook in a bracket, which was securely fastened to the wood on the side of the window, about five feet from the floor. On this bracket was placed a lighted candle between the cords, which were consumed when the candle had burned sufficiently. The ax being then unsupported, fell to do its fearful execution.

I am indebted to Mr. Orth Stein, of this city, for the following illustration, as well as the others in this article. This one shows the suicide in position waiting for the ax to fall.

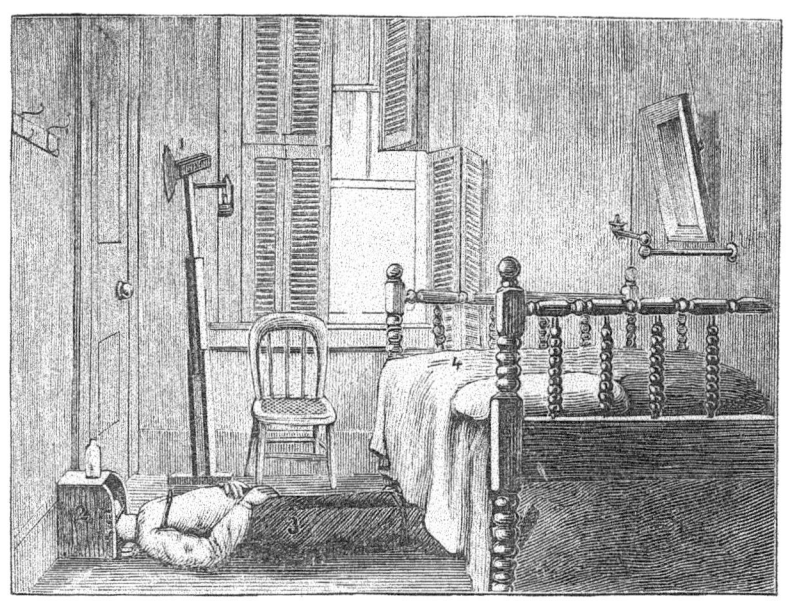

1. Ax on its shaft in elevation; bracket and candle in rear of ax. 2. Box with perforations, and stick holding back Moon's chin. 3. Moon in position to receive ax. 4. Bed partly covering his legs.

The suicide had placed an ordinary soap-box on its side, with its open end just even with the line marked where the ax would fall. The ax consequently, in falling, just grazed the open end of the box, and as the lever was secured at the fulcrum by hinges, it must fall "true." This box contained his head when he lay stretched out on the floor at right angles to the direction of the falling ax. Three pieces of pine board sustained his neck; and to keep his chin out of the sweep of the falling ax, he had supported it by a little wooden rod, one-fourth of an inch in diameter, placed across the box. This rod assisted in preventing the head and upper part of the trunk from being displaced.

But Moon was not wholly indifferent to the fear of pain, and had obtained two ounces of chloroform, with which he saturated a quantity of cotton. The cotton was placed in the box, so that the chloroform could be inhaled after he had adjusted himself by stretching out on the floor at right angles to the path of the guillotine, his head in the box and feet under the bed; his body was firmly fastened to the floor by straps and buckles. While the candle was burning he occupied this position, inhaling the anæsthetic. The flame reaching the cord it was burned through, and the ax fell with fearful force, severing the head completely from the body.

The following illustration exhibits the machine after it had done its work and the corpse removed.

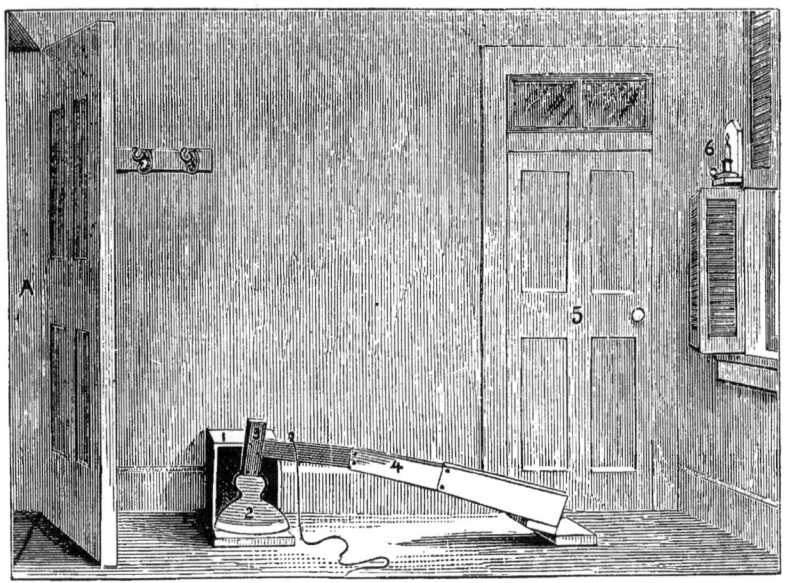

A—Door of room No. 41.  1. Box for Moon's head, with cross-stick to hold back his chin.  2. Ax.  3. Iron bars riveted to ax.  4. Shaft of ax hinged to board-piece screwed to floor.  5. Door to room No. 40.  6. Bracket and candle.

James A. Moon was a man of very fine figure, being six feet two inches in height, and weighing one hundred and ninety pounds. His hair and eyes were brown, and his face exhibited a great deal of character. The annexed illustration 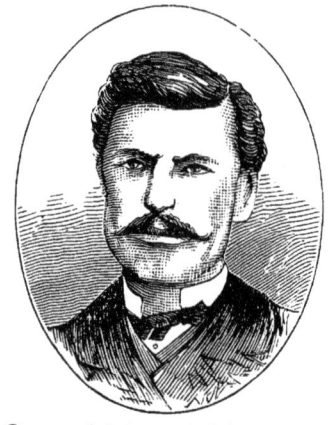 is one made by Mr. Stein, from a picture taken of him at the close of his service in the United States Army in 1865. And although it may seem like prophesying after an event, most persons who examine his counterfeit presentment, will see it presenting decided evidences of insanity; it is the face of a man of unsound mind. He always enjoyed talking about mechanics. It was a hobby with him. One of his neighbors states that he without assistance became an excellent blacksmith, learning the trade during the intervals between working hours on the farm. His mind had a tendency to "run" on methods of causing death. He had great admiration for men who have rendered their names famous as inventors of machines which would cause death suddenly and with dispatch. During a service of three years in the Sixteenth Indiana Battery, he would spend his leisure time in making out of wood, with a penknife only, various articles, exhibiting great ingenuity in design and skill in execution, and presented the products of his labors to his comrades as souvenirs. He had a good education, was temperate in his habits and kind to his family. His intimate friends state that he was thoroughly familiar with the Bible—with both the Old and New Testaments—though a skeptic as to the inspiration of each. All of his acquaintances testify to his habitual genial and pleasant disposition.

The question has frequently been asked, was Moon unconscious at the moment the ax fell? I have thought not. Any one familiar with the administration of chloroform by inhalation, will understand why I think two ounces of the drug poured on an ordinary roll of cotton batting, at a single time, will not produce deep sleep—anæsthesiá. As the bottle was found on the table, at least six feet from where Moon's body was found after death, I conclude that he, being uninstructed as to the use and effects of chloroform, saturated the cotton at the table, having perhaps previously lighted the candle, placed his body in position, buckled the straps over it, placed the rod under his chin, and then the cotton over his nostrils. This must have been his last act. From these circumstances, and the knowledge that chloroform usually causes struggles in vigorous men while passing through the stage of excitement, and the fact that Moon left no evidence of any struggle, I conclude that he was conscious—perhaps somewhat stupefied, but still conscious—while waiting for the candle to burn sufficiently low to divide the cord.

Some idea of the curious workings of this diseased mind, as he busied himself at his night work, may be obtained from the inscriptions placed at irregular intervals, in pencil marks, on the lever; "Kari kari," supposed to be the name he gave his machine; "Patent applied for;" "For sale or to let."

This remarkable suicide affords much food for reflection to all classes. To the physician, especially the psychologist, it is eminently instructive as illustrating the doings of disease in the mind of a man apparently in a good state of health and in the prime of life. Accident has placed me in possession of some general remarks on this case, which I venture to use without the knowledge of the author, Dr. Thomas W. Gordon, one of the Vice Presidents of the State Medical Society of Ohio:

"What curious freaks the creature man shows in this short mundane existence. Most people hold life the chief boon, and yet most of them sacrifice it for a whim, or allow it to be frittered away piecemeal for momentary enjoyments or excitement. Moon is not the only one who has exchanged life for notoriety. Some call it fame, and some pleasure; yet all alike, in a few decades, sink to the same plane. Yet 'his taking off' was startling to the crowd, because of the devilish ingenuity displayed; the steady hand with which he signed the contract, giving his life as a fair exchange for the ephemeral notoriety he could thus obtain.''

LAFAYETTE, IND.

---

# TINCTURE OF CANTHARIDES AND CHLORAL IN ENURESIS.

### BY GEORGE N. MONETTE, M. D.

*Physician to St. Anna's Asylum, New Orleans.*

I have observed with much interest the numerous remedies, and their vaunted therapeutical indications, in the treatment of enuresis in children. Each remedy I tried, but continually failed in benefiting my patients until I had almost despaired of ever curing this habit, so mortifying to girls and boys as they advanced in childhood. Believing the pathological condition an atonic condition of the sphincter vesicæ as well as the muscular structure of the bladder, I tried the tincture of cantharides combined with chloral. The combination fulfilled the indications in reëstablishing the tonicity of the vesical sphincter, as well as modifying the excessive irritability of the muscular coat of the bladder. The tincture of cantharides must not be used in maximum doses, or till strangury is produced, the age and strength of the child being taken into consideration. In enuresis I have used cantharides alone to verify its efficacy, and have also used it to palliate the strangury often present in cystitis, also in cases where enuresis complicated cystitis.

The chloral exerts a palliative or antidotal influence, preventing too violent specific action of the cantharides; hence I deem the combination expedient. I have treated a number of cases of cystitis, in both male and female, this summer, and all have complained of enuresis and strangury. I have used the above remedies with success in these cases, and trust the profession may find them equally efficacious.

NEW ORLEANS, LA.

# Reviews.

---

**Spiritualism, and Allied Causes and Conditions of Nervous De-rangement.** By WILLIAM A. HAMMOND, M. D., Professor of Diseases of the Mind and Nervous System in the Medical Department of the University of the City of New York, Etc. "Ratio quasi quædam lux lumenque vitæ."—CICERO. Illustrated. New York: G. P. Putnam's Sons, 182 Fifth Avenue, 1876.

It was said by the wise king of Israel that, "of making many books there is no end;" and it really seems that Dr. Hammond has set about proving the truth of the saying in good earnest. If ever any man was seized with an itch for scribbling it is he. He would appear from the products, one can scarcely say of his mind, but of his scissors and ink-horn, to be engaged in answering the question, not how many, and what books are necessary for the advancement of the cause of truth and the good of mankind, but what, and how many books, a real frenzy for literary notoriety, may enable a man— sleepless as the insane are sometimes known to be—to pro-duce, without regard either to the promotion of truth or the well-being of men. Of course, his books throughout display this weakness and vanity in the writer. His facts, picked up everywhere, by running the indexes of books, or sweeping the field of his own memory or imagination for them, are not infrequently irrelevant to his subject, and to each other, and without any near relation to the conclusions into whose ser-vice he has drafted them, except such as his own will or the mere chances of his wayward wanderings, may establish between them. His inductions are seldom supported by sufficient instances, sufficiently apt and relevant, while his deductions are quite as unsupported by his premises, and evince an incapacity to reason worthy only of the merest sciolist. Whatever may have been said to the contrary, no book which as yet he has given to the public, within the last ten or twelve years, is entitled to exemption from these observations. None of them contains any considerable indications of thoughtful labor. All of them clearly show that his mind either lacks scope and grasp to take in all the materials pertaining to a given treatise, and consider them at once together, or patience and industry to .calmly survey, consider and arrange them, so as to bring each to its appropriate place and into its proper relation to each other and to all, and so to reduce all to scientific unity. Indeed, if it be conceded that all his materials in any case had been swept into his mind before his labor of reproducing them in book shape commenced, we learn from a glance at the product that they must have been and remained there, until he ejected them, like the contents of the gourmand's stomach, without digestion; for they have come forth, like Ovid's chaos, *rudis indigestaque moles.*

If Dr. Hammond would confine his abortive labors to his own profession, he might be spared the gravest censures to which he is justly entitled; for, in that case, his learned brethren would soon rid themselves of his trashy accumulations, and he would become powerless to harm them, either by getting their money or time, on the meanest of all possible false pretenses—a worthless book. But he has transcended his professional sphere, and become a biographer, journalist, and reformer. He assumes to be an instructor of the general public, the legislator, and the judge. In every relation thus sought to be established, the same restless activity, the same crude and trashy products, and the same arrogant pretension to superior science, have continually startled, astonished, and bewildered the public. "He speaks as one having authority," and yet upon examination he is found to be simply inflated. No bubble on the whole surface of literature so well deserves to be punctured. He is one of the shams that ought to go down; and yet to put him down thoroughly, as thoroughly might be done, would require a thorough review of his different books. This would do it; for then it would appear that he has thus far been kept up only by great activity, pretension and audacity. Our space does not enable us to perform this necessary labor; but we indicate the field, and invoke its occupation by some larger journal and more competent hand. A few instances of some of the qualities of Dr. Hammond's books, to which we have called attention, must suffice for the present. In selecting these, we have limited our choice to two of his many books, namely: "Insanity in its relations to Crime," and "Spiritualism and Nervous Derangement"—the treatise more immediately under consideration.

"Insanity in its relations to Crime," is a brief commentary upon three cases derived from European reports. The space occupied by the reports is considerably more than half the book; and yet no logical relation exists between the cases and the commentary, which would be almost equally intelligible without as with them. But books can not be made, or pages filled without matter; and in this age and country some men make books without paying any very close attention to their contents. But waiving objection to this little book, on the ground of a want of relation between its parts, a few examples will show that in regard to that part of it which is the author's own, we do not do him injustice. He says:

"Clearly intention can not constitute the essential feature of crime, for the best men are liable to err, and *mistake* is frequently more productive of evil results than a *deliberate crime*. It is punished often too with far greater severity than a premeditated legal offense—both by law and society."

It is difficult for us, uninitiated into Dr. Hammond's views and principles as we are in spite of our best endeavors to understand him, to ascertain the sense in which he employs the terms "crime," "mistake," "deliberate crime," and "legal offense." To what civilized code does the author intend we shall go for definitions? In their ordinary sense, the whole passage is senseless jargon. It is founded on a quotation from Beccaria on Crimes, in which that author is endeavoring to show that intention ought not to be the sole criterion upon which the legislator declares an act a crime, but that the consequences of the act to the public must constitute a basis of the recognition of crime in any given act. Upon this most reasonable and almost universally accepted doctrine, Dr. Hammond bases his doctrine that, intention is no criterion of the existence of crime at all—a conception no where sanctioned by Beccaria or any other respectable civilized author. Beccaria was arguing against the meddlesome spirit of the legislator, who, looking to the intention *alone*, would make every act done in pursuance of a wicked or evil disposition a crime, whether it tended to the injury of society or not, and insisting that only those acts which tend to public injury should be so treated. And from such an argument, Dr. Hammond deduces the conclusion that intention is no element of crime at all. He finds an argument against intention being an element of crime, in the fact that if it be so regarded, it will be impossible to avoid "error in regard to its existence or extent;" and adds, "if it is made to consist in intention, there can rarely be any certainty on these points, for a shrewd person may so cleverly conceal his real purpose as to make discovery out of the question." Now, it is notorious that in all great public trials the question of intention is far from being the most difficult; and that, indeed, it is in most instances not difficult at all. The difficulty usually lies in proof of the fact, and the prisoner's connection with it; and when these are established, all the rest is plain. The question of intention is involved in every moral act; and there is none so constantly and satisfactorily determined by men, in their daily intercourse with each other. All actions, from the most trivial to the most grave, that involve a moral element at all, are held to be right or wrong, good or bad, innocent or guilty, according to the intention with which they are done.

His discussion of the nature of law and the origin of crimes is ridiculous. In its course he says: "It is no valid argument against a law simply to demonstrate its injustice. It must be shown to be injurious to society in order to be successfully attacked." It is not then to be taken for granted that injustice is injurious to society! Yet every society is forced to establish or accept the state for its protection against injustice. The state, in fact, is but organized to give expression to man's ideal of justice, which it represents. But the author gravely informs us that when the state contradicts this ideal and destroys it, in one of its laws, society is not injured. The truth is, the first of the two sentences just quoted is a contradiction in itself; for the very notion of "a law" carries with it that of justice, and to deny of it the quality of justice, much more to prove it to be unjust, is to utterly destroy the conception of it as law.

But a complete review of this little book would require that every paragraph should be made the subject of special discussion. The most remarkable portion of the volume is that which relates to the acts of the insane, and our dealings with them as criminal or the contrary. A single quotation on this subject must suffice. After having spoken of the restraints imposed upon the insane in hospitals as punishments, he proceeds:

"Now, the same is true of the insane outside of asylums— and there are many such who pass through life scarcely suspected of being the subjects of mental aberration, but who simply wait for the exciting cause which is to bring their latent susceptibilities into action. Let them understand that insanity does not necessarily license an individual to do what he pleases without punishment, and a power is brought in aid of their wavering intellects which may turn the scale definitely in their favor. It is not only for the safety of society, therefore, that insane criminals should be punished, but for the sake of other insane who are not yet entirely deprived of responsibility."

If anything can be worse in view of reason, or more apt to illustrate the manner of the author than this, it will be difficult to find it. "Insanity does not necessarily license an individual to do *what he pleases.*" Does the insane ever do *what he pleases?* It has been generally maintained, and by none more strongly than Dr. Hammond, that to be insane is to exclude choice, or the notion of "what he pleases" from the movements of the insane. Then again, "it is not only for the safety of society . . that insane criminals should be punished, but for the sake of other insane who are not yet entirely deprived of responsibility." This is truly wonderful. The two classes of insane persons here mentioned embrace all. "Insane criminals" are to be punished, for the sake of society, and to deter other insane persons from becoming "insane criminals." In other words, when the threat of punishment fails to deter an insane man from doing an act that is a crime when done by a sane man, punish him. It will tend to deter other insane men from committing similar acts. It has not had that effect on the man to be punished, however; and if it fail to have thè desired effect on him who witnesses or hears of the punishment, then again he shall be *punished* for the good of society, and to deter others from doing similar acts. And so the law, like the logic of the author, is to go round like the wheel of Ixion in one eternal circle. But, as applied to "the insane criminal," punishment has no meaning, and might be just as properly prescribed for a horse or an ox.

There is scarcely a page in the book where such notions of law and logic do not meet and astonish the reader. And yet Dr. Hammond has frequently insisted that insanity is, and ought to be, exempt from punishment. The instances he gives of discipline in our hospitals for the insane, have no relevancy to the question of punishment of insane persons under the law, to protect society and serve as examples for others of their unfortunate class. Such discipline is part of their treatment, intended for their good.

Dr. Hammond's treatise on "Spiritualism and allied causes and conditions," is of no higher order of composition or preparation, than his "Insanity in its relations to Crime." Both are alike bad. Whatever is bad in the one, finds itself repeated in the other. The jumble of facts, irrelevant materials, and illogical deductions, characteristic, in an equal degree of no other author with whose works we are acquainted, confronts us everywhere. And at last it is difficult for us to say what are the notions of Dr. Hammond in relation to spiritualism. Indeed, as if to add to our embarrassment and confusion, he discusses, we suppose, as "allied causes and conditions," "sleight of hand," dull tricks practiced by shallow deceivers, upon their still shallower dupes, under the name of spiritualism; "somnambulism, natural and artificial;" "saintly influence on animals," "mesmerism of animals," "human automatism," "hysterical anæsthesia," "hysteria," "Jansenist convulsionaires," "New England witchcraft," "the Jerkers," "Rev. Mr. Wesley's ministrations," "Shakerism," "devildancing," "fasting girls," "catalepsy, ecstasy, and hysteroepilepsy," "stigmatization," and other subjects kindred and alien to these. He does not, indeed, find in any one, or all of these diverse crafts and conditions, sufficient evidence to enable him to prove that the phenomena claimed for spiritualism are due to any one or all of them. When it suits his purposes, however, he does not hesitate to insist that any particular phenomenon is produced by one or all of them. In many cases, where his premises are merely potential, and only exist but in supposition, his conclusions are absolute. When he has shown that a given explanation of any phenomenon *may* be true, he does not hesitate to assert that, as the result of his reasoning, it *is* true. Much of his entire book requires the following proposition to be admitted: "Whatever is possible, is actually true." If this be accepted, then "Spiritualism and allied causes and conditions," will stand vastly better than it does. The truth is, Dr. Hammond's facts and arguments do not disprove spiritualism. They only show that it requires further proof, before it is entitled to challenge our full faith. The facts and suggestions which the book furnishes, simply afford ground for a reasonable doubt of the spiritual origin of the very best authenticated phenomena of spiritualism. In other words, they give us an hypothesis, other than that of the spiritualists, which, so far as the facts go, may be sufficient to explain them all. And this is enough for truth, and, indeed, for the argument against spiritualism. It does not satisfy Dr. Hammond, however, for throughout his book he treats this counter hypothesis, which his argument only shows to be possibly true, as absolutely true, and consequently spiritualism as absolutely false.

Take, for instance, his conclusions in relation to the apparition described by Mr. Owen, whose account of it he quotes at length. The story, as told by Mr. Owen, was received by him from all the persons who were with him when the supposed spirit appeared; and he believed what they said, and that the spirit was genuine. It must have been so, unless Mr. Owen was basely duped. The question presented by the case is, was he duped? To enable us to say so, we must be satisfied that some of those present in the room with Mr. Owen, in concert with others not there, practiced a shameful fraud, by introducing a real human being into the room, and by means of the darkness and the use of a dark lantern, so imposed upon his senses as to impress him with the belief that he had seen a spirit. And this is Dr. Hammond's hypothesis. It contradicts the testimony of all present on the occasion. If the appearance was not a spirit, either they were all deceived, or part of them were guilty of flagrant falsehood and fraud. And this is assumed by Dr. Hammond. He maintains that, inasmuch as a door, not in view of Mr. Owen, might have been unlocked and entered by some person who acted the part of the spirit, and as another with a dark lantern might have entered there also, therefore they did so enter. Hence, he triumphantly concludes: "Mr. Owen was therefore egregiously deceived, and the confederates were Miss B——, Mrs. K——, Mrs. D——, and two others unknown, one of whom played the part of the apparition, while the other held the lantern." Thus, our author concludes that whatever is possibly true, is absolutely true, and this in the teeth of human testimony to the contrary. Nay, he goes further; he does not hesitate to accuse several people of fraud and conspiracy without any fact upon which to found his accusation whatever, except a bare possibility and the assumed impossibility of any spiritual manifestation. And even this does not satisfy the demands of his logic. He sounds the minds of the guilty parties, and arrives at their motives. He says: "As to their object, a desire for notoriety, or to play a practical joke, or to accomplish some other desired end, would have been a sufficient motive. . . The conspirators knew how credulous and guileless was the gentleman they selected, or rather who forced himself upon them, as their victim, and they took advantage of their opportunity. And this is the sort of evidence on which the phenomena of spiritualism rests!" Well might the reader inquire, Does the Doctor judge others as he would be judged? Or does he accuse others, thus without evidence, of falsehood, trick, fraud and conspiracy, from the fullness of his own heart?

But his sweeping conclusions embrace a denial of all supernatural phenomena, and of all "miraculous interpositions of the Deity in" behalf of any religion whatever; while with singular inconsistency, he professes profound respect "for the fundamental beliefs of Christianity, to which the civilized world owes so much." Is this profession of respect consistent with a denial of the very grounds upon which its founder placed it? He explains the luminous appearance of a young lady's face by attributing it directly "to a relaxation of all the muscles of the face concerned in expression," and "a suffusion of the eyes and dilatation of the pupils." And thereupon he disposes of the miracle of the shining face of Moses, and the transfiguration of Jesus, in this sentence: "Undoubtedly the instances mentioned in the Bible as transfigurations—(see Exodus, xxxiv:29–35; Matthew, xvii:1, 2; Mark, ix: 2, 3; Luke, ix:29)—were of this character." The conclusion, let it be noted, is beyond doubt—"undoubtedly." Surely, the worst proved miracles ever believed in, stand as well in their proof, as the best of these undoubted conclusions of our Philosopher Hammond.

But we have surpassed our space, and must close. The faults are manifest and manifold which disfigure the works of our author. He constantly oversteps the modesty of nature, and makes a caricature of science; assails religion, which must be supernatural or nothing, while falsely offering it lip service;

and, in as far as he has yet attempted to lead the blind god-
dess justice, either by his testimony or graver discussions, is
a blind leader of the blind, whose goal is the ditch.

The book is handsomely printed by "G. P. Putnam's Sons,
New York, 182 Fifth Avenue, 1876," on magnificent paper.
Knowing its contents, and viewing the superior setting forth
which its publishers have given them, one can scarcely refrain
from quoting the couplet of Byron, describing the funeral
encasements of the remains of King George the Third; but
we do refrain.

---

**An Elementary Treatise on Diseases of the Skin.** By HENRY G. PIF-
FARD, M. D. Macmillan & Co. London and New York. 1876.

The handsome appearance of this volume of nearly four
hundred pages at once attracts attention. The substantial
binding, the fine paper, the large clear type, wide margins,
and excellent illustrations, all give evidence of the care and
good taste shown by the Messrs. Macmillan in the preparation
of their books. The good opinion formed of the book considered as a work of art, will need no modification when it is
studied as a literary or as a scientific production.

In the examination of many of the new works that so constantly demand attention, the conviction is often forced upon
the reader that, starting with a given number of facts, the
chief object of the author has been to cover up and hedge
them about with words, as if the value of a book were in
direct proportion to the number of its pages. A study of
Dr. Piffard's work brings no feeling of this kind, for almost
every page gives evidence of a desire on the part of the
author to present his facts in the fewest words, yet every
statement is clear and distinct.

Another pleasing feature of the book is the evidence it presents throughout of the fact that the author has not simply
studied diseases of the skin, through the observations of
others; for while it is plain that he is entirely familiar with the

writings of the other workers in the same field, it is equally clear that the terse descriptions of disease given, and the effects of treatment presented, are the result of his own personal experience and observation; and it is this feature that makes the work of especial value to the American student.

The volume is presented "as an introduction to the more elaborate works upon dermatology;" but the practitioner who refers to it will obtain more satisfaction than is usually received from an examination of the more comprehensive works.

In the first chapter is given a description of the anatomy of the skin; and the text is well illustrated by plates from Sappey, Frey, Stricker, and others.

"The Physiology of the Skin," "Symptomatology," and "Diagnosis," are presented in the four succeeding chapters, in a brief and simple, yet entirely satisfactory manner.

The sixth chapter is devoted to classification, and of the three systems—the lesional, the structural, and the pathological—the second, or that based upon cause, is selected. While this may not fulfil the conditions "which are required in an ideally perfect classification," it would, if generally adopted in the classification of disease, have the same effect in medicine as the substitution of the natural for the artificial method has had in zoology, botany, etc.

Under the primary group, "Diathetic Affections," interesting and instructive chapters are given on the syphilides, scrofulides, and rheumides. In the latter class are included eczema, psoriasis and pityriasis. These affections are considered as an expression of a diathesis:—the rheumic, a name selected, first, because the etymological signification implies the idea of exudation; secondly, "because the blood condition underlying this diathesis" is believed "to be similar to, if not identical with, that concerned in the production of rheumatism and gout;" a morbid state in which the albuminoids entering the body as food undergo imperfect oxidation, which manifests itself by various affections, among them those of the skin mentioned.

While the teachings of Bence Jones, and others, point to these conclusions, it is evident that Dr. Piffard has thoroughly investigated the subject for himself according to scientific methods. His views will attract attention because of their importance, even if they be rejected.

In the treatment of these affections, arsenic—the medicine generally considered of chief importance—has no prominent place, the author claiming that its reputation is based upon its undoubted control over many of the manifestations of the rheumic diathesis, rather than upon any influence over "the constitutional conditions which underlie them."

Under the principal groups—third, "Reflex Affections," fourth, "Local Affections," and fifth, "Affections of uncertain nature"—every cutaneous disease liable to be met with is described in a clear and satisfactory manner, and the most approved treatment briefly and simply presented.

The affections embraced in the second group—general nondiathetic affections, *i. e.* eruptive fevers, etc.—coming as they usually do under the care of the general practitioner, not of the specialist, are not considered.

A brief notice like this must of necessity fail to do justice to a work of this character; therefore we recommend all who are interested in the study of cutaneous diseases, to procure the book, and see for themselves that it merits all and more than the praise here given.                        J. R. W.

---

An Introduction to Pathology and Morbid Anatomy. By T. HENRY GREEN, M. D. London. Second American from the third revised and enlarged English edition. Illustrated. Philadelphia: Henry C. Lea, 1876.

Space permits us merely to call the attention of the profession to this excellent work, clear and condensed in language, rich in illustrations, bringing under notice the most important matters in pathology, but still only, as its author claims in the title, an introduction; and as an introduction should be used by physicians and students.

## THE REVIEW BY "W. C." OF DR. BARTHOLOW'S LECTURE

on the "Principle of Physiological Antagonism as applied to the Treatment of the Febrile State." A Rejoinder.

The number of the American Practitioner for June, 1876, contains a review of my lecture signed "W. C.," who is, I learn from the list of contributors, William Carson, M. D. Nothing in the lecture satisfies the lofty requirements of the reviewer, and he throughout assumes a confident tone of superiority which indicates that he supposes himself entirely exempt from the errors of judgment and opinion to which ordinary mortals are liable. I have no sort of objection to the good opinion which "W. C." entertains of his own merit, nor to the right of just, even of severe, criticism; but I do object to misstatements of my own opinions, and to the expression of erroneous views which put me in a false position, no matter how solemnly and authoritatively they may be uttered by the reviewer. Beside the right which I respectfully claim, to correct inaccurate statements of my opinions by any reviewer whatsoever, it may not be without utility to discuss some of the points raised in the review in question.

My lecture, as its title—to which I ask the especial attention of the reader—indicates, was intended to set forth a principle—physiological antagonism—and to illustrate the application of antipyretics in accordance with this principle to the treatment of pyrexia. I expressly disclaimed a purpose to go over the whole ground of physiological antagonisms. The title of my lecture would have been a remarkable misnomer, if I had meant to discuss the subject of fever. "W. C.," however, determined at the outset to find fault, and accordingly chooses to assume that in speaking of the heat phenomena, I included the whole process involved in "that complexus of actions to which we apply the term fever." His criticism begins as follows:

"We believe that the author has started out on false or insufficient premises when he endeavors to compress the whole of the phenomena of fever into simply 'increased temperature of the body' or 'a state of preternatural heat,' and that consequently his 'therapeutics' are restricted or constrained."

What I did say is contained in the following extract from my lecture (p. 2):

"In order to a right comprehension of the subject we must have a clear conception of what the febrile state includes. For our present purpose, fever means increased temperature of the body. The rise of temperature above the normal is a result of greater activity of the combustion process. Or, as it has been expressed by Liebermeister (*Handbuch der Pathologie und Therapie des Fiebers*, Leipzig, 1875, page 290), 'the higher temperature of the febrile state is an exaltation of the normal heat-producing process.' It is not necessary to my purpose to admit or deny the existence of Tscheschichin's (*Deutches Archiv f. klin. Med.*, 1867, Band 11, s. 588) heat-regulating center. Whether or not there be an excito-caloric center and a moderating center of combustion in the body, does not affect the inquiry before us; it suffices to accept the definition of fever as a state of preternatural body-heat."

Furthermore, in closing my lecture with a summary of my views on the actions and uses of the various antipyretics, I remark as follows (p. 20):

"When the state of pyrexia is the most important element in the morbid complexus—cold baths, quinia, and digitalis are the remedies to be employed. In the fever of inflammation, is the action of the heart vigorous and the arterial tension high? aconite and veratrum viride are indicated; is the action of the heart feeble and the tension of the vessels low? quinia and digitalis are more appropriate. Is the fever due to putrid ferments, to disease-producing organisms? quinia, salicylic acid are required."

It is evident to any one but a hypercritical reviewer that in discussing the action of "antipyretics," the condition of pyrexia was that part of the "morbid complexus" which chiefly engaged my attention, and necessarily so, and it was no part of my purpose to enter into a general discussion on the subject of fever. Your reviewer, therefore, conveys a wrong impression of my opinions when he states that I "attempted to compress the whole phenomena of fever into simply increased temperature of the body."

I will, in addition to the above quotations, bring forward some independent testimony to show that "W. C." has wilfully misrepresented my position on the subject of a theory of fever. In a review of my lecture published in the New York Medical Journal for the present month (July, 1876, page 77), the reviewer states: "He discusses the principles which should guide us in the treatment of fever, *but avoids committing himself to any special doctrine concerning its mechanism.*" Italics mine. The two reviewers "flatly contradict" each other. Whose statement is to be believed? Under the circumstances of the case, the credibility of "W. C." is open to grave suspicions.

"W. C." finds fault with me because I defer somewhat to the opinions of Liebermeister, and he intimates that I have no other authority for my opinions. He remarks: "He seems to have adopted the extreme views of Liebermeister on fever, though it is known they are not accepted by some eminent authorities of his own country." Such a gratuitous misstatement deserves the severest reprobation, but I will not apply epithets. The following quotation will show how far "W. C." is to be trusted:

"The changes, functional and organic, to which I now call attention are not those due to the growth and multiplication of cacobacteria and other organisms, or to morbific materials (unorganized) circulating with the blood through the organs and setting up, by their presence, morbid processes, but those alterations due directly or chiefly to the abnormal temperature. These anatomical changes have been designated by the German pathologists 'parenchymatous degeneration.' As respects the muscular system these changes have been especially studied by F. A. Zenker (*Liebermeister's Handbuch*, l. c., p. 445), who describes two forms—a *granular* and a *waxy* degeneration. As these changes occur in various febrile diseases and are extensive just in proportion to the degree of fever heat, he concluded that the principal factor in their causation is the temperature. In this opinion he is supported by Lieber-meister. The changes in the parenchyma of organs (*paren-chymatöse Degeneration*) have also been studied by Lehmann (*Ueber das Verhalten der parenchymatösen Entzündungen zu den acuten Krankheiten; Schmidt's Jahrbücher der Gesammten Medi-cin*, Band 139, s. 239, *et seq.*), by Ponfick (*Anatomische Studien über den Typhus recurrens, Virchow's Archiv*, Band 60, 1864, s. 153), by Klebs (*Zur Pathologie der epidemischen Meningitis, Virchow's Archiv*, Band 34, s. 327, *et seq.*), by Liebermeister (l. c.), and by others."

It seems from this extract that I have not simply "adopted the extreme views of Liebermeister on fever." I also call the reader's attention to the fact that this quotation confirms what I have already stated—that for the purpose of the inquiry be-fore me in my lecture, I necessarily considered only the con-dition of pyrexia, or "those alterations due directly or chiefly to the abnormal temperature."

Of the paramount importance of the range of temperature in fever, not only Liebermeister but all other authorities are now convinced. Indeed Liebermeister's conclusions are largely based on the researches of others. "W. C." appears to be entirely unacquainted with the remarkable researches of Sena-tor on the disintegration of the tissues during the fever pro-cess—the urea and carbonic acid waste; the observations of Naunyn on the urea discharge, of Salkowski on the excretion of alkali salts, and of Leyden on the carbonic acid loss. It is true, rather hot polemics have passed between Senator and Liebermeister as to the relation between heat production and heat retention in fever; but all competent authorities are now agreed that increased combustion of tissue takes place in fe-ver. That "W. C." does not approve of the views of Lieber-meister was probably not known in Germany when Ziemssen's *Handbuch* was projected, otherwise the article on typhoid would have been committed to other hands.

In further comment on the relation of the body-heat to the fever process, "W. C." remarks as follows: "Experience will flatly contradict the statement (page 5) that 'there is a distinct ratio between the amount of disturbance in the cerebral functions and the degree of fever heat.' Who has not seen a typhoid fever patient, in one part of his disease, with a temperature of 105°F., at the same time with subsultus tendinum, delirium more or less active, coma, it may be wakefulness, and other serious symptoms of disturbance of the nervous system; and then at another period of the case, with the same temperature (105°F.) without the presence of any of these threatening symptoms?"

Without stopping to question the accuracy of such observations, it is plain to see that my critic entirely fails to comprehend the point at issue. It may be thus stated: Given disturbance in the cerebral functions produced by the abnormal body-heat, the amount of such disturbance will be governed by the range of temperature. This is a question entirely apart from delirium, coma, and other head symptoms produced by other causes than the abnormal heat.

As respects the influence of the cold bath on fever heat, my critic displays his most authoritative manner and exhibits his usual lack of critical acumen. Let me quote his observations: "It would be too sweeping a dictum—even with the interposed qualification—to say that 'it is simply a question, *cæteris paribus*, of the degree of heat and the amount of cooling necessary to abate it' (page 7). The illustration drawn from Wood does not strengthen the assertion, for it is not applicable."

It is incredible that any one should deny that a cold bath will certainly lower fever heat. How far such lowering of temperature will persist and be curative of fever, is another question. Notwithstanding the satisfactory way in which "W. C." disposes of Wood's experiment—by his own *ipse dixit*—I must still maintain that it exactly illustrates the influence of a cold bath in lessening abnormal heat: "An animal heated in a hot-air chamber until the febrile state is induced, is restored to the normal condition by being plunged into a cold bath." "W. C." is apparently unable to discriminate between the physical effects of a bath in abstracting heat, and the therapeutical effects of cold baths in fever. His mind is equally clouded when he comes to discuss the antipyretic effects of quinia. He is unable to separate the antipyretic power of quinia, the subject which I discussed, from its curative property. Who does not know that quinia may lower the temperature without otherwise affecting the course or shortening the duration of fever? It was my purpose to show that its antipyretic effect is applicable by its physiological actions, and that in lessening temperature it antagonizes those processes which maintain the body-heat above the normal. "W. C." exhibits an entire inability to grasp questions of this kind.

Roberts Bartholow, M. D.

NOTE.—The discussion between Senator and Liebermeister may be found in Virchow's Archiv. In Vol. XLV Senator published a paper entitled *Beiträge zur Lehre von der Eigenwärme und dem Fieber.* In Vol. LII, Liebermeister replies to Senator under the heading, *Zur Lehre von der Wärmeregulirung.* In Vol. LIII Senator appears in a criticism of Liebermeister's paper, *Kritisches über die Lehre von der Wärmeregulirung.* To this Liebermeister, in the same volume, responds under the title, *Nochmals zur Lehre von der Wärmeregulirung.*

---

## REPLY TO DR. BARTHOLOW'S REJOINDER.

In my review of Dr. Bartholow's lecture, I stated that the author had started out on false or insufficient premises, when he endeavors to compress the phenomena of fever into simply "increased temperature of the body" or "a state of preternatural body-heat;" "and that consequently his therapeutics were restricted and constrained." In his rejoinder he says that this is a misrepresentation; and thereupon exhibits himself in an unamiable mood. The latter is unimportant, except as a testimonial to the force of the criticism.

We quote from the beginning of the second paragraph of his rejoinder the following language: "My lecture, as its

title—to which I ask the especial attention of the reader—
indicates, was intended to set forth a principle—physiological.
antagonism—and to illustrate the application of antipyretics in
accordance with this principle to the treatment of pyrexia."
In passing, I desire to call the attention of Dr. Bartholow and
the reader, that this is language quite different from what appears at the head of the lecture. Pyrexia has, in medical
usage, a more restricted sense than the words "the febrile
state," and is not found in the title of his lecture.

But we shall allow the Doctor to be his own interpreter,
which he attempts to be in his rejoinder, by quoting from his
language on the second page of his lecture. What is, however, very significant is that he has omitted the first sentence
of that paragraph—by far the most important one. For the
correct understanding of what he said, whether he meant it or
not, I quote it for him; and it will be seen that by taking it
and the explanatory sentences which follow together, that a
fair construction is that he did mean to compress the phenomena of fever into "simply increased temperature of the
body," or "a state of preternatural body-heat." The following is what the Doctor did not quote, as well as the essential
points of what he did quote, from the beginning of the paragraph near the top of the second page: "The problem which
we have now to consider is, what means are available to
antagonize that *complexus of actions* to which we apply the
term fever? In order to a right comprehension of the subject, we must have a clear conception of what the febrile state
includes. For our present purpose, fever means increased
temperature of the body;" . . "it suffices to accept the
definition of fever as a state of preternatural body-heat."
My reading of this, leaving out intervening words of no importance, is that "the *complexus of actions* to which we apply
the term fever" "means increased temperature of the body,"
"a state of preternatural body-heat."

We have further the right to construe the Doctor's language
by the manner in which he has developed and illustrated his
subject. He does this by beginning with an enumeration of

some of the effects of high temperature on the functions and tissues of the human body. We took exception to his interpretation of some of the phenomena appearing in the course of diseases, particularly his dictum that "there is a distinct ratio between the amount of disturbance in the cerebral functions and the degree of fever heat." We said that there were, and are, undoubted facts of clinical experience which would compel us to hunt for some other factor "than excessive body-heat," in order to correctly understand the true meaning of the disturbances in the nervous system. Two of them are as follows: First, that you may have a very high body-heat without any of these symptoms; second, that you can have them all with a low temperature. The Doctor says he meant to say that "given disturbance in the cerebral functions, produced by the abnormal body-heat, the amount of such disturbance will be governed by the range of temperature;" which is plainly a begging of the question at issue, which is that the nervous symptoms are due to the excessive body-heat, when they may exist without it, and may not exist with it. How can the Doctor distinguish when they are produced by the abnormal temperature, and when they are independent of it? In the last analysis, his statement means that the cause is equal to the effect, without telling us how to find out the cause; and we may add, that he may reduce the temperature without relieving the nervous disturbance in many (we do not say all) cases.

We say now, as bearing on the Doctor's construction of the equivalence of "excessive body-heat," that he has included in the conditions to be controlled by his physiological antagonisms phenomena which no power of compression in his theory can bring within the range of undoubted effects of excessive body-heat. In other words, he includes bodily certain disease among his illustrations of the antagonizing control of certain remedies. He confuses and mingles together important phases of symptomatic and essential fever as shown in his illustrations by pneumonia, and puts down "exudation of fibrinous material, the migration of the white corpuscles," as effects of increased temperature of the body. Is he justified in including (which he does), with our present knowledge, parenchymatous nephritis as an effect of high temperature, when it is very apt to come on in the slighter forms of the disease, and is sometimes delayed a considerable period beyond the disappearance of fever?

Our understanding, then, of this lecture is gathered from two sources—the plain language above quoted, and from the manner of treatment and illustration.

We meant to protest, in our review, against the insufficiency of the Doctor's adjustable formulas of physiological antagonisms in the treatment of fever (and in many instances the mere thermic element of it), and against making "excessive body-heat" the equivalent of the "complexus of actions, which we call fever." We protest now against his asserting, as he does in his rejoinder, that it was no part of his purpose to illustrate the principles of physiological antagonisms by their curative powers (see remarks in rejoinder on quinia), but only by their antipyretic actions, when his lecture is published in a course entitled "A Course of American *Clinical* Lectures," and intended, as the precise words are, "to be trustworthy guides to practice." At the same time we recognize the "excessive temperature" of the body in disease as a matter of great importance. He who pays attention to it alone will be miserably disappointed in many instances, while he shall also have signal success in others, which stand, in clinical work, in strict analogy or correspondence with the experimental cases worked out by some well known investigators, particularly Dr. H. C. Wood, Jr. The current season, as well as former ones, has afforded us the most satisfactory results in the antipyretic treatment of "sunstroke" or "thermic fever." The latter term represents an entity of undoubted occurrence in practice, but it does not include all the "complexus of actions which we call fever." You may eliminate it or suspend it by treatment, and yet you do not cure your patient.

The independent testimony quoted from the New York Medical Journal has no reference to any point in dispute between the Doctor and his reviewer.   Will the Doctor quote all of what the New York reviewer says?

That there is some confusion in the application of the Doctor's exact formulas of antagonisms will be apparent when we compare the following passages; first, from page 14 of the Seguin lecture, as follows:

| DIGITALIS. | PNEUMONIA. |
|---|---|
| Contraction of arterioles, and diminished blood supply. | Hyperæmia of part and dilated vessels. |
| Exudation checked or prevented by the heightened tonicity of the vessels. | Exudation of fibrinous materials. Migration of white blood corpuscles. |
| Depression of the temperature. | Elevated temperature. |
| Lessened action of the heart, and increased power.   Arterial tension raised. | Increased action of the heart, and lessened power.   Arterial tension lowered. |

"There are two periods, speaking from the point of view of my personal experience, in which digitalis renders the most important service in pneumonia, viz., during the stage of hyperæmia and exudation, to limit the area of the inflammatory action, and at the period of crisis to maintain the power of the heart."

And second from page 275 of Bartholow's recently published work on "Therapeutics:"

"That digitalis has any power to prevent the depuration of fibrinous material, to prevent or check the migration of the white corpuscles, or to arrest the multiplication of the cellular elements of inflamed parts, seems to the author highly improbable."

The reader will observe the harmony between the two extracts.

# Clinic of the Month.

---

TREATMENT OF RHEUMATIC CARDITIS.—Dr. Peacock, St. Thomas's Hospital Reports, Volume VI, gives the following: The treatment which has generally been adopted for the different forms of rheumatic carditis has been either antiphlogistic—leeching or cupping over the region of the heart, the administration of mercurials, etc., or what may be called expectant—the use of alkalies and salines, etc., as in ordinary cases of rheumatism. I have long almost entirely abandoned the practice of depletion in any form in cases of carditis; for in a disease which, like rheumatism, is so frequently developed in persons not previously in good health or of delicate constitution, I think all depressing measures very undesirable, if they are not imperatively called for, and I believe that the cases do quite as well when the more expectant plan of treatment is followed. When, however, there is much pain in the region of the heart, the application of a few leeches sometimes affords great relief. Having also seen pericarditis developed in a person under full mercurial action, I can not think that mercurials are by any means so useful as was supposed by Dr. Latham, though they are probably valuable adjuvants in the treatment when judiciously administered, tending to check the outpouring of exudation and to assist the absorption of the effused materials.

I generally adopt, or continue if previously in use, the ordinary rheumatic remedies—the alkalies and salines—such as the bicarbonate, tartrate, citrate, or nitrate, of potash; the liquor ammoniæ acetatis, etc., and exhibit small doses of hydrargyrum cum cretâ with Dover's powder, applying at the same time blisters over the region of the heart and following them by poultices. When the liquid effusion accumulates, the iodide of potassium is generally combined with these remedies, being given at first in small doses, and the doses being generally increased, as otherwise from the ready elimination of the iodide by the kidneys, it is of little use. If the patient be very restless or delirious the Dover's powder is given in full doses, or some more powerful anodyne is administered. When the patient's strength begins to fail stimulants are ordered. It is always somewhat difficult to decide when the time has arrived for the exhibition of stimulants, and it is well to commence their use in very small quantities—not more than a teaspoonful of brandy, for instance—and to increase the doses and repeat them more or less frequently, according to the effects produced. If the remedy answers there will be very obvious improvement in the condition of the patient; he will be less restless and excited, and the pulse will become fuller and firmer; and when judiciously given, I believe there is no class of cases which derive more benefit from the administration of stimulants than the acute inflammatory affections of the heart.

During the progress of the case I continue the administration of the slight mercurial and the iodide, and repeat the application of blisters and poultices over the region of the heart, or paint the surface with the tincture of iodine, till the symptoms and signs of active disease subside. The patient is also kept in bed till convalescence is well advanced, and he is only allowed to lie on the outside of the bed or on a couch till he has gained strength and all danger of relapse has passed away. In a large proportion of cases, the patient becomes anæmic toward the end of the attack, and quinia and iron are then given. When after considerable time has elapsed, there is still some uneasiness in the region of the heart and pains are felt in the joints and other parts of the body, advantage may often be derived from the administration of small doses of iodide of potassium, bicarbonate of potash and colchicum, combined with bark or quinia and iron. In such cases also relief is often obtained by the application of belladonna plasters over the præcordia, or by simply covering the surface with some warm material.

Of late years I have generally adopted in cases of rheumatism, whether simple or complicated, the blister treatment as recommended by Dr. Herbert Davies. I believe the blisters to be very efficacious in arresting the inflammation in the joints, and, when several are employed simultaneously or in rapid succession, in relieving the constitutional disturbance also. The benefit which results from the treatment is, I think, in direct proportion to the freedom with which the blisters are applied; and, though the first effect is generally to increase the febrile disturbance and raise the temperature for a few hours, the most remarkable amendment, both local and general, ensues. I have been repeatedly told by patients that the pain caused by the application even of four or five blisters at the same time, is far less than that which they had experienced from the disease. In a recent instance a man, whom I had twice previously treated for acute rheumatism, in the one attack by blisters and in the other by general means, told me that he was much more completely and more rapidly relieved by the blister treatment; which was therefore again employed in his third attack. The blisters are applied around the limb above all the affected joints, and the surfaces are poulticed till they entirely heal. Though I have generally employed the ordinary anti-rheumatic treatment in conjunction with the blisters, when the patients have been much exhausted, from the long duration of the symptoms before admission into the hospital, or from their being the subjects of old heart disease, or being weakened by any other cause, as by prolonged nursing, I have sometimes relied exclusively upon the blisters, and have never had reason to doubt the propriety of having done so. In some cases, however, of very severe rheumatic fever, I have thought, on reviewing the cases, that the constitutional treatment might with advantage have been more freely used in combination with the local measures.

In reference to the effect of the blister treatment upon the development of the cardiac complications of rheumatism, I believe it is both preventive and curative. As the heart and other internal organs become affected almost always in the earlier and more active stage of the disease, any treatment which tends to shorten the duration of this stage must lessen the liability to the occurrence of such complications; and I have no doubt that more rapid and complete relief of the local inflammation is obtained by blistering than by any other means. I think, however, that the treatment does more than this. I have seen, in cases in which complications were very decidedly threatened, the progress of the internal disease apparently entirely arrested by the application of blisters to all the affected joints at the same time.

ON THE PROCESS OF FEVER.—Dr. J. Burdon Sanderson thus concludes a paper on this subject, Practitioner, June:

A satisfactory explanation of the nature of fever and of its relation to the febrile process is not at present possible, because we are not as yet possessed of the necessary physiological knowledge. We have stated that two possibilities are open to us. One is, that fever originates in disorder of the nervous centers, that by means of the influence of the nervous system on the systemic functions, the liberation of heat at the surface of the body is controlled or restrained, so that "by retention" the temperature rises, and finally that the increased temperature so produced acts on the living substance of the body, so as to disorder its nutrition. The other alternative is that fever originates in the living tissues, that it is from first to last a disorder of protoplasm, and that all the systemic disturbances are secondary. In both hypotheses it is tacitly assumed that fever is the product of a material fever-producing cause contained in the blood or tissue juice, the morbific action of which on the organism is antecedent to all functional disturbances whatever. At bottom we are all humoralists, and believe in infection. It is not until we have to say where and how the infection acts that questions arise.

The facts and considerations we have had before us are, I think, sufficient to justify the definitive rejection of the first hypothesis in all its forms; for, on the one hand, we have seen that, no disorder of the systemic functions, or of the nervous centers which preside over them, is capable of inducing a state which can be identified with febrile pyrexia; and, on the other, that it is possible for such a state to originate and persist in the organism after the influence of the central nervous system has been withdrawn from the tissues by the severance of the spinal cord.

We are, therefore, at liberty to adopt the tissue-origin of fever as the basis on which we hope *eventually* to construct an explanation of the process. But if we attempt to do so *now*, we shall at once find ourselves in face of an unsolved physiological problem, that of the normal relation between temperature and thermogenesis, for the elucidation of which it is necessary to investigate much more completely than has yet been found possible, the influence of temperature variations on those chemical processes in living tissue, with which thermogenesis is necessarily associated. The little that has been already accomplished in this direction is sufficient to show that the living substance of our bodies is, if I may so express myself, delicately sensitive to variations in the temperature of its environment, so that very slight deviations from the normal may produce effects of surpassing magnitude.

APHASIC AMBLYOPIA AND AMAUROSIS.—Dr. Galczowski, in a paper upon amblyopia and amaurosis occurring in those affected with aphasia, *Archives Générales*, June, presents the following conclusions:

First. That the amblyopiæ of which the aphasic complain, are due rather to a failure of memory and an amnesia of letters and words, than to a diminution of acute vision.

Second. That in a certain number there will be found amblyopia with hemiopia of the right side of the two eyes.

Third. That in quite exceptional cases, there is papillary atrophy in one eye, habitually the left.

Fourth. The amblyopia can be cured and vision return more or less completely.

A New Method of Treating External Aneurism.—
Walter Reid, M. D., R. N. Staff Surgeon, Royal Naval Hospital, Plymouth, in a short monograph, gives the result of
treatment of a case of popliteal aneurism with Esmarch's
bandage. Genuflexion was tried, also rapid compression by
one of Carté's compressors applied to the femoral artery at
the pelvic brim, the Esmarch bandage was resorted to, the
theory being that if every blood current in the limb could be
arrested, that absolute stagnation of the blood left in the
aneurismal sac must be produced, and its coagulation follow
as a consequence.

"Accordingly," the author says, "I proceeded the next
day to apply Esmarch's bandage from the toes upwards to the
aneurism in the popliteal space. Here it was passed lightly
over the tumor, and then carried on rapidly as high as the
junction of the middle with the lower third of the thigh.
The elastic tubing was then wound round the limb over the
highest turn of the bandage, which was now removed. The
entire circulation below the tubing was thus arrested, and the
limb, all but the aneurismal cavity, emptied of its blood.
The parts assumed a death-like pallor, and gradually lost temperature."

After fifty minutes the elastic tubing was removed, and a
Carté's compressor applied to the femoral at the pelvic brim,
to prevent the blood current from washing away the newly-
formed clot in the sac. A few minutes afterwards the compressor was removed, and no pulsation could be detected in
the aneurism, which felt quite hard. The patient himself applied the compressor at intervals for twenty-four hours. The
collateral circulation established itself at once, but the pulsation never returned.

The author thinks the success was due to the novel method
of treatment, although previous compression might have had
some iufluence on the result, and that one can empty the limb
of its blood and yet keep the aneurismal sack full. He gives
the following conclusions in regard to coagulation:

First. That at a reduced temperature *in vacuo* coagulation
is hastened.

Second. That atmospheric air being simply excluded in a stoppered bottle, the temperature not being reduced, coagulation is retarded.

Third. That all communication with atmospheric air being prevented, the temperature not being reduced, coagulation is much retarded, and hence the influence of a cold death-like condition in the limb aided in producing a sure and speedy coagulation in this case.

A note of the case, eight months after the cure, says there is a small lump in the left popliteal space, which can only be distinguished when compared with the opposite side. The femoral pulsates as far as Hunter's canal, below which it is occluded. The patient reports one leg as good as the other. The author remarks that the method is at least simple, and requires neither surgical dexterity nor expensive apparatus for its trial, and that it is as safe, and perhaps safer, than any method hitherto known to surgery.

PRECAUTION IN REFERENCE TO PUERPERAL FEVER. — Dr. Henry Gervis, in a paper upon puerperal fever, St. Thomas's Hospital Reports, Volume VI, New Series, thus refers to this topic: Although not believing puerperal fever, so called, to be a specific fever capable of transmission except through the actual transfer of septic products, I have seen too many instances of the kind to doubt that the medical attendant may be the involuntary agent in so transferring it. Whenever, therefore, a medical man is in attendance on a woman suffering from puerperal fever, and it devolves upon him to use the uterine douche, or in any way bring his fingers in contact with the secretions of her genital passage, he runs considerable risk of transferring septic poison to any other patient he may attend. And conversely, any medical man who has to dress an erysipelatous or sloughy wound, or come in close contact with cadaveric poison or other source of sepsis, runs some risk, without at all events the greatest care, of inducing septicæmia in any lying-in woman he may attend, if by chance she present any absorbent surface accessible to the poison. As to how long a medical man who has become infective may so continue, it is most difficult to decide. I have known it continue in the case of medical friends until the hope of ever being otherwise was well nigh despaired of, in spite of all kinds of baths and ablutions; but were my advice asked under similar circumstances now, I should certainly recommend the plan of disinfection by iodine suggested by Dr. Wynn Williams.

CRAYONS OF TANNIN.—In the *Annales de Gynécologie*, May, we find the following formula for the preparation of crayons of tannin: To fifteen grains and a half of tannin add a drop and a half of glycerine, and make a crayon nearly four inches in length. Crayons thus made will keep their forms for months; they may be lengthened or shortened as required, after simply warming them in the fingers, and yet are sufficiently firm to be passed into the uterine cavity without breaking them. In consequence of their ductility, they may be lengthened so as to make them into astringent bougies, and then introduced into the urethra will be an efficient substitute for tannin injections.

DYSPEPSIA A GASTRITIS.—M. Leven, in a paper read before the Paris Academy of Medecine, May 16th, *Archives Générales*, recounted experiments upon the dog, whose stomach presents the most marked analogy with that of man, giving the animal food that could not be digested, and finding two hours after the evidence of a more or less severe phlegmasia; and concludes that dyspepsia is not a mere functional disorder, not a gastralgia or neurosis, but is really an inflammation of the mucous membrane and subjacent tissue. According to him, too, simple ulcer of the stomach is always due to an anterior dyspepsia, and does not result, as Virchow has suggested, from thrombosis or embolism. He has tried to produce these ulcerations by injecting the arteries of the stomach with powder of lycopodium, but never succeeded: the numerous arterial amastomoses of the stomach readily compensate for the obstruction of a vessel.

# Notes and Queries.

SELF-ABUSE IN WOMAN.—Dr. Pouillet has recently published a carefully prepared essay* upon this subject, and though there are statements in it as to the extent to which self-abuse in the female sex exists, that may be quite true in France, they are very far from true in this country. While it is believed that this vice is far from common with us, yet it does exist. The translator happens to now know of five cases in girls under eighteen; and quite recently he has been consulted in the case of a married lady, the mother of two children, of good social position and of excellent character, and who would be willing to submit to any treatment promising a cure; and a brief study of Pouillet's work, though dealing with one of the most loathsome of human depravities, may be useful.

The author observes that of all vices, of all turpitudes, that can justly be termed treason against nature, preying upon humanity, menacing its physical vitality, and tending to destroy its intellectual and moral essence, the greatest and the most widely diffused is masturbation. The vice exists in both sexes, at all ages of life, in all places, and in all classes of society.

Pouillet, though indorsing the criticism of Lallemand upon the unfitness of the term Onanism, quoting the familiar Bible story, still retains it, defining it as an act against nature, made by means of a living organ—the hand or tongue—or by any instrument whatever, for the purpose of producing the venereal spasm. In alluding to the assertion that self-abuse is natural, he refers to the manifestations of the vice in dogs and monkeys.

* Essai Médico-Philosophique sur les Formes, les Causes, les Signes, les Consequences et le Traitement de L'Onanisme chez la Femme. Paris, 1876.

That the vice among women is one of at least great antiquity is shown by the seventeenth verse of the sixteenth
chapter of Ezekiel; by the story of Sapho and the Lesbian
girls who despised men and sacrificed alone to Venus, and
who were surnamed *tribades*, from the method in which the
venereal orgasm was produced; by the conduct of the Roman
women under the Emperors, so bitterly denounced by Juve-
nal; by the numerous instruments for self-abuse, of bronze, of
gold, etc., found in the excavations of Pompeii and Hercula-
neum: these *priapi* or *phalli* of ancient times, have their
counterparts in China at the present day, in similar instruments of a gum-resinous mixture, somewhat flexible and
flesh-colored.

In the middle ages manualization, as Pouillet terms it, was
probably in part the cause of nervous epidemics—epilepsy,
hysteria, chorea, catalepsy, ecstacy, *furor uterinus*, etc.—so
generally regarded by canonical judges as manifestations of
sorcery.

The vice is probably more common to-day than formerly,
but more concealed. One reason for this belief is found in
the literature of the age; two well known romances—one by
Gauthier, the other by Belot—have as their point of departure, their vital knot, *tribadia* or masturbation in common:
novelists do not invent vices, they merely reflect those that
society offers.

The two divisions of masturbation made are *vaginal* and
*clitoral*, the former being less frequent and is almost always
solitary; and the latter presenting itself under three forms—
first and most frequent, the individual performs friction of the
clitoris herself; second, another does the office; and third,
*bestial*—too abominable to be further explained—which is said
to be far from rare in large cities.

We have not time to follow the author in his exposition of
the causes, physical, intellectual and moral; want of cleanliness, certain eruptions on the external sexual organs, such as
eczema, psoriasis, etc., and especially vulvar pruritus; some
medicines and condiments, cantharides, phosphorus, savin,

absinthe vere, etc., pepper, cloves, cinnamon, musk, vanilla, etc.; the rectum loaded with scybala, or tormented with oxyures; dancing, riding on horseback, prolonged sitting, the use of sewing machines;* lascivious images, statues, paintings, romances, plays, obscene gestures, the contagion of example, "boarding schools are frequently centers of infection," hereditary influence, impotent or abhorred husbands, widowhood, etc.

The author regards the consequences of Onanism as more serious than those of venereal excess; they are sometimes mortal, often terrible, always injurious.

In considering the treatment of the affection, Pouillet devotes considerable space to the prophylaxis, dividing the preventive means into physical, social, intellectual, and moral. He especially interdicts girls seeing obscene or voluptuous statues, reading romances or vulgar books, visiting theaters, hearing any licentious conversation, and advises assiduous daily intellectual toil, and cultivating a taste for art.

We have often thought that those whose ardent imaginations were liable to bear them away into the darkness of impurity of thought, desire or deed, would do well to ponder and practice the wise words of the wisest of men, whose own life had been terribly tainted with licentiousness, Keep thy heart with all diligence, for out of it are the issues of life.

But prevention having failed, persuasion should be tried, the development of noble sentiments recognized, shame, dread of exposure, should be appealed to, and the fearful consequences of the vice pointed out. The subject should be required to exercise the body until fatigued, and to retire early to bed, and rise early. If the patient is married, the maternal sentiment should be appealed to—the danger of sterility or of diseased offspring made known. .

In the case of children, it is necessary to constantly watch

---

* We wonder that the author in this connection has not referred to the fact that a Greek law forbade women to be weavers, for precisely the reason which may be urged in certain cases against the use of a sewing machine.

them, and even to resort to corporeal punishment* whenever detected in manualization.

Infibulation is spoken of only to be condemned. The camisole, while of great utility in the male, is of much less value in the female, since by the movement of one thigh upon the other, or by rubbing the external organs of generation upon the edge of a bedstead or of the table, voluptuous excitement may be produced. Pouillet suggests a bandage similar to that worn by Circassian girls, that shall completely close the vulva, leaving space for the escape of urine and the menstrual flow.

Clitoridectomy is so repugnant that it should only be resorted to in the last extremity, and then after the concurrence of able consultants.

The author states that no medicines have any marked effect upon masturbation. It is possible that camphor, turpentine, the bromide of potassium, monobromide of camphor, etc., by their general sedative influence, may have an effect upon the genital organs, lessening their vitality, and therefore may be tried with the treatment previously advised.

DR. L. P. YANDELL'S REPORT ON DERMATOLOGY.—The report on dermatology made to the Kentucky State Medical Society last April, by Dr. L. P. Yandell, Jr., and published in the May number of the American Practitioner, has been issued in pamphlet form. We regard it as an admirable paper, most useful and suggestive. The general propositions that he has maintained, viz., that chronic skin affections chiefly originate in the strumous diathesis, while the acute are malarial in source, constitute when fully established a most important advance, and will wonderfully simplify the therapeutics of these diseases. But are these propositions true? Medical observation must decide. But we believe that among the physicians of the west and south there will not be any great dissent, and that the general professional acceptance of Dr. Yandell's views is probably merely a question of time.

---

* In the cases of the girls to which reference has been made, a cold plunge and shower-bath have proved most useful.

INTERNATIONAL MEDICAL CONGRESS—PHILADELPHIA, SEPT. 4–9, 1876.—The International Medical Congress will be formally opened at noon on Monday, the fourth of September. The sessions of the Congress and of its Sections will be held in the University of Pennsylvania, Locust and Thirty-Fourth streets. The general meetings will be held daily, from 10 to 1 o'clock. The sections will meet at 2 o'clock. Luncheon for members of the Congress will be served daily in the University building from 1 to 2 o'clock.

On Wednesday evening, September 6th, Dr. J. J. Woodward, U. S. A., will address the Congress on the Scientific Work of the Surgeon-General's Bureau.

The public dinner of the Congress will be given on Thursday evening, September 7th, at 7 o'clock.

The registration book will be open daily from Thursday, August 31, to Saturday, September 2, inclusive, from 12 to 3 P. M., in the Hall of the College of Physicians, northeast corner of Thirteenth and Locust street, and at the University of Pennsylvania on Monday, September 4, from 9 to 12 M., and daily thereafter from 9 to 10 A. M. Credentials must in every case be presented.

Letters addressed to the members of the Congress, to the care of the College of Physicians, northeast corner Locust and Thirteenth streets, Philadelphia, during the week of meeting, will be delivered at the University of Pennsylvania.

The Secretaries of State and Territorial Medical Societies are requested to forward without delay to the Chairman of the Committee on Credentials—I. Minis Hays, M. D., 1607 Locust street, Philadelphia—lists of their duly accredited delegates to the Congress. Delegates and visitors intending to attend the Congress are earnestly requested individually to notify immediately the same committee. This information is desired to facilitate registration, and to ensure proper accommodation for the Congress.

Members intending to participate in the public (subscription) dinner of the Congress will please notify the Secretary of the Committee on Entertainment, J. Ewing Mears, M. D., 1429 Walnut street, Philadelphia.

THE EXCITABILITY OF THE HEART.—In a recent note on the excitability of the heart, read before the Académie des Sciences, M. Marey shows that this organ, at each phase of its revolution, undergoes changes of temperature which modify its excitability. Experiments demonstrate that the excitability of the heart, like that of other muscles, augments and diminishes with variations of temperature, and his experiments also demonstrate that the excitability of the heart changes at different phases of its revolution. This leads us to ask whether the temperature of the heart does not vary at different instants of its revolution, and also whether the succession of these variations is not such that the period of cooling corresponds to the phase of least excitability?—and further experiments have enabled him to return an affirmative reply to both these questions. The heart increases in temperature while it executes its mechanical work, and cools down as it relaxes. The moment when the heart is coldest, and consequently least excitable, is that when it has accomplished its period of cooling down. This will be the *début* of the systolic phase, and experiment is now in full accordance with theory. (Lancet.)

AN AMERICAN DERMATOLOGICAL ASSOCIATION.—A meeting for the organization of such an association will be held in the University of Pennsylvania, Philadelphia, on Wednesday, September 6, at 6 P. M. Doctors Bulkley and Fox, of New York, Wigglesworth of Boston, L. P. Yandell, Jr. of Louisville, and J. E. Atkinson of Baltimore, unite in the call.

DR. FLINT'S ARTICLE IN THE JANUARY NUMBER OF THE AMERICAN PRACTITIONER.—This will be found republished in the *Archives Générales* of July.

A DESERVED HONOR.—William R. Warner & Co., of Philadelphia, have received the prize medal of the Chilian World's Fair, for the superiority of their soluble sugar-coated pills.

# The American Practitioner.

## SEPTEMBER, 1876.

Certainly it is excellent discipline for an author to feel that he must say all that he has to say in the fewest possible words, or his reader is sure to skip them; and in the plainest possible words, or his reader will certainly misunderstand them. Generally, also, a downright fact may be told in a plain way; and we want downright facts at present more than any thing else —RUSKIN

## Original Communications.

## A CASE OF PODELCOMA.

### BY G. W. H. KEMPER, M. D.

## WITH MICROSCOPIC EXAMINATION OF THE DISEASED STRUCTURE.

### BY HENRY JAMESON, M. D.

Podelcoma, from πους, ποδος, a foot, and ἑλκωμα, an ulcer, is a malady affecting the feet, and sometimes hands, of the inhabitants of intertropical countries; and known by various other names, such as "Madura foot," "fungus disease of India," etc.

It is rarely seen without the tropics, and has been little studied either in this country or Europe. Miller, of Edinburgh, gives an elaborate treatise upon this subject; and in the Transactions of the Medical and Physical Society of Bombay, No. IV, for 1861, an essay is published by Dr. Carter, giving the true nature of the disease for the first time. This constitutes the principal literature upon the subject.

The extreme rarity of the disease in this country has induced me to give a detailed report of a case which recently came under my notice. This case was seen by a number of physicians, among whom was Professor Parvin, and all state that they have never before seen a similar case. In a recent conversation with Professor Dawson, of Cincinnati, he stated to me that he had never seen a case of podelcoma. The following detailed report gives the essential features in the case:

Mr. Harry Bowman, a native of Ohio, aged twenty-four years, by occupation a dry goods clerk. He has a nervous temperament, with a clear and delicate skin, yet gives no history of a scrofulous taint in the family, neither has he suffered from venereal disease. He consulted me on the nineteenth day of May, 1876, and gave the following account of his case:

About the middle of December, 1875, the right foot became swollen, reddened and painful: there was no constitutional disturbance, and it was thought to be rheumatism, and was treated with domestic remedies. At the expiration of three weeks from the beginning of the attack, the entire sole of the foot was so tender that he could bear no weight upon it. This condition continued until about the middle of the following April, when, after an intense itching of the bottom of the foot, several blebs about the size of a split pea made their appearance.

When I first saw him, some of these blebs had enlarged and otherwise changed their character; they were five or six in number, and were about half an inch in diameter. The cuticle, which was of a dirty white color, was intact, except at the center of each bleb, where a round opening existed with well defined borders. From these open centers issued daily about half an ounce of glairy fluid resembling the white of an egg, which was exceedingly offensive—a true meligeion. This discharge did not contain purulent matter, nor was pus present at any time during the course of the disease. There was but slight constitutional disturbance at any time.

Such was the condition of my patient at his first visit, after

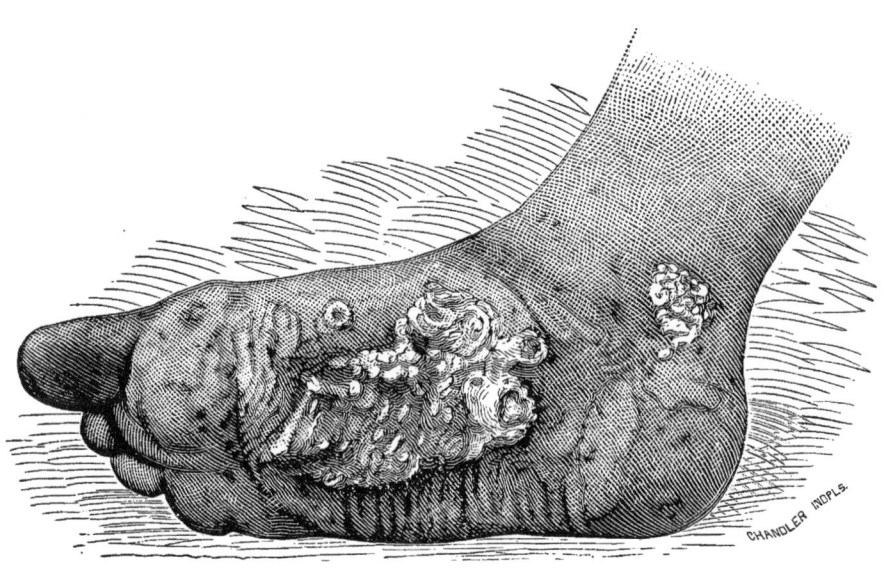

*Fig.* I.

which the ulcers gradually enlarged until they were separated only by undermined bands of integument; and still later, they were lost in one large ulcer at the inner side of the arch of the foot, as seen in Fig. 1. This was followed by the formation of a second, a little below and posterior to the internal malleolus, which was characterized by the same peculiar growth and offensive discharge as the first. A third and smaller ulcer appeared over the first metatarsal bone, and still later a fourth upon the bottom of the heel. The whole foot, including the toes, was greatly swollen and exquisitely painful; the slightest pressure over the diseased or healthy portion was sufficient to cause acute suffering.

Before his first visit to me, the usual routine of domestic remedies had been tried without even temporary relief. The constantly increasing pain drove him to seek medical advice. At this time I ordered a dressing composed of equal parts of acid nitrate of mercury and simple cerate, to the ulcers, with a continued application of flaxseed meal poultice to the foot.

May 21st. Since the last date his suffering has been very acute. He sleeps but little, notwithstanding the free use of opiates. I ordered laudanum to be used freely upon the poultices, and half grain doses of morphia to be given as often as prudent for the relief of pain.

May 23d. The patient has only had temporary relief while under the influence of opiates. In addition to the local measures named, I directed the foot to be painted with tincture of iodine three times daily. He was also given iodide of potassium, in doses of fifteen grains three times a day. Hydrate of chloral was tried in large doses on the night of the 22d, without much benefit.

June 2d. There is no perceptible improvement, the ulcers have gradually increased in size and are constantly painful, and at times severely so. I applied chromic acid thoroughly, and after the thickened cuticle was destroyed the tar ointment was used. This proceeding so increased his suffering that he was relieved only by the free use of injections of morphia into the calf of the leg, and immersion of the foot in warm water.

June 5th. The condition of the foot is somewhat improved. He has had less pain for the last two days, and rested better at night. Nitric acid was applied to the ulcers instead of the chromic, on account of the intense suffering produced by the latter.

June 11th. The smaller ulcers have not increased since the last date, and the larger one has decreased its diameter nearly one-half. The healed portion presents a smooth appearance. For two nights he has suffered greatly with pain, which seemed to originate in the cicatrix, passing up the limb to the spine. It was paroxysmal and manifested periodicity, recurring each night about eleven o'clock. With a view of counteracting this tendency, I administered large doses of sulphate of quinia. Notwithstanding the disposition of the ulcers to heal, the foot yet remains greatly swollen and very tender on pressure. Hypodermic injections of morphia give only partial relief.

June 15th. The suffering is yet so acute that at times signs of opisthotonos are present, and chloroform was administered for relief. The cicatricial tissue has broken down, and the ulcers are larger than at any previous time. His general health has steadily but markedly declined. For the past month his rest has been greatly disturbed, and his appetite has gradually and almost entirely forsaken him.

The means named, as well as others not mentioned, having been thoroughly tried, with no prospect of success, and in view of the fact that my patient's strength was failing, I advised amputation, which met with his hearty approval.

June 16th. Assisted by Drs. Winton and James, Drs. Boyden and Leech also being present, I amputated the leg at the junction of the lower and middle thirds, so as to avoid the diseased tissue above the ankle-joint. Esmarch's bandage was applied, commencing above the ulcers, and about two ounces of blood were lost.

June 19th. The healing process is progressing rapidly in the stump, his general health is improving, and all indications are favorable to speedy and permanent recovery.

MUNCIE, IND.

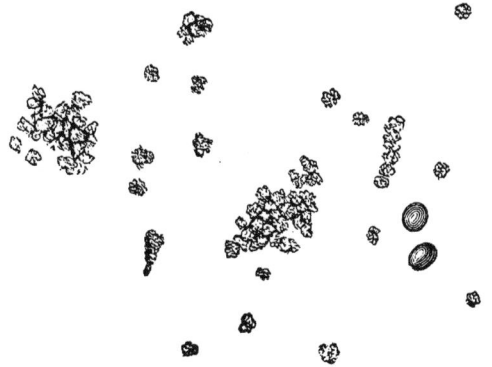

*Fig. 2.*

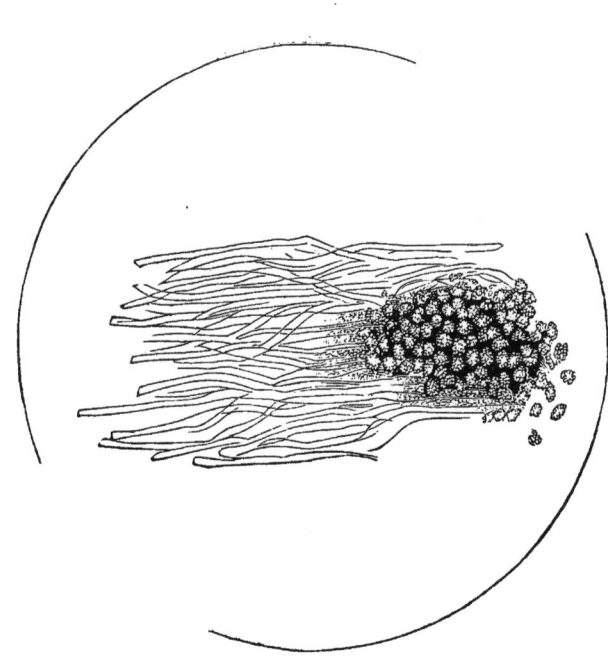

*Fig, 3.*

*Dr. G. W. H. Kemper—Dear Sir:* The external gross anatomical changes which existed in the foot at the time of amputation have been so clearly described in your report of the case, and moreover their having undergone certain changes due to immersion in alcohol, which impairs in a measure their value, they will simply be noticed before giving the appearance of the tissues upon dissection.

The larger ulcer, which is admirably represented at Fig. 1, was depressed below the general surface at least one-fourth of an inch, having sharp and well defined borders, was covered with a white fluffy substance. This substance was friable, breaking down readily under the scalpel, and presenting to the naked eye the appearance of mould or fungus, evidenced by difficulty in determining the position of its surface. This difficulty is probably due to a peculiar method of reflection or absorption of the rays of light by some of the various species of fungi. A probe being passed over the surface, discovered several openings passing down into the deeper tissues of the foot, but in no instance coming in contact with dead bone.

The smaller ulcers were probed in a like manner, and the openings were found to pass tortuously between the deeper muscles.

Upon laying the foot open, these canals could be distinctly traced, and were found to involve nearly all of the deeper muscles, which in many places were completely disintegrated, giving place to masses of the same material found upon the surface of the ulcers.

When examined with the one-fifth inch objective, with the B eye-piece, magnifying about two hundred diameters, which was ample to bring out the structure of this substance, it presented numerous granulated bodies, as seen at Fig. 2. They were rough and irregular in outline, yellowish in color, and refracted the light in such a manner as to give them a brilliant hue. These tubercles, variable in size, were massed together in mulberry-like groups, but bore no special relation to each other, except in one instance, when they assumed a chain-like form, as seen in the right side of the field in Fig. 2.

It was further noticed that the tortuous canals leading from the ulcerous surfaces, lead into cavernous openings in the bodies of the muscles, and these loculi were filled with a mass of the white tubercles, as represented at Fig. 3, which also serves to illustrate the relation of this material to the normal tissues. These minute spores were accompanied nowhere with any other anatomical element, which is strong evidence in proof of mycetoma. Vegetable parasites subsist upon the wasting substances of the body they attack; and were they simply present, taking no part in disintegration, we would certainly find associated with them the débris of the wasting tissue. That these white tubercles are vegetable spores there can be no doubt; but as to their identity with the *chionyphe Carteri* of Berkley, which is productive of the Madura foot, we can not be absolutely certain, as the identity of the different species of vegetable spores can not be established by any description given of their forms and appearance. "There is no branch of science whose synonomy is more burdensome. It is almost a hopeless task to attempt to identify the species of authors by description alone, the plant itself being necessary for comparison." The protean character of a single fungus would require long and continued observation to properly classify the many forms assumed during its brief existence. To this is due the contrariety of belief of different authorities concerning vegetable parasites.

Notwithstanding the difficult task of properly locating these ever changing organisms, we can but conclude that they are identical with those that are described by Carter and others; and while there may be points at variance in the clinical history of the case and the morbid appearance of the tissues, yet the essential factor in the disease seems to be the presence of this minute spore, with the power of reproducing itself in the living tissues, and sustaining itself by their destruction.

Many questions of interest suggest themselves in connection with this case:

First. As to the origin and introduction of the mycelium, for it will be remembered that in many cases the symptoms are manifested internally long before the integument is attacked, which might lead to the error of belief in their spontaneous generation in the blood. "We need not resort, however, to the unsatisfactory theory of spontaneous or accidental origin, if indeed we are able to conceive of any vast assemblage of organized structures, permanently reproductive and identical through centuries, being the result of chance." The delicate mycelium penetrates the hardest wood, and the vegetating fibers are so extremely minute that they find ready entrance through the pores of the densest substance.

Second. The conditions which must be present to favor their propagation, and the means by which they may be destroyed and these conditions counteracted.

INDIANAPOLIS.

---

## SOME OBSERVATIONS ON THE NATURE AND TREATMENT OF CHOLERA INFANTUM.*

BY B. D. KEATOR, M. D.

The term cholera infantum, as generally used, includes too much—so much as to embrace nearly all the stages of both diarrhœa and dysentery. In this paper I would restrict the term to that disease of young children occurring during the hot season, perhaps more frequently in large towns or cities, characterized by both vomiting and purging. The disease may approach slowly, with slight diarrhœa and occasional vomiting; but more often it comes on suddenly, with few premonitory symptoms; the vomiting, if not arrested, being soon followed by cold extremities, pinched features, sunken eyes, pallid countenance, spasmodic symptoms, great restlessness, moaning, turning the head on the pillow, approaching

---

* Read before the Champaign County (Ill.) Medical Society, at its meeting in Tolono, June 15, 1876.

coma, and finally death from exhaustion or a condition known as hydrocephaloid.

As we seldom have cases of genuine cholera infantum before the thermometer has stood for some days between 80° and 90° Fahr., the remote cause of the disease appears to be extreme heat, operating on the impressible nervous systems of children; and the approximate cause is found in some sudden alternation of temperature, as hot days attended by cool showers or followed by cool nights.

During this hyperæsthetic and impressible condition of system, more immediate exciting causes will be found in errors of diet, dentition, torpidity of the liver, acidity of the stomach, vitiated or decomposed bile, retrocession of heat-rash, etc.

Dr. McBride, of Berea, Ohio, in an able article on this disease (Lancet and Observer), believes this last—heat-rash—to be the sole cause of the disease. While this can not be conceded to be strictly so, yet according to my observation many of the most sudden and alarming cases come from this cause. Time and again have children been brought to me with this rash, who, in a few days after, were attacked suddenly with cholera infantum. In such cases the irritability of the stomach will prove very persistent, and the skin, from the first, present a more blanched and exsanguine appearance than usual.

Another able writer, Dr. J. P. Mann (New York Medical Journal, Vol. X, No. 1), believes the cause of the disease to be decomposition of bile in the gastro-intestinal track.

A majority of the physicians of my acquaintance with whom I have conversed on the subject, attribute the disease to torpidity of the liver, which plainly needs a little mild chloride of mercury, or hydragyrum cum cretâ, for its obstinacy. That there is an absence of the yellow, or so-called ''bilious'' appearance of the stools, is often, but not invariably, true; but whether this is the cause or a result of the disease, might be a subject for discussion. The icterode hue of countenance, common in cases of arrest of biliary secretion, is not generally found.

To return: It would thus appear that while extreme heat

may be fairly regarded as the remote cause of the disease, the proximate cause may vary. The disease can often be arrested by timely and judicious treatment in its first stages; but if not, the acute form generally proves fatal in a time varying from a few hours to a few days; or else, the vomiting ceasing, it passes into the chronic form, the duration of which is very indefinite.

According to a recent work (Steiner's Compendium), "the pathological changes—most frequently found post mortem, affecting the stomach, small intestines, and occasionally the ascending colon—consist in injection and swelling of the mucous membrane; and when the course of the case is very rapid, extensive destruction of the epithelial coat: ecchymoses are also sometimes seen. Acute enlargement of the mesenteric glands and general anaemia of the organs, especially of the brain, which often also gives evidence of fatty degeneration and œdema; hyperæmia of the kidneys, and in occasional cases acute parenchymatous nephritis." Though "most frequently" it appears there is found anæmia of the brain, yet not always, for "the brain is sometimes found congested with serous effusion into its ventricles." (Maxson.)

Where the head symptoms come on early, before there has been much drain on the system by diarrhœa, we should investigate as closely as possible, and endeavor to ascertain whether the brain and its membranes are in a hyperæmic or anæmic condition, and conduct our treatment accordingly. It appears to me there is too much tendency towards regarding all these head symptoms of cholera infantum as the result of cerebral anæmia, and thus leading not infrequently to injudicious treatment.

As preliminary to touching upon the treatment of this disease, I would not fail to mention the flannel bandage, to be worn about the abdomen as a means of prevention; and to protest against the weaning of children (except through necessity) during the season of the year when this disease prevails. In a case of real cholera infantum, in which there are both vomiting and purging, it has always appeared to me that the vomiting did more immediate harm than the purging. It appears to be in some way directly connected with the development of cerebral difficulties, and hence our first aim should be to allay the gastric irritation. For this purpose, small doses of hydrargyrum submuriate, triturated with white sugar and placed upon the tongue, often prove effectual. Some prefer to add a little plumb. acetate, and both are used with considerable success. The cerium oxalate, in doses of one-sixth to one-fourth of a grain, repeated at short intervals, I regard quite as successful, if not more so. . But the best remedy of all, in my opinion, is creasote or carbolic acid with an alkali. Add to a goblet of water two or three drops of creasote and a pinch of sodium bicarbonate. Of this give a teaspoonful often as required, withhold all drink for a time, place a sinapism weakened with flour over the stomach, and you will generally succeed. Or, in place of this, a drop of creasote added to an ounce and a half of lime-water, and given in teaspoonful doses, will answer as well.

If there is evidence of torpidity of the liver, half to a grain of hydrargyrum submuriate, guarded by as much Dover's powder, may be given once in six or eight hours, until the function of that organ be restored. I say this *may* be done, and I have often done it; but of late I have a better remedy. Whether there be decomposition of bile in this disease, as supposed by a writer before quoted (Mann) or not, I can not say; but I can certify that the remedy he proposes is an excellent one, almost specific. Here is the formula:

R. Aloes socot pulv., . . . ⎞
   Potassii sulphat., . . . ⎬ āā ʒi
   Sodii bicarbonat., . . . ⎠
   Caryophyl. pulv., . . . ʒss

Mix, and divide in twelve powders. For use, put one of the powders in a cup, and add three tablespoonfuls of hot water. Dose, one teaspoonful, warm as it can be taken every half hour, until bright yellow bile appears in the stools.

This is the original, with directions; but I use it somewhat differently. I keep it on hand in quantity, using it both for adults and children for all bilious symptoms. In cases of cholera infantum, put a teaspoonful of the powder and a tablespoonful of sugar in a teacup, and fill with boiling water. When cool enough to use, give one teaspoonful every fifteen or twenty minutes, withholding drink until vomiting ceases, then every hour until it acts on the bowels as before mentioned. Though having the appearance of a nauseous dose, I find this to remain on the stomach when scarcely anything else will.

But to return: After the vomiting is checked, our attention should next be given to the diarrhœa. The practice of giving astringents and opiates, with the intention of suddenly checking the diarrhœa, is, I am satisfied from experience, decidedly harmful not to say dangerous.

Opium, or even morphia, may be given in most cases with benefit, but in such minute doses as to secure and keep up, as long as required, its soothing and stimulating influence without reaching its stupefying and narcotic effects. If the brain is in a condition of anæmia, what will better tone and send the blood to its empty vessels than stimulating, not depressing, doses of opium?

The effect of subnitrate of bismuth, combined with small doses of Dover's powder—say three to five grains of the former and one-fourth to one grain of the latter—is sometimes very satisfactory. It appears to exert a soothing and quieting influence on the irritated mucous membrane of the stomach, and thus diminishes general nervous excitement. A convenient form of administration is to add it to the ordinary chalk mixture, in the proportion of thirty grains to the ounce of chalk mixture, with the addition of paregoric in some cases. This, according to the old adage, must be "shaken before taken."

The only astringents allowable in the early stage of cholera infantum proper, in my opinion, is zinc oxide. This, besides its astringency, is a nervine, and like the bromides lessens cerebral hyperæmia, and is, on the whole, one of the best remedies we possess for this disease. Not only will it quiet general nervous irritability, but, like the bismuth subnitrate, it has a soothing influence directly on the irritated gastro-intestinal mucous membrane. There may be some who will take exceptions to this, but such is my opinion after an extensive use of it. To neutralize acidity, as well as prevent the possible formation of zinc salts, in the stomach, it should be combined, when used in this disease, with sodium bicarbonate, in about the proportion of eight grains of the sodium salt to each drachm of the zinc.

The actions of creasote and carbolic acid are nearly the same, but what difference there is appears to be in favor of the creasote in this disease. The beneficial effect of these medicines is not limited to the arrest of vomiting; but they appear to be among the best means of checking the diarrhœa also, and from their antiseptic properties of preventing fermentation in the stomach, as well as tending to lessen the destructive changes likely to occur in the mucous membrane. In using carbolic acid, the following formula from Professor Davis, of Chicago, is a very excellent one:

R. Crystal carbol. acid, . . . . . grs. iii
Glycerine (Bower's), . . . . ℥ss
Paregoric, . . . . . . . ℥i
Water, . . . . . . . . ℥iss

Mix. Dose, twenty drops every half hour, until the vomiting ceases; then every two hours. (*Vide* Half-Yearly Compendium, January, 1873.)

A favorite formula with me for administering creasote and morphia in proper doses is as follows:

R. Creasote, . . . . . . . . gtt. xvi
Morphia sulph., . . . . . . gr. ii
Ess. peppermint, . . . . . ʒi
Syr. rhei. aromat., . . . . . ʒx
Glycerine (Bower's), . . . . ʒx

Mix. To a child of one year give from ten to fifteen drops in a teaspoonful of milk, every two hours while awake. If in the vomiting stage, only a few drops, frequently repeated, with lime-water and milk, withholding drink.

Much benefit is often obtained in this disease by the use of mucilages; especially should they be given during the use of creasote or carbolic acid. Among these I prefer salep, twenty grains to four ounces of hot water; and next gum arabic.

After the first stages of the disease have passed by, the discharges often become less frequent but more copious, the disease passing into a chronic stage. Here the treatment must be tonic and supporting. Now, with the exception of iron, in cases where it is plainly indicated, no tonic can come in competition with salicin, given in half to grain doses to a child one year old, three or four times daily. It appears to be not only better than quinia, in restoring appetite and aiding digestion, but is the best remedy we have in moderating the diarrhœa, which it does in a gradual and apparently natural way, without the development of the complications following its arrest by ordinary astringent treatment.

We meet with cases of this disease, in its chronic form, which baffle all our skill to arrest, and our only hope is to bridge them over to the approach of cool weather. Such cases I would trust to good nourishment, port wine, and salicin. Whenever the discharges become purulent, or there is any evidence of intestinal ulceration, I have found potassium chlorate, combined with a little Dover's powder, worthy of much confidence.

In those cases which supervene on retrocession of heat rash—*lichen tropicus* of Dr. McBride, and which I am confident constitute a large percentage of the worst cases we meet with every season—our aim should be to determine the blood to the surface, recall the rash if possible, and so relieve the congested mucous membrane of the stomach and bowels. For this purpose, no single remedy equals belladonna. Dr. McBride gives it in half drop doses of the fluid extract, until the cuticular circulation is reëstablished. This dose was for a child of one year. I would advise, in addition, that the child have a warm mustard bath, or be enveloped in a shawl or other woolen piece, wrung out of warm mustard water, and cooling drink be given.   In such cases, we often find the mucous membrane of the mouth very red and hot, and the child ready to swallow anything in a liquid form, be it even a nauseous dose of medicine, for the sake of drink.   In these cases, nothing appears to give so immediate relief as scraped ice, in half teaspoonful doses, or in the form of ice cream.

As it has been shown that the brain has been found, post mortem, in opposite conditions, the treatment should, so far as possible, be adapted to the condition present in each case.   If there be evidence of cerebral hyperæmia, the best remedies, according to my observation, are the bromides and zinc oxide.   The bromides must be given, in such cases, in sufficient doses to control spasm and compel sleep.   I have had recoveries from apparently hopeless cases of this character, by keeping the patients asleep by the use of potassium bromide, for several days in succession, only disturbing them at proper intervals for the administration of nourishment in the shape of milk or sweet cream.   We thus give the oppressed brain the rest it needs for recuperation.   Warm footbaths, and frequent bathing of the head with cool water, are also proper additional means.

On the contrary, as is more often the case, if the brain give evidence of anæmia, belladonna, from its action on the extreme capillary circulation, and nux vomica, from its power to arouse nerve energy, are the most reliable means at our command. Although opium and belladonna are antagonistic, in some respects, yet it appears to me that when alternated in the proper dose of each, they have been co-workers for good in cerebral anæmia.   The head should not be elevated, and should be kept at a warm, even temperature by a woolen cap.   These means should be aided by nourishment in the shape of brandy and cream, or pounded raw beefsteak and wine.

TOLONO, ILL.

# REDUCTION OF DISLOCATION OF THE HIP-JOINT BY MANIPULATING THE FEMUR OVER A FULCRUM PLACED IN THE GROIN.

### BY GEORGE SUTTON, M. D.

In the April number of the American Practitioner, on page 225, are rules for the reduction of dislocation of the hip-joint by making the femur a lever and manipulating it over a ful-crum placed in the groin. In the second rule occurs a typo-graphical error which I wish to correct. I am made to say, ''If the dislocation is into the ischiatic notch, the femur is to be flexed over the fulcrum, which movement will lift the head of the bone out of the ischiatic notch, and at the same time raise it high enough to pass the rim of the acetabulum; the knee is then to be moved *inward*.'' This should read, ''the knee is then to be moved *outward* to place the head of the bone over the cotyloid cavity; which, by so doing, will enable the surrounding muscles to effect the reduction.'' So glaring a mistake would readily be detected and probably be regarded by most persons as a typographical error. Whether this mis-take was made by myself or the printer I do not know, as I find, on examination, that it does not occur in the copy of the manuscript I have in my possession.

Since the paper alluded to was published, I received a pro-fessional call from Ohio county, and reduced another disloca-tion of the hip-joint without difficulty by manipulating the femur over a fulcrum. The dislocation was of the ischiatic variety, of four weeks' duration, and had resisted all the efforts made to effect its reduction. The case was about to be aban-doned, but the two physicians in attendance—Doctors H. T. Williams and W. H. Sullivan, prominent physicians of Rising Sun, the county seat of Ohio county—hearing of the facility with which several dislocations of the hip-joint had been re-duced at Aurora, by the aid of the fulcrum, after all other means had failed, addressed me a letter on the 26th of April last, inviting me to meet them in the case of a dislocation of the femur, if I did not think it one of too long standing, as they informed me the bone had been out of place twenty-eight days. Being anxious to avail myself of every opportunity to try this mode of reducing dislocation of the hip-joint, I at once accepted the invitation and visited Rising Sun the next day, April 27, 1876, accompanied by my son, Dr. Harley H. Sutton.

We found the case as represented, the head of the femur lodged in the ischiatic notch. Originally the head of the bone was on the dorsum of the ilium, but in the efforts at reduction the bone had slipped into the ischiatic notch, from which the attending physicians could not remove it.

We proceeded to effect the reduction. From the length of time the bone had been dislocated, and the complete failure of all efforts employed to remove it from the ischiatic notch, we anticipated difficulty. Consequently I had two pads or fulcrums made of different sizes, one a piece of muslin rolled up between two and three inches in thickness, and about fifteen inches in length; the other, made of the same material, between three and four inches in thickness. Strings were tied around each to prevent unrolling. A broad board was procured nearly two feet in breadth and about ten feet in length. There were two beds in the room; these were drawn near enough together to place an end of the board on each bed. Comforts were spread on it, a pillow placed in position, and the patient lifted on to this board. This arrangement places the patient in a very convenient position for the manipulations of the surgeon, and enables both the surgeon and assistants to be close to the side of the patient, and is much better than having to manipulate on a broad bed, or in the stooping position on the floor.

Assisted by Drs. Williams, Sullivan, G. V. Stevenson—medical gentlemen of Rising Sun—and Dr. H. H. Sutton, and other gentlemen who were in the room, we proceeded to reduce the dislocation. Dr. Sullivan administered chloroform. The patient, however, did not come under its influence well, and unfavorable symptoms appearing, we placed the smallest fulcrum in the groin, one end of which was held by Dr. Williams and the other by Dr. H. H. Sutton. I then flexed the thigh over it; the patient struggled considerably, and Dr. Sullivan again administered the chloroform, which in a few moments partially produced the desired effect, without this time alarming symptoms. The limb during the time had been kept slightly flexed over the fulcrum. I now increased the flexion, which by lever power raised the head of the bone at once out of the ischiatic notch, and also high enough to pass over the rim of the acetabulum. I then flexed the leg upon the thigh, and with my right hand on the bottom of the foot pushed the knee forward toward the sternum, to place the head of the femur on a level with the cotyloid cavity. I then with my left hand moved the knee outward, and while doing so moved it upward and downward, which, from the lever power that I had, broke up the adhesions and enabled me to move the head of the bone along the line by which it could most readily return to the socket. While making these movements, which required but little force, I slightly raised the knee—the leg still abducted—and felt the bone glide into its proper place.

The thigh could now be moved in any direction without difficulty, the toes no longer turned inwards, and the limb was of the proper length. Dr. Williams measured the distance of the trochanter from the superior spinous process of the ilium, and found no difference from that of the opposite leg. The dislocation was reduced. The time required to effect the reduction was probably between five and ten minutes. The patient has since recovered, and is again attending to business.

The difficulties which two experienced physicians had met with in their attempts to reduce this bone—the length of time (four weeks) the limb had been dislocated increasing the complications of the case, the ease with which all obstacles were overcome, the adhesions broken up, and the reduction accomplished, even while the patient was only partially under the influence of chloroform—makes this not only a test case, but presents facts which, I think, prove beyond all doubt the value of this mode of reducing dislocations of the hip-joint. We claim for this method the power of controlling, guiding, and raising the head of the femur; consequently by this plan we avoid the danger of rolling the bone around the outside of the cotyloid cavity, also of changing one form of dislocation into that of another, and producing unnecessary contusions, lacerations, or injury to the parts. We also claim for this mode the best means of guiding the head of the bone along the *only* line by which it can return to the socket, and the best means of raising the head of the femur over the rim of the acetabulum, by which we overcome one of the principal difficulties to the reduction of dislocation of the hip-joint. And if the head of the bone does not readily pass through a rent in the capsular ligament—"button-hole rent"—we claim for this plan the best mode of enlarging this rent, by which the femur can again return to its proper place.

The full particulars of the above case, with observations on the value of manipulating the femur over a fulcrum in reduction of dislocations of the hip-joint, were presented in a report to the Indiana State Medical Society, at its last meeting, from which the above is an extract.

This now makes the fourth case in which dislocation of the hip-joint has been reduced with remarkable facility, after all other means had failed, by manipulating the femur over a fulcrum. Up to the present time we have no failures to report. Three of the cases have been on the dorsum of the ilium, and one into the ischiatic notch.

Since making this last reduction, I change the second rule of the series presented in the April number of the Practitioner, so as to read as follows:

"If the dislocation is into the ischiatic notch, the femur is to be flexed over the fulcrum, which movement will lift the head of the bone out of the ischiatic notch, and at the same time raise it high enough to pass over the rim of the acetabulum; then the leg is to be flexed upon the thigh, and with the hand on the bottom of the foot, the knee is to be pushed forward toward the sternum to bring the head of the femur on a level with the cotyloid cavity; then the knee is to be moved outward to place the head of the bone over the acetabulum, and enable the surrounding muscles to effect the reduction."

AURORA, IND.

---

## AMBLYOPIA FROM RETINITIS PIGMENTOSA.*

BY T. D. MANNING, M. D.

M., aged thirteen years, applied in June, 1875, for admission to the Texas Institute for the Blind, but the spring term of that institution being well nigh over, she was not received until the next September. The surgeon in charge obtained, however, at the time the following history: From childhood, and especially after beginning school, which was at an early age, the patient complained of "weak eyes." At first the trouble was not so much actual dimness of sight as inability of the eyes to bear prolonged use. At the close of a day at school, her eyes were fatigued and easily suffused. This condition gradually increased until there was perceptible failure of sight; and finally, two months previous to applying at the institution, the trouble culminated in actual blindness throughout a greater part of the field of vision in the left eye, and inability to read ordinary print with the right eye. The eyes had a vacant look, as if nothing was seen distinctly, while a convergent strabismus was noticeable in the left eye. The ophthalmoscope revealed a widespread pigmentary deposit throughout both retinæ; the extent of deposit being about

* The accompanying paper is but an abstract of that read by its accomplished author at the meeting of the Texas State Medical Association in April last.— D. W. Y.

equal in the two eyes. Large dark masses, composed of granular or "irregular-shaped spots," with prolongations following the course of the retinal vessels, occupied most of the face of each retina. Tension was not notably increased in either eye; but anæmia of the left retina was perceptible.

Although necessity of immediate attention to the diseased organs was urged by the surgeon in charge, the patient was not seen again for four or five months, when, in November, the left eye was found to have only qualitative perception of light from the temporal side; the right eye could distinguish No. L Snellen, at twelve feet from the temporal side, the field of vision being exceedingly narrow. Many of the retinal vessels of the left eye were apparently obliterated, while the retina of the right eye showed a decided paleness. Hemeralopia was now distinctly marked, and headache coming on at night prevented sleep. The headache was probably due, as Von Gräfe has pointed out, to the failing sight, and is produced by the intent endeavor of the patient still thoroughly to realize the visual impression.

Although things seemed so hopeless, it was determined to give the patient the benefit of an iridectomy in the right eye, removing at least one-fifth of the iris through an upward incision in the sclero-corneal junction. No pain or other trouble followed, and when, at the end of four days, the bandage was removed, the patient immediately declared she could see better by far with either eye than before the operation. Two months later, it was found that she could read ordinary print with her right eye; and at the expiration of three other months, she was able to read the finest print with that eye.

The left eye, before considered as entirely amaurotic, and beyond any relief whatever, had also gained somewhat, though very little. This little gain, however, coupled with a return of pain on that side, led to an iridectomy on the left eye; and while it effected no improvement in its sight, it gave permanent relief of the pain in the orbital region. The operation was not as thorough as was desired, the iris not being removed up to its ciliary attachment; yet the failure to increase vision was due, no doubt, to atrophy of the optic nerve, as shown by the ophthalmoscope.

I need scarcely remark that the prognosis in this affection is extremely unfavorable, and no special treatment further than to protect the eyes from bright light and over-taxation is insisted on. The disease—retinitis pigmentosa—is evidently characterized by a decided torpor of the retina; the retinal vessels diminish in caliber, and many of the smaller branches are apparently obliterated. Schweigger has pointed out that this torpor of the retina "is due to the fact that on account of the diminution of the caliber of the arteries, an insufficient amount of blood is supplied to the retina;" and all writers agree that the pigmentation of the retina follows the contraction of the arteries, and is not the direct cause of blindness. The iridectomy was undertaken with the view of relieving this torpor by causing a determination of blood to the retina. No unusual tension was perceptible, which we know was the cardinal point with Von Gräfe when he operated for the relief of glaucoma.

The foregoing is the only case within the knowledge of the writer where retinitis pigmentosa has been treated by iridectomy, done as in incipient glaucoma, and more particularly where no abnormal tension could be discovered after the most careful examination.

I am aware that no single case can go far toward establishing anything; and in that now under consideration, it is possible, perhaps, that such improvement as occurred was a coincidence rather than a result. But the fact can not be questioned, that while previous to the iridectomy sight was very limited in one eye and wholly absent in the other, the patient expressed herself, immediately after the operation, as being improved, and came eventually to read ordinary print with the right eye, and experienced some, though very slight benefit to the sight of the left eye. Since no adequate explanation has yet been given of the good that follows iridectomy in glaucoma, I may be pardoned for offering none for the good done by the same operation performed in retinitis pigmentosa, where, in the single case reported, ocular tension was not present.

The patient has a brother three years her junior, whose eyes seem to be going as hers went. The pigmentation in his appears to be equal to that observed in his sister's, though he still preserves good sight on first impression. A double iridectomy will be done for him with the hope of saving vision in both eyes.

WACO. TEXAS.

---

# SYPHILITIC DISEASES OF THE THROAT.

### BY RICHARD C. BRANDEIS, M. D.

These affections have always been considered as the most dangerous forms of constitutional syphilis, and cause the patient more distress, and the physician more anxiety, than almost any of the complications of this disease. They have generally been treated as identical diseases; but, for the sake of clearness, we will divide them into three classes, viz:

First. Simple syphilitic angina, which is the least dangerous, and which generally affects the parts at or about the isthmus of the fauces.

Second. Syphilitic pharyngitis.

Third. The ulcerated, perforating affections of the soft palate.

The first, or the simple syphilitic angina, is the most common form of the disease. It rarely attacks all the tissues included in the isthmus of the fauces, but more commonly one or the other parts, generally the tonsils, not so often the arch of the palate, appears as commonly on one side as the other, and not infrequently attacks both tonsils simultaneously. At certain times it makes its appearance very soon after the primary symptoms of syphilis are first detected, which I noticed to be a very frequent occurrence in the syphilitic wards of Professors Zeissel and Sigmund, in the General Hospital of Vienna, during my stay there in the years 1871 and 1872. Occasionally I have observed the same thing since I have entered upon private practice.

On examination, we will find grayish white patches deposited on the congested mucous membrane, which, in the more marked cases, have the appearance of distinct exudations very similar to the appearance produced by a gentle cauterization of a mucous membrane. The affected parts are greatly congested, and this is particularly noticeable in case the tonsils are the seat of the disease. In the more severe cases, we observe a yellowish white exudation (membrane) situated on a very much congested portion of the isthmus, which gradually disappears from its border, and which will leave a slight superficial excoriation. I have never seen any true ulcerative action in any of this class of cases, which helps to distinguish it from the second and third divisions. Those ulcers, however, which are sometimes seen in this region may be considered as secondary to some pharyngeal or soft palatal trouble, or may even have extended upwards from the larynx.

I find in my case-book, June 3, 1875, the results of a post mortem examination of J—— T——, aged forty-two years, who died from the effects of a fall, which gave rise to concussion of the brain: "There was seen a deep ulcer, the size of a silver half dollar, which extended upward from the root of the tongue, the right valleculus, affecting the tonsil, the anterior and posterior pillars of the fauces, and reaching up to the uvula, which was very œdematous. This ulcer was bounded by a pale border varying in width from one to three lines. In the region of the tonsil, there were only a few wartlike remains of that gland to be seen. The epiglottis was almost entirely destroyed, as were the arytenoid cartilages, some dense cicatrices being the only things to mark their former seat. The posterior wall of the pharynx was very much swollen and œdematous." In this case, I have no doubt that the origin of the ulcer was at the epiglottis, from which it spread in the direction above mentioned.

In very severe cases we sometimes find shallow ulcerations
on the soft palate, on the palatal arches, and rarely on the
tonsils, which, however, never grow any larger than when
they made their first appearance. The base of these ulcers
is covered with the yellowish exudation already spoken of.
After they have been cured, their site is marked by slight
excavations. I have seen this condition in but two instances.
It will easily be understood why there is an almost entire.
absence of subjective symptoms when we consider that the
sensitiveness of a mucous membrane diminishes in inverse
ratio to the distance from the external cutaneous covering,
and that the ulcerations are very superficial, and the inflammatory process very mild, in character. Only when the yellowish white exudation makes its appearance do the patients
complain of burning and pressure in swallowing, which is
probably due to the excoriation. The condylomata which
make their appearance on the isthmus of the fauces, may be
considered as a variety of these affections; they generally
appear on the lower border of the soft palate and on the
uvula, and at times must be removed with the scissors. We
must not confound these with the *papules* and *plaques muqu-
euses* of Ricord, who regards the affection just treated of as
one of the secondary symptoms of syphilis, and as a substitute of the exanthematic syphilides of the skin.

The second and more dangerous form of angina is the pharyngitis syphilitica. The seat of this disease is generally on
one or the other, or both, sides of the pharynx, and more
rarely in the middle of its posterior wall; sometimes it extends
downward to the orifice of the œsophagus, behind the larynx,
and only the experienced observer will be able to determine
the nature of the case after learning all the subjective symptoms, and hearing all about the previous primary affection,
and examining the hyperæmic condition of the posterior wall;
only then will he be able to diagnose an ulcer of the pharynx,
and recognize its callous borders. This form is generally limited to the mucous membrane, but occasionally extends to the
submucous cellular tissue; and if the base of the tongue be

depressed and the patient yawns, and the soft palate is lifted up with a sound, an oval, serrated phagedænic ulcer will be seen on the posterior wall of the pharynx, very red and swollen. This is often covered by a layer of tough, yellowish white mucous, not very adherent and easily removed, when the ulcer will be easily recognized. The surrounding parts are generally, more or less, hyperæmic. The depth of the ulcer may vary from one-third to one-half a line, but appears deeper owing to the swelling of its margin. This form of pharyngitis always makes its appearance without presenting any subjective symptoms, but is soon followed by pricking and burning pains, which are always increased during deglutition; there is also dryness of the mouth, and on examination the ulcer already mentioned will be discovered. The callosity of the parts can readily be detected on touch, and the patient complains of pain if the part is pressed upon.

This disease is not alarming *per se*, but only on account of the danger of affecting the adjacent organs. Those ulcers which are situated low down are apt to extend to the larynx, and those situate near the soft palate are apt to extend to that part. If the disease is restricted to its original seat, it rarely affects the voice, which fact can readily be explained. Only the most superficial ulcerations, which do not require any treatment, disappear without leaving any traces behind, while the more marked ulcers leave a cellulo-fibrous cicatrix behind them, which sometimes occupies a considerable space, and may then produce a constriction of the pharynx, with all its disagreeable consequences. It is not very probable that this disease may, if it extends deeper, also affect the vertebra, as has been suggested. The probability is that, if there be both pharyngeal and vertebral disease, the latter was prior to the former affection.

Third. The most dangerous form of *angina syphilitica*, which is always a secondary symptom, is that which occurs on the soft palate, which destroys that part with great rapidity, and which gives rise to various deformities. Owing to its destructiveness, the attention and anxiety of the profession has been aroused, and we are thus enabled to give an accurate account of the evil results which may follow. This disease is so insidious in its approaches that it not infrequently has advanced to a considerable extent before the patient has become aware of its presence; and it may, in the very shortest time, extend from a simple perforation of the soft palate to a total destruction of the same, as well as the inner and outer nasal tract, thus leaving behind it ineradicable deformities. In the majority of instances the nasal passages are affected, although it not infrequently occurs that the soft palate alone is the seat of the disease; and moreover it appears that the starting point of this affection is generally situate on the floor of the posterior nares, from whence it extends to the *septum narium*, and to the soft palate.

In case it first arises on the upper surface of the soft palate, the ulcer will not be as violent in its onslaught, and will more readily remain stationary than otherwise. The anterior surface of the palate is then highly congested, sometimes assuming a purplish tinge. The patients complain of severe pains, which are most intense during deglutition, and the posterior wall is hardened, ulcerated, and the least touch is very painful. The ulcer extends in area and depth very gradually, and sooner or later we notice an elevation of the epithelial layer of the anterior surface of the soft palate, through which numerous whitish yellow granules can be discovered; this elevation may become globular in shape. Within the next twenty-four hours this epithelium is destroyed, and a funnel-shaped ulcer is apparent, the smaller opening of which presents itself in the roof of the mouth. This soon increases in size, and assumes a very irregular and jagged shape. The margin is thickened and œdematous, and has the appearance of amyloid degeneration. If the circumscribed congestion does not diminish, we may rely upon it that its progress will be very rapid, and an energetic interference is very much needed. If the ulcer heals in this stage, which can be foretold if the congestion becomes less, then there will remain an oval perforation of the palate, which will ultimately heal up and cicatrize,

and leave no further unpleasant symptoms behind. In healing, if the ulcer had attained any considerable size, the uvula
is drawn to one or the other side.

This disease often extends from the posterior palatal surface
to the posterior wall of the pharynx. We then have, in addition to the symptoms just described, those already mentioned
in connection with *pharyngitis syphilitica.* Both parts are
swollen and inflamed; they approximate each other, and
fibrous bands may extend from one to the other. The soft
palate will thus become adherent to the pharynx after healing
has set in, and the former arch of the palate and *isthmus
faucium* will, after the destruction of the uvula, acquire a tri-
angular form. If the ulcer has destroyed the greater part of
the soft palate, it will be drawn further back, and will be converted into a dense, firm and unyielding bridge of cicatricial
tissue. The communication between the nose and the mouth
is thus cut off, and the patient will only be able to breathe
when the mouth is wide open, if there be no perforation of
the palate, or a small opening in the cicatrix, which latter is
found in almost every instance.

The most alarming and hideous form of this disease is that
in which the ulcerative process extends to the nasal mucous
membrane and the septum of the nares. After the patient
has been troubled for some length of time with a feeling of
dryness in the nasal cavity, an offensive purulent discharge
will suddenly make its appearance, which not only annoys
the patient but those around as well. A sinking of the cartilaginous portion of the nose will soon manifest itself, so that
we will have a deep furrow between the tip of the nose and
the inferior border of the nasal bones; the continuity of the
bridge of the nose is thus interrupted, which will enable us to
differentiate between this and congenital deformities. This
deformity, so commonly observed, seems to be due to the
destruction of the cartilaginous or bony portions of the septum of the nose. although most patients deny that there was
ever any separation or discharge of fragments of bone. We

must not place too much reliance on these statements, however, because without the knowledge of the patient little particles of ulcerated bone or cartilages are often hawked up; the septum of the nose is generally perforated, if not entirely gone.    In only one instance do I remember that a patient showed me a small fragment of dead bone which he had removed from his nose, and it proved to be one of the turbinated bones, and was sufficient in itself to enable me to determine as to the syphilitic character of the disease.    This form is the more marked if the disease extends to the floor of the nose, and terminates in perforation of the palate, as sometimes occurs.    The basilar process of the occipital bone can sometimes be recognized if sufficient light be thrown through the perforation, and syphilitic patches can also be discerned.    If this process proceeds unchecked the entire nose may be destroyed.    But the further discussion of this subject would carry us beyond the legitimate limits of this paper.

In all the varieties of the ulcerative affections of the soft palate, we meet with the nasal voice, which varies in character with the severity of the attack, and is in itself a most lamentable result of this disease.

A peculiarity of the different forms described is their proneness to relapse.    They manifest themselves under all methods of treatment, from simple antiphlogosis to the most thorough course of mercurialization.    They appear to be most common after the use of the iodide of potassium, and then oftener if this be given in pill or solution than when used in substance. I have occasionally seen them after a course of the proto-ioduret of mercury.

LOUISVILLE, KY.

# A CASE OF INTESTINAL FISTULA—RECOVERY.

BY E. P. GILPIN, M. D.

William Jenkins, an intelligent mulatto, aged nineteen years, was admitted into the Indianapolis City Hospital, April 14, 1876, with the following history:

About a year ago he had been crushed between two logs, so as to break several ribs and force a splinter into the left side on a line with the ensiform cartilage. Being strong and healthy he made a good recovery, and soon resumed his work on the farm, although sometimes troubled by what he thought were pieces of splinter in his side. Ten days previous to admission he felt a "lump" in the left side of his abdomen, which was very painful; and three days after his abdomen was much swelled, accompanied by severe colicky pains, and on the following morning an abscess opened in the left iliac fossa, which he said discharged "blood, matter and filth." From that time until his admission to the hospital—one week—he had no passage by the rectum, but passed pus, gas and feces through the abdominal opening. He states that some physicians, in making an examination, passed a probe four or five inches into the bowel.

*Present Condition.*—Found an opening in the left iliac fossa, about three-fourths of an inch in diameter, from which feculent gas, pus and feces escaped. A little internal to the opening can be felt a moderately firm tumor, the size of a goose-egg, not sensitive to pressure. There is some deformity of the chest from the fractured ribs, and considerable enlargement of the liver. Pulse and temperature normal.

Intestinal fistula being diagnosed, he was ordered to be kept on his back, a compress was applied to the opening, and an enema of warm soap-suds administered, which was to be repeated every three hours until free evacuation occurred. After the second injection the bowels moved, and were kept open while he remained. Nutritious fluid diet was given, but no solid food, and opiates sufficient to keep the patient comfortable.

On the second day the abdomen became very tympanitic and painful; the pulse and temperature, however, remained normal, and on removing the compress there was a free escape of fetid gas, followed by immediate relief. After this the compress was left off, and although there was frequent escape of gas, there was none of feces. At the end of a week there was no discharge of any kind, and the opening gradually grew smaller till May 8th, when he was discharged at his own request almost entirely well.

This case is reported for two reasons, first, because it is not a very common lesion; second, to show the happy result of a slight aiding of nature's efforts.

INDIANAPOLIS.

---

# SUCCESSFUL REMOVAL OF AN EXTRA-UTERINE FETUS.

## BY E. T. EASLEY, M. D.

Frances Twitchell, aged thirty-four years; married, mother of three living children; duration of pregnancy, twenty-four months; position of child, directly across the front of the abdomen, head in right iliac fossa, back to pubic symphisis. Incision in the line of the linea alba, extending from an inch above the umbilicus to within an inch of the pubes. The cyst—dense, fibrous and tough—was not adherent in front, but had contracted extensive adhesions below. The child, of good size and well preserved, was adherent intimately at *all* points to the cyst. Liquor amnii absorbed; placenta nearly atrophied; the cord a mere string. The child was broken up and extracted piece by piece, a tedious dissection; and the cyst cavity sponged out and cleansed with a chlorinated wash.

The edges of the cyst were stitched to the abdominal wound by a fine uninterrupted suture, and the whole closed by deep interrupted sutures made to include the cyst walls. Free drainage was kept up from the lower end of the wound, and the cyst cavity constantly cleansed with antiseptic solutions, until it has gradually become obliterated by suppuration and granulation. I succeeded in excluding all exudation, hemorrhage or fluids, from the peritoneal cavity.

The patient is now in better health than since this pregnancy occurred. The operation was undertaken on account of the exhaustion and irritation of rapidly recurring attacks of pelvic and abdominal pain, and at the urgent desire of the patient and her friends. Doctors Watkins, Southall, Cross, Dibrell and Smith were present, and ably and judiciously assisted.

LITTLE ROCK, ARK.

[Dr. Easley is to be congratulated upon this successful operation. By a letter received from him this month (August), we learn that the patient remains in perfect health.

Dr. Parry, in his admirable monograph upon Extra-Uterine Pregnancy, observes that in case of the death of the fetus, gastrotomy is indicated if septicæmia, peritonitis, or exhaustion endangering life should supervene; it will be noticed that Dr. Easley had, therefore, excellent reasons for the operation. His method of operating and the after-treatment are alike to be commended.—*Editors of American Practitioner.*]

---

## AN EXAMPLE OF THIRD DENTITION.

BY W. J. CARTER, M. D.

Mr. I. M., aged twenty-two years, came to my office July 3, 1876, to have the first upper molar tooth of the left side extracted, which he said had been aching severely for the past two weeks. The tooth was drawn with great difficulty after the third trial, traction being made with all the power of both hands. The first effort slightly elevated one edge of the tooth, the second lifted it almost out of the socket, but the sequel proved it was not completely out, for the third pull was as hard and prolonged as the previous ones. The tooth came away entire, except a small longitudinal sliver of the outer prong which adhered to the alveolus, thus accounting for the great force required in the operation. The patient, who is perfectly reliable, informed me that this was his third set of teeth. The first set appeared when he was five or six years old, and was a full set of thirty-two teeth. The second set was also one of thirty-two teeth, and was shed when he was ten years old, following which the present set gradually made its appearance. Subsequently the young man's mother confirmed the above statements of her son. Three years previous to this time, Mr. M. informed me that a dentist in Indianapolis made three successive efforts to extract the corresponding tooth on the opposite side, which resulted in crushing the crown of the tooth.

Never before having met with a similar case, either in my practice or reading, I communicate it to the profession, thinking it may be of some interest physiologically, and of some practical value especially to the cross-roads portion of the profession, who are obliged to pull teeth as well as give physic.

Mount Jackson, Ind.

# Reviews.

---

A Treatise on Surgery, its Principles and Practice. By T. Holmes, Surgeon to St. George's Hospital. With four hundred and eleven illustrations, chiefly by Dr. Westmacott. Philadelphia: Henry C. Lea. 1876. 8vo. 960 pp

Mr. Holmes's treatise on surgery has by this time pretty well gone the rounds of the press, and has received even more than the amount of encomiums usually bestowed on works written by distinguished authors and issued by powerful publishers. Its style has been praised, its plan pronounced perfect, and as a text-book for students especially it has been declared the best in the language. Flaws in the work have been detected by an occasional reviewer, but these have been considered only such as are inseparable from human handiwork. We confess that we have been greatly puzzled by the general reception of this work by the press. Discounting the natural amiability of medical reviewers and the ease with which praise is bestowed, and all other circumstances which induce to make a favorable notice of a work so much more probable than an unfavorable one, we can scarcely account for the praise which has been bestowed on Mr. Holmes's book. The task of reviewing the work in the journals has, no doubt, in many instances, been committed to competent and independent surgeons, and that they should have found in it a tithe of what they declare they have found, is to us a matter of unqualified surprise.

Mr. Holmes says, in his preface, that he has attempted to represent the present condition of surgery, as it is practiced in his country, by a treatise which shall not be unworthy to rank with the other excellent text-books of the day. Certainly his ambition should have been satisfied in writing just this sort of book. The ponderous and expensive volumes of his System of Surgery, filled though some of them are, in certain departments at least, with sawdust, have presented him to the profession as one supposed to be familiar with all of surgery. His treatise on the surgery of children, by odds Mr. Holmes's best performance, had stamped him as a specialist of excellent quality, and immediately gave him very high rank; and he could well afford to direct his last effort to that most important class of readers, the undergraduates of medicine. He says:

"It is not only the immense number of topics, and the endless details of all these, though necessarily some of these topics must be less familiar to any single surgeon, however wide his experience, than others are, and though it is hardly possible that some of the details should not escape the writer's attention, but added to this the necessary conditions of space press hardly upon the writer of a surgical work."

This is not very clear, but means, as the context shows, that nine hundred pages are not enough to give more than a brief abstract of the subjects which the author supposes to be indispensable in a text-book. And right here lies, in our opinion, Mr. Holmes's great mistake. His "System" is certainly boiled down in the work under notice, but the process has failed to produce a text-book in surgery as signally as would the compression of La Place's mechanics result in a suitable book for the use of beginners in mathematics. We agree with our author that the task is a difficult one. The difficulty, however, does not, as he seems to think, lie in the necessity for economizing space, but in curbing one's ambition to dip into all matters connected with subjects at once so numerous and so vast.

Mr. Holmes has made the common error of writing with the double object of reaching practitioners and students alike. Of his style, we are reluctantly obliged to admit that we have failed to detect that brilliancy with which he has been accredited. We have quoted above one of Mr. Holmes's worst sentences, it is true, but throughout the book, and notably after the opening chapters, there abounds a looseness of expression calculated to awaken in the mind of the reader the idea that too much writing had overtaxed the powers and destroyed the enthusiasm of the author.

To one among many of Mr. Holmes's statements we must take decided exception. We can not agree that his treatise represents the present condition of surgery. We are sure that he labored to make it so; but that he failed can, we think, be shown in a very few words. Take, for example, the chapters on syphilis. These are certainly notably behind the times. Again, he would trust a fractured thigh in a child to a leather collar, which he says is better than the immovable apparatus, as it can be removed at pleasure. And later, he exhibits all the paraphernalia for the treatment of fractures generally, which seem bound to live until at least some great conflagration shall destroy the plates of the last century.

In the chapter on dislocations he introduces, it is true, Bigelow's methods, but *parenthetically* only; and then he pictures the pulleys of Cooper's days, which, if chloroform and manipulation are to go for anything, can but be regarded as useless.

Of hernia he says (page 618): "If the contents of the sac have, from any cause, become adherent to its interior, it ceases to be reducible, and is then called *irreducible* or *incarcerated;* and if besides this, the herniated viscera are constricted, so that the circulation of the contents of the intestines is suspended, it is said to be *strangulated."* We are unwilling to believe that Mr. Holmes regards "irreducible" and "incarcerated" as convertible terms, or that he thinks strangulated and incarcerated hernia the same.

But we will not pursue this part of our notice further. We have not the space, nor our readers the time, to go into details.

Mr. Holmes says he has not failed to refer to American and continental surgeons, so far as his information and space would allow. We are amiable enough to set down the small part which the labors of our countrymen are made to play in the work, rather to the want of space than to anything else.

In conclusion, we are constrained to say that we do not share Mr. Holmes's hopes in thinking his book deserving to take rank with some other excellent text-books in our schools. It has been said that comparisons are odious. But we can scarcely believe that our author will feel hurt when we say that among English books Mr. Bryant's Surgery is a better work for students—for students and practitioners alike; and that Mr. Erichsen's faultless volumes are in almost every single respect—in scope and in detail, in style and in finish—its superior. We even hope that we will not be thought sectional or deficient in the catholic spirit of the reviewer, when we venture the opinion, which we do only after a very careful comparison of the two books, that Ashhurst's Surgery is a very greatly better work than Mr. Holmes's. Indeed, with Ashhurst for the student and Erichsen for the practitioner, we see no opening yet for further lessons, certainly not for any contained in the treatise which it has been our ungracious task thus to notice.

Mr. Holmes should have been content with his great labor, the System of Surgery, and with his altogether admirable work on the Surgical Treatment of Children's Diseases. These two were as much as any one man could fairly be expected to do well in his day and generation.

---

Micro-Photographs in Histology, Normal and Pathological. By Carl Seiler, M. D. In conjunction with J. Gibbons Hunt, M. D., and Joseph G. Richardson, M. D. Philadelphia: J. H. Coates & Co. Published monthly at 60 cents per number.

No doubt the above periodical will be a valuable aid to physicians in the study of microscopy, so important now in the department of medicine.

In the June number, among other photographs is one of a transverse section of bone, showing beautifully the Haversian canals, with the surrounding lacunæ and canaliculi. This shows how well and accurately the work is done.

# Clinic of the Month.

HYSTERICAL AFFECTIONS OF THE EYE.—Dr. George C. Harlan, Surgeon to Wills Hospital, Philadelphia, (Medical and Surgical Reporter, August 12,) thus speaks of these:

Though the term "hysterical" is a vague and indefinite one, which most of us would rather not be called upon to accurately define, still it has a conventional meaning, and, by common consent, is made to include a large class of cases in which there may be decided or even alarming symptoms without real disease. The expression is used here in its broadest sense, as it is not my intention to undertake a discussion of psychological pathology, but merely to call attention to a class of eye symptoms which I believe are not sufficiently dwelt upon in the text-books, and which I feel sure are very often misinterpreted in practice. I have more than once met with interesting, but rather mysterious, cases which had been reported in good faith by experienced surgeons, but which seemed to me to be clearly of this character; and, without doubt, a large proportion, if not all, of the magical cures of blindness by galvanism, that we occasionally hear of, may be referred to this class of cases. The hysterical affections of the eye that have come under my notice have appeared to me to include three kinds of patients:

First. Those who are the subjects of a kind of moral insanity, or at any rate of an insane perversity, who deliberately simulate a disease for months or years; who, in short, may be called hysterical malignerers; and who, to be cured, need only to be exposed.

Second. Those who really believe themselves to be affected as they profess to be, and are honestly anxious to be cured;

who are subjects of hysterical paralysis; and whom it would, perhaps, be unjust to accuse of acting a part.

Third. Those who are subject to irregular nervous action, to paralysis or spasm without assignable cause, but in whom there is no question of mental or moral complication.

Almost any derangement of vision may be counterfeited. A little girl of eight years complained that every object that she looked at seemed covered with diagonal white lines, the direction of which she indicated with her finger. As the ophthalmoscope revealed a normal fundus, a favorable prognosis was given. This was made more positive the next day, when the white lines changed to blue, and was justified by the early disappearance of the difficulty.

In the second class of cases we have more or less retinal anæsthesia, with anomalous and variable symptoms, changing, perhaps, at each examination.

In the third class of cases the parts affected have been the retina, the muscle of accommodation, the external muscles of the eyeball, and the elevator of the upper eyelid.

It is not very uncommon to meet with patients who have apparently perfect eyes and full acuity of vision, but who say that the test letters become blurred and unrecognizable after they have looked at them for a few seconds. That this is due to an exhaustion of the sensibility of the retina, which disables it from the sustained performance of its function, and not to an irregular action of the accommodation, is shown by the fact that it persists when the eye is fully under the effects of atropia. A partial failure of the accommodation may occur in nervous persons, either alone or in connection with other symptoms. Very satisfactory results may sometimes be obtained from the use of weak convex glasses, in the case of ladies who are quite young and entirely emmetropic. Exception may be taken to including the opposite condition of accommodative spasm among hysterical affections, because it usually occurs in connection with some error of refraction. In a very large proportion of cases, however, the subjects are delicate women, and the error of refraction is a very slight departure from the normal standard, such as would not be felt by a person of fair average strength and nervous equilibrium. In other words, it is only the exciting cause, a strong predisposition existing in the temperament of the individual. These cases are of quite frequent occurrence in ophthalmic practice. Irregularity in the action of the external muscles of the eyeball, particularly insufficiency of the internal recti in convergence, is not uncommon in patients of this class, and frequently complicates their other ailments. A young married lady, a painfully hysterical subject, could scarcely use her eyes at all, though they were perfectly healthy and emmetropic, and the acuteness of vision was normal. The external muscles seemed, as it were, to have dissolved partnership, and each to act on its own account when she attempted to converge. Their irregular and variable action made anything like an accurate measurement of their force impossible.

The following is one of several cases in which there was occasional double vision from spasmodic action of one of the external muscles: Miss M., a little below par in general health, and of extremely nervous temperament, complained that frequently, without warning and without special exciting cause, as at the dinner table or at the opera, everything suddenly appeared double, and at the same time it was evident to her that she had lost control of the movements of one eye, which felt as if forcibly turned to one side. On closing the lids and pressing the ball for an instant, the symptoms would disappear. The acuteness of vision was normal, the balance of the external muscles for distant sight correct, and refraction nearly emmetropic. The correction of a hypermetropia of $\frac{1}{48}$ did not prevent the recurrence of the annoyance.

There is one more affection to which I wish to call attention; it is of especial interest, because, though in this class of cases of little moment, it may be in others a symptom of very grave lesions. I refer to a temporary paresis of the elevator of the upper lid. There is a great difficulty, sometimes an impossibility, of opening the eyes when rousing from sleep. Some patients are able to raise the lid naturally after several vigorous efforts of the will, while others are obliged to raise it with the fingers, and to rub or bathe it before acquiring control over its action. This occurs always on awakening, whether in the morning, during the night, or after a nap in the daytime, and is naturally the occasion of much uneasiness. I have notes of four such cases occurring in delicate ladies, and evidently of a hysterical character. Two recovered entirely, though not very quickly, under the use of tonics; a third lived at a distance, and I saw her only once; and the fourth is still under treatment. In the last the affection is of long standing, and is peculiar in the fact that for many months it was confined to one eye. The patient, about eighteen months ago, had difficulty in opening the left eye on awakening, the trouble lasting at that time for a few weeks only. About a year ago it commenced again in the same eye, has persisted since, and during the last few months has involved the right eye also, though to a less degree. Always when tired or weaker than usual she has the annoyance to a much greater extent; at times she is almost free from it. Her health is very feeble; she has had attacks of ague, etc., and is subject to functional palpitation of the heart and nervous prostration. There have never been any brain symptoms. The only example of this affection that I have seen in the case of a man, rather confirms the view of its hysterical character.

HEAT AND ITS INFLUENCE ON MORTALITY AT DIFFERENT AGES.—The weekly returns of the Registrar-General showed that the unseasonably moderate temperature which prevailed during June was very favorable to the public health. In London, for instance, the annual death-rate during the five weeks ending July 1st, averaged only 19.1 per thousand, whereas, under the influence of the seasonably hot weather which prevailed during the first three weeks of July, the death-rate successively rose to 19.8, 22.1, and 28.1 respectively. Thus, in the third week of July the mortality exceeded by forty-seven per cent. the average mortality in the five weeks of moderate temperature; in other words, six hundred more deaths were registered in the third week of hot weather than the average number in the five weeks ending July 1st. There need be no hesitation in attributing this excessive mortality almost exclusively to the intense heat which prevailed during the first three weeks of July. If we exclude the deaths from diarrhœa, which are especially sensitive to temperature, the fatal cases of other zymotic diseases were remarkably stationary throughout the eight weeks under notice. It will be interesting, therefore, to note the effect of heat upon the deaths recorded in the different groups of ages adopted by the Registrar-General in his weekly returns.

It may be first noted that the deaths of persons aged under twenty years registered in London, in the five weeks ending July 1st, averaged 613, whereas they had increased to 1215 in the third week of July. This increase was equal to ninety-eight per cent. On the other hand, the deaths of persons aged upwards of twenty years averaged 665 in the five cool weeks, and were 663 in the third week of hot weather. The heat does not appear to have unfavorably affected the mortality of adults or elderly persons in the aggregate; the mortality between the ages of twenty and forty years, indeed, showed a decline of thirteen per cent., while that of persons aged upwards of forty years had only increased five per cent. Having ascertained that the whole of the increase of deaths due to heat occurred under twenty years of age, it will be useful to notice the excess in the subdivisions of this vicenniad, which, in the Registrar-General's weekly returns, are three. Among young persons aged between five and twenty years the increase due to heat was eighteen per cent.; among children aged between one year and five it was twenty-three per cent.; while among infants under one year of age the increase was so great as 185 per cent. The deaths of infants under one year of age, which had averaged but 288 during the five cool weeks ending July 1st, rose to 822 in the week ending July 22d. Of the 600 deaths in the latter week which may be called the excess due to heat, no less than 534 were of infants under one year of age. Diarrhœa was the direct cause of most of these deaths of infants, as the deaths from this disease, under one year of age, which had averaged but sixteen in the five cool weeks, increased to 386 in the week ending July 22d. The increase of deaths of infants from other diseases due to heat was, however, well marked, and was equal to sixty per cent. Seasonable weather, whether it be cold in winter or heat in summer, inevitably raises the death-rate. Its effect upon the mortality at different groups of ages is not, however, the same. Cold in winter is most fatal to elderly persons, and to adults who are more especially exposed to its influence. Intense summer heat, however, is only fatal to infants and in a less degree to children, while it exercises but slight effect upon the mortality of adults or elderly persons. The fatal effect of heat upon the death-rate of infants is, however, in great measure the natural result of ignorance and neglect of parents, who sacrifice their children to uncleanliness, improper and unwholesome food, and carelessness as to the prompt treatment of diarrhœa. There is scarcely any form of mortality which can with greater justice be described as preventable than that due to infantile summer diarrhœa. This annual epidemic is a sad commentary upon the intelligence and social condition of our working classes. (Lancet.)

THE USE OF AROMATIC SULPHURIC ACID IN NECROSIS. — Dr. E. Cutter (Boston Medical and Surgical Journal) gives the following:

April 10, 1875, Dr. A., of Worcester, requested the writer to remove the necrosed alveolar process of his wife's sister. She was of middle age, pale, thin, weak, anxious, and worn. She had suffered much with her teeth. Her upper right middle, and two lateral incisors were found to be loose, and their lower edges hanging below the line of their fellows. There was a fungoid, spongy swelling over the front of the diseased process. When this was pressed, pus freely exuded from several openings, and also from a softish, elastic swelling as large as a hazel-nut, situated at the dome of the hard palate inside the mouth. The loosened teeth could be freely moved in every direction with the thumb and fingers. The roots of the teeth distinctly grated against the sound alveolar process. There was a complete separation of the teeth and the bone. Dr. A. said that he had thought of using the aromatic sulphuric acid, but that the disease was so extensive and the separation so complete that he regarded it as useless to try to save the teeth in any way. It appeared to the consulter, however, while the surgical extirpation would be effective and justifiable, that if free incisions were made into the swollen and spongy gums there would be an evacuation of the contents of the dilated capillaries and abscesses; that a healthy action would be promoted by relieving this unnatural distention, and that the necrosed bone might be slowly removed by the stimulation of the aromatic sulphuric acid topically applied without destroying the teeth. It was thought that then the periosteum would lay down new bone in place of the old, and refasten the teeth in their old place. It was agreed to employ the following:

$$\text{R}\quad \text{Aromatic sulphuric acid,}\quad . \quad . \quad . \quad . \quad \text{Ʒj}$$
$$\text{Aquæ,}\quad . \quad . \quad . \quad . \quad . \quad . \quad . \quad . \quad \text{Ʒj}$$

By means of a half-ounce syringe supplied with a small ivory tip, one inch and a half long, and one-eighth inch in diameter, the acid solution was injected at first twice a day and afterwards once a day. About two drachms were used at each injection. The syringe tip was deeply buried into the soft tissues through one of the openings. Pus would freely exude from the other openings, even from that in the top of the mouth, after each injection. Tonics were administered; a diet of animal food and unbolted wheat was rigidly maintained.

From the outset of this departure a marked improvement in the soft tissues occurred. But the teeth remained loose and dangling, and Dr. A. thought their recovery doubtful. It was resuggested that it would be an easy thing to remove them at any time if they did not reset, but that the process of replacing old with new bone was of necessity a slow one.

In about forty days the outer incisor became solidly fixed in its old site. Then the next incisor also tightened. The middle incisor tightened slowly. In November following it could be very slightly moved, but its edge was a little below the line of the other teeth. The other two incisors were as stiff as they ever were. A few spiculæ of bone were removed from the front of the alveolar process during the period of the treatment. In the meantime the general health of the patient improved greatly. She gained in weight, color and strength. At the present time (July, 1876) she is entirely recovered.

We think it is reasonable to connect the result in this case with the means employed, the acid, the tonics, and the food.

Dr. Atkinson, of New York, has reported some remarkable instances of cure of necrosis by this agent used in its full strength, it is said. It hastens the disintegrating and separating processes, and at the same time destroys the germs of parasitic micrographic growths in the dead and dying bone. According to Dr. Atkinson, it does not act unhealthily upon sound tissues whose vital connections are unimpaired. No substances stand higher than the mineral acids as antiseptics and destroyers of bacteria, amœbæ, and vegetations of animal secretions. Were it not for their caustic effects, they would long ago have supplanted carbolic acid.

MR. WALTER REID'S METHOD OF TREATING ANEURISM.— Last month we gave a notice of this method. In the Lancet of August 5th, we find a communication from Mr. Reid, in which he mentions the death of the patient, and gives the post mortem examination:

The cause of death, as ascertained by post mortem examination, was hypertrophy of the heart, associated with bronchitis, effusion into both pleuræ, and cirrhosis of the liver. There was no internal aneurism, and the coats of the large vessels appeared to be sound.

The remains of the aneurism in the left popliteal space were removed and examined. The tumor, when cleared, was of the size and general form of a small walnut. The artery was occluded for two and a half inches of its course by fibrous tissue, and from the lower half of this portion the aneurism sprang. The popliteal vein was pervious throughout. Numerous collateral branches could be seen running into the artery above and below the occluded portion. On making a section of the tumor in the long direction and from the side opposite the artery towards the vessel itself, the following appearances presented themselves: The sac was well defined, being thicker where it joined the artery than elsewhere. The center and also that portion of the cavity adjacent to the vessel were occupied by an amorphous, non-laminated, coffee-colored substance, of the consistence of cheese, which showed no signs of organization or of vascular connection with the surrounding parts. That portion of the circumference of the cavity of the aneurism opposite its mouth was occupied by several layers of laminated fibrine. Some of these were partially separated from the others and approximated towards the center, the interspace thus caused being filled by the amorphous substance, which, however, was of a looser character than that already described.

The amorphous, non-laminated substance could be nothing else than the remains of an ordinary blood coagulum, and, since the aneurism was originally the size of a hen's egg and finally that of a small walnut, it could only have represented a small proportion of the original bulk of the clot. The fibrinated laminæ were probably due to the attempts which I made at cure by compression, and the displacement of some of these resulted from the contraction of the sac upon them subsequent to the cure. I think so, because the coagulum in the interspace was soft and loose, and seemed to represent a portion of the more fluid parts of the larger mass which had been expressed from it, likewise by the contraction of the walls of the sac.

In my pamphlet, which was written a month previous to the death of the patient, I attempted to show that the aneurism was cured by the rapid coagulation or death of the blood consequent upon its complete stagnation in the sac. I think that this explanation is well borne out, not only by a consideration of the phenomena of cure, but also by the post mortem appearances. I beg here to acknowledge the numerous communications that have reached me from surgeons, generally expressing an intention to try this method on the first opportunity. I am accordingly in hopes that it will ere long be determined as to whether the success which may follow its application shall only be looked upon as a rarity, or whether it may be destined to revolutionize the whole surgical treatment of aneurism, and enable us to treat the disease in certain situations with the regularity and precision of a physical experiment.

HYPOPHOSPHITES OF LIME AND SODA IN PHTHISIS.—Dr. M. Charteris (Lancet, July 29), after giving the history of some cases in which the hypophosphites were administered, says:

These cases are faithful examples of the use of the hypophosphites in phthisis, either in the form of lime or soda. That the medicine is not inert, its power of checking nightsweats evidences, and also its influence in giving tone to the system, if by this is meant increase of appetite and general cheerfulness. Without expressing a definite view on the subject, I have been somewhat forced to the conclusion that if the hypophosphites did no good, they certainly did harm, and in some measure hastened a final issue by increased fever, as indicated by a higher temperature. While acknowledging the benefit derived from their use, as testified to by patients themselves and by competent witnesses, I am of opinion that they should by no means be used indiscriminately, and that when given their effect should be carefully watched by daily thermometric observation.

In further alluding to the difference of temperature in the sides affected in phthisis, the following results have been noted: In one extreme case, following an attack of pleurisy of the left lung, and where the right was unaffected, the average increase of the evening temperature for a month was .96°, or very nearly a degree. In another, where the right lung appeared alone affected at the apex, the result of ten observations showed a difference of .38° in the morning and .40° in the evening. In another case, at present in the hospital, and where there are absolutely no other physical signs of phthisis except weakness and emaciation, the following facts have been recorded as the result of temperatures taken morning and evening, and extending over a period of ten days: Evening, left side, average 101.86°; right side, 101.56°· Morning, left side, 100.36°; right side, 99.96°. Health certainly gives no variation like this, and no other-disease simulates phthisis so much as enteric fever. A case of enteric fever was admitted into my wards on the same day as the one last mentioned, and the temperature was taken carefully on both sides, with the result of finding no appreciable difference, the average being on both sides 99.4° in the morning and 101.2° in the evening, and, as convalescence was reached, 98.2° in the morning and 99.6° in the evening.

PLEURAL EXUDATION EMPTIED THROUGH THE MOUTH.— The following case is communicated by Dr. Fronmüller from the hospital in Fürth: John S., aged twenty-one years, belt-maker, has suffered a long time from a severe cough, with profuse expectoration, general emaciation, hectic fever and night-sweats. He observed one evening, while he was stooping over to pull off his boots, that on account of very limited respiration and from an impulsive cough, a very large quantity of a clear, yellowish fluid gushed out of the mouth. Some days afterwards, on the 19th of November, 1875, he entered our hospital. Physical examination disclosed far advanced tubercle of the lungs, especially at the right upper lobe, and a rather extensive exudation into the right pleural sack. On more than one occasion the experiment of stooping over being repeated by him, he discharged every time a moderate quantity of a clear, yellowish-green fluid. This fluid much resembled the white of an egg, with all the properties of an exudation from the lung covering. On the sixteenth day after his admission the patient died. At the autopsy there was found an exudation into the right pleura; the right lung was suppurated greatly, and broken through with cavities. The largest of these cavities—about the circumference of a chestnut—was found in the middle lobe, in the nearest proximity to the pleura, where it communicated with the pleural exudation. On the other side of this cavity a communication had taken place with a large bronchus at its point of bifurcation. The mucous membrane of the stomach and intestines was pale but normal: there was chronic nephritis; spleen and liver were normal. (*Memorabil.*, July, 1876.)

LANGENBECK'S SURGICAL TREATMENT OF HERNIA.—In the *Memorabil.*, July, there is a communication upon M. Langenbeck's treatment of hernia. He operates without opening the sac, is careful in breaking up all adhesions, and has lost only three cases in fifty-nine operations.

For the radical cure of hernia, his method of operating gives excellent results. A flap of skin as thick as possible, and corresponding in length and width to the hernial opening, is made from the abdomen. For an inguinal hernia, the base of the flap extends from the symphysis pubis to the pubic tubercle, and the flap extends upward and outward an inch and a half or two inches; for a femoral hernia, the flap is made from the *fossa ovalis*, and is about half as long; for an umbilical hernia, from any direction except near the suspensory ligament of the liver, or *ligamentum teres*. After preparing the flap, the finger is introduced through the canal or opening, to make room for it; then the flap is introduced either by the finger or an instrument; it is not twisted, but only laid deeper in its natural position in the abdominal wall. The external wound is closed by twisted sutures, and cold applications made for only a few hours.

HOT WATER IN UTERINE THERAPEUTICS.—Dr. Hyatt (Virginia Medical Monthly, August) has an excellent article on this subject. Dr. Hyatt recommends hot water in various uterine diseases, as originally suggested by Dr. Emmet, and in pelvi-peritonitis and pelvi-cellulitis. He has also had success with it in metrorrhagia. In this last application, however, Dr. Hyatt has been anticipated by Trousseau.

SALICYLIC ACID AS AN ANTISEPTIC.*—As lately Professor Salkowski, of Berlin, did not agree with the results of the experiments by Kolbe, by which the antiseptic qualities of salicylic acid seemed to be established, but questioned them, and referred to benzoic acid as giving better results (*Berliner Klinische Wochenschrift*, 1875, No. XXII,) it shall not be the object of this article to controvert the theories of the former, but simply to gather together the results of previous investigations and experiments with the salicylic acid, and make a rapid review of Kolbe's investigations to determine their weight and character. Farther experiments must be deferred to determine which of the acids shall gain preference, both technically and in operative employment. I have found such satisfactory results from the salicylic acid in my specialty that I can not believe it will be displaced by the benzoic.

Salkowski brings up the high price of salicylic acid as an objection to its use; but since this has been so much reduced by Kolbe's methods of production, it has become a small item of difference. In the conclusion of Salkowski's article, he says that Kolbe's services should not be underrated, because his investigations have, if nothing more, drawn attention to the aromatic combinations. It must be said, however, that these investigations were made with a perfect knowledge of the character and properties of the benzoic acid. There can be no doubt but that salicylic acid—the medical treasure introduced by Kolbe, which is now the subject of so much discussion, and the usefulness of which is confirmed by Professor Theirsch—is drawing more and more attention, not only from the professionally educated part of the community, but also the producing classes are following the development of its properties and virtues with the deepest interest. The undoubted confirmation of its antiseptic properties points to early and important changes in the production of many of the necessaries of life. Especially we may mention the conservation of wines, beer, and meats; also the management of

* From the Vierteljahrsschrift für Zahnheilkunde, page 20, 1876. By Prof. H. Humm. Translated from the German by Dr. G. V. Black, Jacksonville, Ill.

wounds and suppurating surfaces with salicylic acid in substance or in solution, and the treatment of three epidemics
which depend on fungoid growths, both in man and beast.

The knowledge and the production of salicylic acid, is not
of recent date.    It was first obtained only from salicin, which
was discovered by Regatelle in 1826, but earlier by Fontana,
an apothecary in Laziza, near Verona, in 1825.    It was obtained from salix pentandria and salix fragilis.    According to
Lasche, salicin can also be obtained from other varieties of
salix, as salix purpuria, salix helix, salix lambertina, and not
only from the leaves but from the female flowers and the
young twigs.

Salicin crystallizes in small, four-sided, brilliant milk-white
prisms, or small white scales.    It is of an intense bitter and
astringent taste, is not changed in the air, dissolves readily in
water or alcohol, but is not soluble in ether and the essential
oils; melts a few degrees above 100° C., and is decomposed by a few degrees higher heat.    It is not an alkaloid,
but in its chemical relations is indifferent.    By sulphuric acid
it is changed into a dark brown mass (retilin), and according
to Marchand, its formula is C 28, H 38, O 15.    (Journal for
Practical Chemistry, 1842, Vol. XXVI, p. 385.)

According to Piria, salicyl is the radical of salicin.    With
hydrogen it forms a hydrate of salicyl, which is a reddish oil,
readily soluble in alcohol and ether, and behaves with alkalies and metaloids like the hydrogen acids.    When salicyl is
treated with melted potassium, the salicylic acid is formed.

It is this formerly known, but almost unnoticed acid, which
has of late attracted such universal attention, not merely from
the chemist but also from the physician and artisan.    For this
we must thank Kolbe, Theirsch, Newbauer, and others, for
their very interesting and complete investigations; especially
the first, who, in company with Lanteman in the year 1860,
in a course of investigations of salicylic acid as a derivative,
discovered the salyl acid, which he described as isomeric with
benzoic acid.    Soon afterward Kerkule pointed out the possibility that there were other acids isomeric with the benzoic,

which he based upon an hypothesis of his own in regard to the chemical constitution of benzoyl. His conclusions were taken up by a number of chemists, and it was held that the finding of one acid isomeric with the benzoic threw the whole fabric of the chemical constitution of the aromatic combinations together (in one isomeric line), and they were therefore unstable. A correct decision as to whether salicylic acid is identical with the benzoic, or isomeric with it, is of the utmost importance. This has induced Kolbe to again take up the work formerly done by himself and Lanteman, especially as the argument brought forward by Richenbach and Beilstein seems not to be so conclusive as might at first be supposed. In the meantime it was no light task for him to more clearly prove his opinions of 1860 and defeat Kerkule's argument. This was largely the fault of circumstances, since it was exceedingly difficult to bring together the necessary materials for the required amount of salicylic acid without too great a cost. This difficulty resulted in directing him to the finding of a cheaper mode of producing the acid. The gaultheria oil contained but a very small per cent. of salicylic acid, and seems poorer latterly than formerly, and is therefore too costly for the preparation of very many pounds. Kolbe was, therefore, led to reinvestigate the plan previously described by himself and Lanteman, by which salicylic acid was prepared artificially from phenol and carbonic acid in the presence of sodium, to determine whether or not it could be simplified or perfected to such an extent that a cheaper acid could be produced. He succeeded in producing by this means a very considerable quantity of the salicylic acid, which, at the present price of sodium, would not be dearer than that produced from gaultheria oil.

During these experiments, Kolbe was surprised to find that by apparently the same manipulations the amount of salicylic acid obtained was sometimes quite large, sometimes very small. In finding the key to this mystery, he was led to a new plan of production. Upon dissolving sodium in hot phenol, in a current of dry carbonic acid, salicylic acid is formed, and with it always, more or less, carbonate of soda and phenate of soda. Kolbe now found that the richer the production of salicylic acid, the less of the compounds above mentioned were found. He afterward observed that a product which was especially rich in phenate of soda, and poor in salicylate of soda, produced a large amount of salicylic acid when treated anew with carbonic acid under a higher heat. Upon this discovery, he determined to again try the plan of producing salicylic acid from phenate of soda and carbonic acid, which had formerly yielded but a very trifling amount. After many experiments he succeeded in determining the conditions, and so completing and simplifying this process, that from phenate of soda and carbonic acid, the theoretically reckoned amount of salicylic acid could be obtained without difficulty, and at small cost, which was done in an iron retort, prepared for the purpose, in twelve hours, without much attention during the process, producing eight to ten pounds of salicylic acid. A saturated solution of phenol and soda is evaporated in a shallow iron vessel, and the resulting mass—phenate of soda—is then dried over a light heat, with continued stirring, and afterward rubbed until it is reduced to a dust. This is then (when large amounts are used) put into an iron retort, and slowly heated in an oil, metal or air-bath, until it has reached about 100° C.,* then a light current of carbonic acid is passed through it. The temperature is gradually raised, reaching 180° C. some hours afterward. Some time after the introduction of the carbonic acid phenol begins to distill over; later in larger quantities. At last the temperature is raised to 200° C., 250° C., and the operation is ended. When under this temperature, with the continued passage of the current of carbonic acid, no more phenol passes over. In regard to the process of the formation of salicylic acid, Kolbe says he had at first supposed that one molecule of carbonic acid inserted itself into one

---

* Degrees of the Centigrade thermometer may be reduced to Fahrenheit thus, 100° C $\times 9 \div 5 + 32 = 212$.

molecule of phenate of soda, and so formed one molecule of salicylic acid, according to the following formula:

$$C_6 H_5 Na.O + CO_2 = C_6 H_5 O COO Na.$$

But I now perceive that the process runs otherwise, which I could not before understand. That by the influence of carbonic acid on strongly heated phenate of soda, a large quantity of quick crystallizing phenol distills away from the phenate of soda, which, as I have lately determined, is just one-half of the phenol used in preparing the phenate of soda. The contents of the retort, after the reaction is ended, *i. e.*, after the continued passage of the current of carbonic acid until the heat has attained 250 C. as described, is by a good resulting operation of a grayish white color, it is salicylate of soda, the so-called basic. The following formula expresses the chemical changes during the operation:

$$\left. \begin{array}{l} C_6 H_5 \, Na \, O \\ C_6 H_5 \, Na \, O \end{array} \right\} + CO_2 = C_6 \left\{ \begin{array}{l} H_4 \\ COO \, Na \end{array} \right\} Na \, O + C_6 \, H_5 \, HO.$$

| Two mol. phenate of soda. | Salicylate with two equiv. of sodium. | Phenol. |

With two molecules of phenate of soda in the presence of carbonic acid, one equivalent of hydrogen is displaced by soda, which results in the formation of phenol and a phenate of soda containing a double portion of sodium, which last immediately combines with the carbonic acid, producing the salicylate of soda, thus:

$$\left. \begin{array}{l} C_6 \, H_5 \, NaO \\ C_6 \, H_5 \, NaO \end{array} \right\} = C_6 \, H_5 \, HO + C_6 \left\{ \begin{array}{l} H_4 \\ Na \end{array} \right\} NaO + CO_2 =$$

| Two mol. phenate of soda. | Phenol. | Dinatrum phenol. | Carbonic acid. |

$$C_6 \left\{ \begin{array}{l} H_4 \\ COO \, Na \end{array} \right\} NaO$$

Salicylate of soda with two equivalents of sodium.

This last combination bears a temperature of 300° C., without decomposition; dissolves readily in water with a dark brown color. On the addition of hydrochloric acid the salicylíc acid is precipitated in the form of a thick curd. This is dried on a linen cloth, or the mother liquor pressed out as well as possible. Through recrystallization and other methods of purification, the salicylic acid may be obtained perfectly pure. If it is wished that it be obtained chemically pure and snow-white, it is dissolved in methyl alcohol or ethyl alcohol, which is removed by heating in a pure solution of caustic soda, precipitating with hydrochloric acid and thoroughly washing the precipitate.

The salicylic acid prepared in this way is isomeric with that prepared from the willow bark. When not rectified, its color is a light yellow from a small portion of phenol. It is in powder, crystalline, or in needle-like crystals. Slightly soluble in cold water, more largely soluble in warm water, melts at about 60° C., and by a slight elevation of this temperature is decomposed into phenol and carbonic acid. For the reason that salicylic acid may be formed from carbolic acid and carbonic acid, and is also decomposed into the same compounds by light heat, Professor Kolbe came to the conclusion that it would, like the carbolic acid, prevent decomposition, or possessed antiseptic properties. The conclusion was verified by experiments by himself and Professor Theirsch. Amygdaline was dissolved in water, and a small percentage of salicylic acid added and well mixed, and an emulsion of sweet almonds added; after a quarter of an hour there was not the slightest smell. In a similar way a number of experiments were tried with small additions of salicylic acid, and there was no smell of the bitter almonds for several hours, and by the addition of a little greater proportion of the salicylic acid no smell was detected for twenty-four hours.

Ground mustard in lukewarm water soon gives out the smell of mustard-oil, but fails to do so when a slight amount of salicylic acid is added. A small portion of salicylic acid, added to a solution of sugar, prevented yeast from working. A solution of sugar already in the process of fermentation was stopped by a small amount of the acid.

One thousand grammes* of beer, to which 0.8 to 1.0 grammes of salicylic acid was added, showed no sign of spoiling after fourteen days' exposure; also less than the one-thousandth part of salicylic acid is sufficient to prevent beer from spoiling for a long time. The small amount of 0.04 per cent. of salicylic acid added to fresh milk, is sufficient to prevent its souring at a temperature of 118° C. Fresh meat, with salicylic acid rubbed upon it, does not spoil for weeks in the open air. Fresh eggs, that were soaked for an hour in a water solution of the acid, lost nothing in taste or smell in four months, and could not be told from fresh eggs.

The salicylic acid, by common room temperature, is dissolved by distilled water in the proportion of one to three hundred. This solution is called salicyl water† by Professor Theirsch, and possesses remarkable antiseptic properties. Urine to which the acid is added in this proportion, or in larger quantity, does not decompose, and still contains uric acid after nine months. Blood and pus are kept in the same way. A large amount of albuminates are precipitated from the serum of pus by salicylic acid, as is also done by one per cent. solution of carbolic acid. Fresh and granulating wounds are in no wise injured, nor is any inflammation caused by washing with salicyl water. By long washing of wounds with salicylic acid, it may be detected in the urine. Instead of washing with salicyl water, Professor Theirsch advises the application of the acid in substance to suppurating wounds or mortifying parts to the thickness of 0.2 to 0.5 centimeters, for the reason that in washing with the solution the effect will not reach to sufficient depth. After many and continued experiments, Professor Theirsch is of the opinion that the salicylic acid possesses all the virtues of carbolic acid without its objectionable features.

Newbauer and Kolbe have made further experiments for determining the antiseptic properties, which are of importance to producers of wine and beer. Newbauer tried the following

* One gramme equals 15.444 grains.
† Salicyl wasser.

experiments with chemically pure salicylic acid: Fifty C. C.*
of clear filtered unfermented wine, which had been heated to
65° C., was mixed with salicylic acid, and a small amount of
wine ferment added to it. The same quantity of the same
wine was mixed with a like quantity of wine ferment without
the salicylic acid, for comparison. In the last, fermentation
proceeded as soon as the ferment spores had begun to increase—in a few days; while in all experiments there was no
increase of the ferment spores, and absolutely no fermentation
in that to which the salicylic acid had been added. In order
to determine the amount of salicylic acid required to destroy
or prevent the operation of a certain amount of wine ferment,
the following line of experiments (beginning on the morning
of November 17th) were tried. To each one thousand liters†
of unfermented wine, the following quantities of salicylic acid
were mixed; first, none; second 12, 24, 36, 48, 60, 72 and 96
grammes. Each of these received one C. C. of active wine
ferment, which was found to contain 0.0049 grammes of dried
ferment cells. The ferment used was sacchromyes ellipsoi-
dens, with a small amount of sacchromyes apiculatus, fresh
grown, and entirely free from other fungous seeds. On the
morning of the 19th (two days), the wine having no salicylic
acid (No. 1) was in active fermentation; No. 2 also showed a
weak fermentation, not nearly so active as No. 1, but apparently normal; Nos. 3 and 4 first showed signs of fermentation
on the 20th; No. 5 showed the first signs of fermentation on
the afternoon of the 23d, and on the 25th the fermentation
was proceeding very feebly; No. 6 showed the first gas bubble on the 27th, and a very slow fermentation followed; No. 7
showed the first gas bubble on the 2d of December; No. 8
was perfectly clear at the end of four weeks, the ferment cells
which had been added had sunk to the bottom, no growth
had taken place, no gas bubble had been formed; not the
slightest trace of fermentation could be discovered, although
the amount of ferment had been ample.

* Thirty-one cubic centimeters equals one ounce.
† One liter equals 2.1135 pints.

[TO BE CONTINUED.]

# Notes and Queries.

STOLTZ ON MENSTRUATION.—The ovarian theory of menstruation having recently been ably controverted, we opened the last issued volume of the *Nouveau Dictionnaire de Médecine et de Chirurgie Pratiques*, which has just been received, anxious to know whether the most recent French authority would discredit the researches and reject the conclusions of Negrier, Coste and Raciborski. Stoltz is the author of the article on *Menstruation* in this volume, the twenty-second of the series; and we wish those who have been in so much haste to follow a few wandering German lights, or from occasional exceptional cases, such as conception without menstruation, and periodical hemorrhage from the womb after the removal of the ovaries, have been in haste to assert as a general truth that ovulation and the monthly flow are independent phenomena, would carefully read Stoltz's views. He states that the theory of periodic ovulation to-day deserves the most reliance, since it rests upon numerous observations, is completely in accordance with observations made in animals, and finally is the simplest and easiest of comprehension. Ovulation is not only *spontaneous*, that is independent of sexual excitement, but still more, is subject to the law of periodicity. Menstruation is the sign of ovulation, at the same time that it is a consequence of ovarian activity. The disposition to procreation is continuous in the male, while fecundity is intermittent in the female, alike in the human race and in animals; though certain German writers have sought to make women differ from other females in regard to reproductive power.

DISCUSSION UPON THE PUERPERAL SOUFFLE.—In the Paris Academy of Medicine there has recently been quite an interesting discussion upon a souffle, first pointed out by Kergaradec in 1822, and denominated by him *placental*, a title which it still unfortunately holds with some obstetricians. The discussion grew out of a paper by M. Glénard, of Lyons, who presented a new explanation of the souffle, attributing it to pressure upon the epigastric artery, and denominated it epigastric. But Glénard has had to acknowledge himself mistaken, and now deserts the epigastric, carrying his theory to an artery connecting the ovarian and uterine artery on each side, and baptized by him the anastomotic; but it is doubtful whether the theory can live more securely in its new retreat than it did in its first home.

The objections to the *placental* theory are that the souffle persists after the delivery of the placenta, does not cease after section of the umbilical cord, there is no important branch of the umbilical artery specially designed for the nutrition of the placenta; and, finally, the souffle is isochronous with the fetal heart.

The epigastric and the placental theories being rejected, there remain the iliac and the uterine theories. Bouilland is the author of the iliac theory, and ably sustained it; while the uterine theory—that which meets with most general acceptance—originated with Dubois, and has been firmly supported by Depaul.

AN ENCYSTED OR ADHERENT VESICAL CALCULUS.—Dr. W. H. Park, of Tyler, Texas, encountered an adherent calculus in one of his late lithotomies. The patient, a male, was aged twenty-five years. On reaching the bladder the operator found two calculi, one small and free, the other very large, encysted or adherent to the bladder high up and behind the pubes, and so far away that neither the finger nor scoop could be used in detaching it. It was after much difficulty seized with the forceps, crushed and removed in fragments. The bladder was largely encrusted with phosphatic matter around the site of the stone; and the removal of these crusts with the finger and scoop, added to the time occupied in extracting the larger calculus, made the operation extremely tedious, notwithstanding which, however, the patient made a quick and good recovery.

THE CRITICISM OF DR. BARTHOLOW'S LECTURE BY DR. CARSON AGAIN.—The last number of the American Practitioner (August) contains my rejoinder to the criticism of Dr. Carson, and his reply. I might comment on the singularity of the rejoinder and the reply appearing in the same issue; but I am pleased that the papers should stand side by side. I am quite content to leave the questions thus far discussed to the judgment of all unbiassed readers. Your reviewer has, however, brought forward a new question entirely. He quotes from my recently published Treatise on Materia Medica and Therapeutics, in order to make it appear that I contradict myself on the subject of the action of digitalis. You must allow, I think, that he has exceeded his privilege as a reviewer of my lecture, and now makes issues that wear a personal aspect. I am glad that he has thus more decidedly even than before shown the *animus* of his criticism.

I have now the serious accusation to make against Dr. Carson, that he quotes me wrongly, and in a way that is perfectly abominable. I formally declare that he has falsified the text of my work; and I demand now, in the presence of all your readers, that he confess this shameless license. That there may be no doubt, I quote the passage and indicate the word in italics, which he has substituted:

"That digitalis has any power to prevent the *depuration* of fibrinous material, to prevent or check the migration of the white corpuscles, or to arrest the multiplication of the cellular elements of inflamed parts, seems to the author highly improbable." (*A Practical Treatise on Materia Medica and Therapeutics:* New York, D. Appleton & Co., 1876, p. 275.)

If any one will take the trouble to refer to the volume and page as above given, he will find that I say *deposition*, which gives a wholly different meaning.

The opposition of opinion which Dr. Carson affects to discover in my views as expressed in my lecture and in my treatise, exists only in his own mind. In my lecture (p. 14), to illustrate the antagonism in the action of digitalis and the morbid process in pneumonia, I place the following in juxtaposition:

| DIGITALIS. | PNEUMONIA. • |
|---|---|
| Exudation checked or prevented by the heightened tonicity of the vessels. | Exudation of fibrinous material. Migration of white blood corpuscles. |

In my lecture I state that the heightened tonicity of the vessels may, by checking exudation, and the migration of the white blood corpuscles, "limit the area of the inflammatory action." I show in my work that digitalis can hardly affect the power of amœbiform movements possessed by white blood corpuscles, or prevent the multiplication of the cellular elements of inflamed parts. This is a power distinctly possessed by quinia. The same result—as respects fibrinous exudation, or the passage through the vessel walls, of leucocytes—may be, in part at least, secured by the property which digitalis has of raising the tonicity of the vessels. The same idea precisely is expressed in my work in the sentence immediately succeeding the one quoted by Dr. Carson:

"That it [digitalis] may be useful to combat some of the symptoms—high temperature, ischæmia of the arterial system from pulmonary obstruction, and low tension of the vessels—may be well admitted." (l. c., p. 275.)

I, of course, am not to blame, if Dr. Carson is unable to appreciate these elementary truths. A reviewer should have a little common sense as well as common honesty.

Dr. W. C. is like a certain hefty medical writer in our city, who is constantly discovering fallacies in physical diagnosis, when he is merely discovering his own ignorance.

*Cincinnati, August* 22.          ROBERTS BARTHOLOW.

THE POPE'S SECRET SURGEON.—The death of Dr. Vincenzo Sartori left vacant the post of "secret surgeon" to the Pope, and that has just been filled up by the appointment of Dr. Ceccarelli, who has for some years acted as surgeon extraordinary. For his introduction to the Vatican Dr. Ceccarelli was indebted to Monsignor de Mérode, whose fractured leg he skillfully reduced, and who, out of gratitude, got the Pope to consult him, although His Holiness had already two competent medical advisers in Drs. Viale-Prelà and Constantini. Regretting as he does the death of Sartori, who was nearly contemporary with himself, and whose sagacious judgment he often had recourse to in other matters besides his bodily infirmities, the Pope has had good ground to be satisfied with his new "secret surgeon." His health was never better than at present. The same restorative treatment is observed. The strong capon-soup, followed by a glass of "the best of Rhenish wine" (sometimes alternating with Romanée, Conti, or Cyprus of the Commandery,) sustains his strength. In the prevalent heat he avoids the gardens of the Vatican, and takes his daily walks in the spacious and equably ventilated halls of the palace itself. He visits regularly the "Gallery of the Geographical Maps," where he traces the movements of the belligerents at the seat of war, in which he takes a lively interest. He surprised his attendants the other day by mounting the stairs that lead to the gallery in question without the aid of the staff, which is generally his support and invariably his companion. (Lancet.)

THE CONVENTION OF MEDICAL COLLEGES.—Our able cotemporary, the Atlanta Medical and Surgical Journal, says:

"Let every school send one or more delegates to the next convention, and let them go prepared to make concessions, and to adopt in good faith whatever the majority in council, after mature deliberation, may decide is best for all." If this excellent advice is followed, we may hope soon to see a forward movement along the whole line of the profession.

HAY FEVER.—The Boston Medical and Surgical Journal (August 24th), in a notice of Dr. Wyman's work, and Dr. Beard's upon hay fever, thus refers to the latter volume:

Dr. G. M. Beard, in a recent publication on hay fever or summer catarrh, claims that the two forms of catarrh occurring in June and September are identical, and, moreover, that there is an intermediate form, beginning in July, which has not been previously described. He also states that all forms of the disease in all countries are essentially the same, and all dependent on one cause, a functional disease of the nervous system, a neurosis. Dr. Beard arrives at this conclusion from the analysis of the answers to fifty-five questions with regard to the residence, temperament, hereditary predisposition, date of attack, exciting causes, nature of symptoms, etc. These questions were distributed quite extensively in the form of a circular, and answers were received with regard to some two hundred cases. One half only of the cases, however, were observed by himself or by other physicians, and in view of the liability to errors of diagnosis in cases reported by unprofessional observers, it seems as if a smaller number of cases more thoroughly investigated might be of greater scientific value. Though the author hardly settles the problem as to the nature of hay fever so satisfactorily to our mind as he appears to have done to his own, many points of interest are developed. With regard to the localities in which hay fever is liable to occur, cases are recorded from most of the States east of the Rocky Mountains, south as well as north. Some regions supposed to be exempt from autumnal catarrh are said to contain many cases of hay fever. This may be accounted for by the fact that the two diseases have different limits, or future research may show that the supposed limits require modification.

This book is in the main corroborative of Dr. Wyman's previous work. It is interesting to notice that, of the two hundred cases collected, twenty-seven were of the early or June form, nineteen of the so-called July form, and one hundred and fifty-two of the autumnal variety. With regard to the existence of a July group Dr. Wyman says: "If this be so, the separation of the June and September groups is established. Any two groups between which there is a third must be separate. A description which confounds June cold and autumnal catarrh does not exactly suit either separately, either in the time of attack, the causes of paroxyms, the geographical distribution, or the means of relief. It may be observed that Dr. Phoebus records no distinct group in July, although he mentions that a few cases thus occur."

The theory of the nervous origin of the disease is more satisfactory than any of the other hypotheses, and is in accordance with Dr. Wyman's original suggestions, which are quoted above, but are not alluded to by Dr. Beard.

In the way of treatment, a mild galvanic current, applied both centrally and locally, is said to have proved of immediate benefit in two cases, but the particulars are not given. Dr. Hutchinson, of Providence, reported a case treated in a similar manner, in the Journal of November 5, 1874, which Dr. Wyman criticises by saying that the supposed cure coincided with the natural time of disappearance of the disease. Dr. Hutchinson, however, in a later communication, attributes a permanent beneficial effect to the galvanization, since the symptoms in 1875 were much milder than in previous years.

M. Vulfranc Gerdy, who was for a long time inspector of Uriage, has left a sum of money to the Academy of Medicine of Paris, to found a kind of school in which young medical men, with suitable salaries, shall, for four consecutive years, repair to such watering places as shall be pointed out to them, study and collect cases, and report upon them to the Academy. Satisfactory reports will be specially rewarded.

DOCTORS VS. DEVILS.—Lieutenant Masters, R. N., has discovered that the natives of Terra del Fuego believe in devils, and that they are the departed spirits of members of the medical profession. The main object of their religious ceremony is to keep these devils at a distance from them.

TEST FOR ASCERTAINING THE PRESENCE OF BLOOD IN CLOTH OR IN LIQUIDS.—For physicians and clinical instructors the following method of discovering the presence of blood may be useful, especially in the examination of urine: it combines simplicity with absolute certainty. Mix in a test-tube two cubic centimeters of tincture of guaiac with an equal volume of oil of turpentine, and then add a few drops of the urine which is to be examined. If it contains any blood, even in minutest quantity, the whole mixture at once shows a more or less intensely blue color, sometimes a deep indigo, while this coloration is produced neither by normal urine nor by urine containing albumen or pus. If you wish to ascertain whether stains in linen, wood, etc., contain blood, you proceed in this way: Dissolve five grammes of guaiac in one hundred cubic centimeters of absolute alcohol, and filter the solution; then mix five cubic centimeters of this solution with the same volume of rectified oil of turpentine, and put into this mixture the small piece of linen, wood, etc., the suspicious stains of which have been previously treated with warm diluted acetic acid. The presence of blood will at once show itself by a blue color.

COD-LIVER OIL AND FERROUS IODIDE.—The following formula has been published in the *Nieuw Tijdschrift voor de Pharmacie in Nederland*, by a commission appointed by the Netherlands Pharmaceutical Society, to examine secret remedies and specialties: Iodine, one part; pulverized iron, one part; pale cod-liver oil, eighty parts.

Triturate the pulverized iron in a mortar with the iodine and one-fourth of the oil, and heat the mixture in a water-bath, with constant stirring, until the brown color of the iodine has entirely disappeared and given place to a deep purple color, showing that the ferrous iodide has been formed and dissolved. Then add the remainder of the oil, mix carefully, and after standing decant into dry bottles, which are to be completely filled, closed immediately and kept sheltered from the light.

# THE AMERICAN PRACTITIONER.

## OCTOBER, 1876.

Certainly it is excellent discipline for an author to feel that he must say all that he has to say in the fewest possible words, or his reader is sure to skip them; and in the plainest possible words, or his reader will certainly misunderstand them. Generally, also, a down-right fact may be told in a plain way; and we want downright facts at present more than any thing else.—RUSKIN.

## Original Communications.

## DISEASES OF THE PANCREAS.

### BY J. E. LOCKRIDGE, M. D.

Heretofore most of the systematic writers on the practice of medicine have treated very slightly the diseases of the pancreas. Some, like Barlow, have ignored them entirely; the classical Sir Thomas Watson, rather than "slight" this organ, devotes just eleven lines to its diseases, but winds up by saying, "I do not know of any remedies" for these complaints. Flint and Wood each gives about one and a half pages to their consideration. It is not my purpose to write a treatise on these complaints, but rather to enter a mild protest against two propositions that all of these writers seem to lay down; these are, that diseases of the pancreas are very rare, and when they do exist the diagnosis is most difficult, if not impossible.

In considering the first of these propositions, I will say that I can see no good reason why we might not expect to encounter diseases of the pancreas as well as almost any other of the adjuvant organs of digestion; and that, too, both primarily

VOL. XIV.—13

and secondarily. Anatomically, it resembles the salivary glands, and in physical properties its secretion is almost identical. The organ derives its blood supply wholly from the hepatic, splenic, and superior mesenteric arteries, and hence trouble at these fountains would be likely to affect it secondarily. In the last ten years of my experience it has been my lot to encounter disease of the organ, in some form, quite frequently; but during the first ten years of my experience I met with not a single case to my present knowledge, because, having been taught that they were "very rare," I doubtless overlooked many cases. Sir Thomas Watson writes that "perhaps he has seen eight or nine cases of cancer of the head of the organ in his experience;" I, with not one tithe of the experience or skill that he possesses, have seen quite that number of either cancer, simple hypertrophy, or chronic inflammation of this organ. I am forced to believe that many cases have run their course, either to a favorable or fatal termination, without their real nature ever having been suspected. From having been called in consultation in these cases, and by having them come under my care after having passed through the hands of other physicians, I have learned that they are most apt to be mistaken for the following complaints, taking them in the order in which I here place them: dyspepsia, so-called "liver disease," scirrhus of the pylorus, and hypertrophy of the greater curvature of the stomach, aneurism of the abdominal aorta, enlarged spleen, floating kidney (left), and an accumulation of fæces in the transverse colon from obstruction. This brings us to the attempted refutation of the second proposition, that the diagnosis is next to impossible.

In the outset it would be well to enumerate a set of symptoms that generally accompany affections of this organ; but, by way of parenthesis, I might as well say that there are only two symptoms that are pathognomonic of pancreatic diseases, and these are a tumor situated between the pit of the stomach and umbilicus, and which has been ascertained by elimination to be in the pancreas; and the other symptom is the constant

passage through the bowels of the undigested fatty portion of
the food; for it is the known function of the pancreatic juice
to emulsify fats, and render them suitable for imbibation by
the lacteals. But there are scores of other symptoms, some
of which I will enumerate; a fixed pain, or rather soreness on
pressure over the epigastrium, a disposition to lie on the right
side, because the dorsal *decubitus* is rendered painful by the
weight of the stomach; and on the left side by that of the
liver; the patient is generally affected with a train of gastric
or dyspeptic symptoms, such as pyrosis, gastrodynia, nausea,
and vomiting, which for the most part come on a few hours
after eating; there is often inordinate action of the heart, without alteration in structure or rhythm; there is, on very close
examination, a deep-seated tumor just above the umbilicus,
fixed and roundish, hard and somewhat nodulated in scirrhus,
but rather oblong and elastic in simple hypertrophy; there is
jaundice, or at least an approach thereto, from pressure on the
common duct; there is generally aortic pulsation, and sometimes a *bruit*. As the disease, or diseases, advances, there is
emaciation and general malaise; the bowels are either consti-
pated or loose, as the case may be; there is generally an absence of fever, and the tongue is generally coated with a white
fur denoting feeble digestion, and the appetite is generally
moderately good.

I will now attempt to lay down some rules for the differen-
tial diagnosis of the diseases of the organ in question, from
those of some of the other organs and parts of this anatomical jumble, with which they have often been confounded. In
the case of some of them it is comparatively plain sailing,
but in others, I am willing to admit, that it is as difficult as
possible. But in none do I consider it impossible, if we take
ample time, and bring to bear on the case all of a reasonably
good anatomical and physiological knowledge.

As previously indicated the superficial observer is almost
sure to mistake disease of the pancreas for dyspepsia. He
encounters a case with the usual symptoms of dyspepsia, and
either for a want of tact in detecting anatomical changes, or

much oftener from a failure to examine the region *at all* for these changes, he goes to work and plies his remedies with vigor, and directs his treatment altogether to the stomach. He never suspects that he has an hypertrophy, chronic inflammation, or scirrhus of the pancreas, to deal with. After six months or a year, more or less, the patient may *by chance* get well, or his physician may send him off to some mineral spring which happens to possess powerful deobstruent properties, and by this means a cure may be effected. But more often he goes from doctor to doctor, if he does not go to the graveyard in the meantime, until at last he meets with one who detects the true nature of his case, and institutes the proper treatment.

Here is a case in question. Early in June of the present year, and just before I left Virginia, a gentleman came to consult me from a neighboring county. He told me that he had enjoyed almost uninterrupted health until the first day of last January, at which time he took a bad cold which almost ran into pneumonia before he got over it; and during this time, and for some weeks afterwards, the glands of his neck were very much swollen. After using iodine on them for some time the swelling entirely disappeared, but still he was not well. When I saw him he was complaining of soreness in the region of his stomach; his appetite was quite good, but yet he had lost forty pounds in flesh, and was still losing; he complained of considerable uneasiness after meals, yet he seemed to digest his food very well; he had rather an inordinate desire for fat meat, but there was no evidence that the fat passed through undigested, or at least he had not observed anything of the kind; there was inordinate action of the heart, the pulse counting one hundred and twenty to the minute, yet the heart was perfectly sound in structure and rhythm. On examination I at once detected a deep-seated tumor between the pit of the stomach and umbilicus; the tumor was pulsating and attended with a faint *bruit;* it was rather oblong in shape, somewhat elastic, and was really less painful under pressure than a line or circle of soreness which

surrounded the tumor, and which was caused by its encroachment on neighboring parts or organs. Now for the differentiation of this tumor. It was not in the stomach, for there
were really no symptoms of indigestion that would imply that
there was a large portion of the stomach involved in organic
disease, for the tumor was at least three times the normal size
of the pancreas; there was no pyrosis, or water-brash, but
rather a sensation of encroachment. It could not be in the
liver, for whilst there was rather a jaundiced hue of the skin,
which was caused by pressure on the common bile duct, yet
the tumor was in the median line and the liver was felt in its
normal position, and without tenderness or alteration in size.
Of course the left kidney and spleen were out of the question;
for a floating kidney—two cases of which I have seen, both
on the right side, and both in the female—is quite easily made
out from its shape and smoothness, and want of tenderness
on pressure; and the median position and circumscribed character of the tumor distinguished it from an ague-cake.

We come now to the consideration of this, and other such
cases, as regards their discrimination from aneurism of the
abdominal aorta at the most common seat, where it is weakened by giving off the cœliac axis; this, perhaps, is the most
difficult in most cases to determine. Both tumors are deep-
seated; in both there is generally pulsation; in both there is
commonly a *bruit* of some kind. The pancreatic tumor is
generally longest transversely, whilst the aneurismal is most
often fusiform, and is therefore vertical; the practiced ear will
generally distinguish the simple *bruit de souffle* of the pancreatic tumor, caused by its pressure on the aorta, from the well
known aneurismal purr. If the fingers of both hands be
gently but persistently insinuated down on either side of the
tumor, if it be a pancreatic tumor, it can be raised from its
contact with the aorta and the pulsation will cease, as well as
the bruit; but in the case of an aneurism the tumor is more
fixed, and the pulsation will continue laterally, as well as ver-
tically. Still further, if the patient be placed in the genumanual or "all-fours" position, the diseased gland will gravi-

tate from the aorta, and the *bruit* will cease unless it be an aneurism.

In my preceding remarks I have been dealing, for the most part, in negations and eliminations; but now let us inquire into the purport of some of the positive signs of pancreatic diseases. The jaundice and gastric symptoms are produced in part by direct pressure; but in many cases I am disposed to attribute the origin of these symptoms to the direct pressure of the tumor on the semilunar ganglion and solar plexus of the sympathetic nerve, with which both an enlarged pancreas and aortic aneurism would come in contact; and I have seen both these maladies produce precisely analogous symptoms on each of these neighboring organs. It is very easy to explain this nervous catenation through the irradiating fibers of the solar plexus and its connection with the pneumogastric. So great was the tumult of the heart in the case of the gentleman, whose case I have been carrying along with me in these remarks for the sake of differentiating the diagnosis, that he could scarcely believe but that his heart was awfully diseased.

Another symptom of vast importance in the diagnosis, is the inordinate desire for fat meats. This is of easy explanation. The emulsifying process and consequent absorption of the fatty ingesta by the lacteals is in abeyance for the want of healthy pancreatic juice, and the economy is simply crying for this element of nutrition, and hence the appetite for the fats. Another point of importance is the very *deeply-seated* location of the tumor, which should of itself almost reduce the case to the diagnosis between it and aneurism; and of this I have spoken very fully, but will have occasion to allude to it again.

But do not let us lose sight of the case which I have taken along as a sort of *vade mecum* in this paper. This gentleman had been treated for four or five months by several very intelligent physicians for dyspepsia, but without any improvement, but on the other hand a progressive loss of flesh and strength. They had not discovered the tumor in the hypogastric region, and the patient informed me that neither of them had even examined or *touched* him in this region. From the fact that the family was evidently a scrofulous one, I diagnosed the case as strumous enlargement of the pancreas; and although, from some indications about the case, I could not give a very favorable opinion as to the result, yet the gentleman seemed relieved that the cause at least of his ailment was probably discovered, for I placed his own hand on the tumor, which he could plainly discover, and feel the aortic pulsation quite plainly. I made the following prescription, which I directed him to use indefinitely, as I was about to leave the state; and the understanding was, that if he needed further aid he was to address me in this city. I have not heard from him, and conclude that he is improving at least. I ordered him to paint the tumor three times a day with tincture of iodine, and take the following:

R. Syrup iodide iron, . . . . . . $\bar{3}$ij
Fowler's solution, . . . . . . ʒiv
Corrosive sublimate, . . . . . grs.ij
Quinia, . . . . . . . . . grs.xx
Water, . . . . . . . . . $\bar{3}$vss

M. sig. Take one teaspoonful, three times a day, after each meal.

I will briefly review two or three cases of other forms of the disease that have fallen under my observation, and then close by referring to a case or two in which the trouble consisted principally in diagnosing *from* pancreatic disease.

In 1870 I was called in consultation in the case of a young man who was within a few days of his death from a progressively wasting disease which had existed for several months. The most prominent symptoms were those of dyspepsia, for which complaint he had been treated by several physicians until within a week or two of my call, when, owing to the extreme emaciation, a tumor was discovered in the region of his stomach. As to the nature of this tumor, and its location, there were just about as many opinions as there were doctors employed in the case: one thought it was in the stomach, another contended that it was a tumor of the liver, and a third, of very considerable experience and fair reputation, thought that it was a chronic abscess situated in some of the organs or tissues in that vicinity, and he seemed to be strengthened in this belief from the fact that there was another small tumor situated in the inguinal region. Owing to the extreme degree of emaciation of the patient there was but little trouble in handling the tumor, which, however, was very painful under pressure; it was situated against the spinal column, roundish in shape, hard and distinctly *nodulated;* it was attended with the usual gastric and hepatic symptoms; there was an unmistakable cancerous cachexia about the appearance of the patient, besides he had lost a number of relatives with cancer and consumption. From the very deep-seated location of the tumor, it was obviously not in the liver; in the absence of any kind of a *bruit,* or decided aortic pulsation, an aneurism was out of the question. So the differentiation was evidently between scirrhus of the pylorus of the stomach and cancer of the head of the pancreas. Although there was occasional vomiting, and sometimes too of a dark-colored material, yet there was not that regular and persistent and scarcely ever-ceasing ejection of partially digested food that is always met with in cases of scirrhus and occlusion of the pylorus. I will just say here, once for all, that neither in this case, nor any other, have I had the opportunity to witness the admixture with the fæces of undigested and unemulsified fat; but I have more often met with an inordinate appetite for fatty food. This man's appetite was reduced to *nil.* This man died in about one week, and the post mortem, at which I was not present, revealed cancer of the head of the pancreas, with a small abscess forming on the liver from mere pressure, and a small abscess in the vicinity of the cæcum.

On one occasion, seven or eight years ago, I was consulted by a strong blacksmith for what he called dyspepsia. There was uneasiness and some soreness under pressure in the region of the stomach, a good deal of trouble during digestion, but a pretty fair appetite, and a *very good* appetite for fat meat;

he complained of a constant feeling of fullness in his stomach, and withal too much ill at ease to carry on his trade. On examination I found a considerable enlargement of the pancreas, which I diagnosed as chronic inflammation of the organ, and directed him to paint the skin over the tumor three times a day with tincture of iodine, and gave him ten grains of iodide of potassium three times a day. In a few days the tumor began to gradually melt away, and in three or four weeks it was entirely gone and all the dyspeptic symptoms with it, and he went to work and has never been sick a day since to my knowledge.

In 1870 I was called in great haste to see a very strong laboring man, and found him suffering most excruciating pain in the vicinity of the pit of the stomach; it was evidently a "fit of gravel" of some kind. I at first suspected the passage of a gall-stone, but there was *no jaundice*, nor was there the nausea and vomiting of bile usually met with in such cases, and the pain was too much toward the median line of the body for a gall-stone; I diagnosed pancreatalgia from the passage of a calculus, and under the usual anodyne treatment the man was out in a day or two.

Before quitting this branch of my subject I must make a passing remark about the purely functional troubles of this organ. Their direct diagnosis must be hypothetical; but the best way I know of to confirm the supposition is the administration of pancreatine in some form; and these are, in all probability, the cases in which the pancreatic emulsion "acts like a charm." Indeed this remedy should be used in all cases of organic disease of the organ for the purpose of assisting digestion, until curative agents shall have had a chance to effect a cure. My experience with this remedy has not been sufficient to warrant any positive opinion as to its efficacy in such cases.

I will close this paper by giving as succinctly as possible a history of two cases of other complaints in which the diagnosis from pancreatic disease, and some other affections in that vicinity, was as difficult as possible. About a year and a half ago I was consulted by a gentleman in a neighboring county about a train of symptoms which had been treated as dyspepsia by several physicians for about two years. The patient was about fifty years of age, of rather low stature, but very corpulent, weighing then something over two hundred pounds, his healthy avoirdupois being two hundred and sixty pounds. His principal complaint was a sense of constant uneasiness in the stomach, with a variety of dyspeptic symptoms; one very prominent one I noticed was a very frequent eructation of gas. Although he is now a good citizen and prominent christian gentleman, yet I noticed from the flat appearance of his nose that the bones had been destroyed by syphilis or some other ravaging disease; and in fact, upon inquiry, he candidly informed me that in his younger days he had had tertiary syphilis and had been a hard drinker. Upon very careful examination I detected a *very deep-seated* tumor, but owing even to his present obesity any tumor beneath the layer of adipose tissue would necessarily be deep-seated. The difficulty in locating this tumor was extreme: but in the absence of any jaundice the liver was eliminated from the count; a total absence of any *bruit* enabled me, in a measure, to exempt the pancreas and aortic aneurism. From the syphilitic taint, and from the fact that he had once been a hard drinker, I was enabled, with a pretty fair degree of certainty, to diagnose a thickening of the walls in the greater curvature of the stomach. I put him on the following prescription and in two weeks he began to feel better, and in three months the tumor had almost entirely disappeared and the dyspeptic troubles with it, and he had gained fifteen pounds in weight. I directed him to paint the skin over the tumor three times a day with the tincture of iodine, and take the following:

    ℞ Iodide Potassium, . . . . . . ℥v
        Corrosive sublimate, . . . . . grs. iij
        Fowler's solution, . . . . . . ℥iv
        Comp. sp. lavender, . . . . . ℥ij
        Water, . . . . . . . . . ℥vj
    M. sig. Take one teaspoonful, three times a day, after

each meal. I saw this gentleman a year afterwards, and he was entirely well.

One more case, and an interesting one too, and I am done. In April, 1873, a robust young man came to consult me about a very severe pain in the region of the stomach, attended with gastric disorder and inordinate action of the heart. This pain had existed for six weeks, during which time he had lost fifteen pounds, he usually weighing two hundred and fifteen pounds. For about the four preceding years I had been treating this man for what I at first supposed was neuralgia of the head. At different times I had tried every conceivable remedy for neuralgia without ever having given him the slightest relief, except the most temporary. The pain was fixed always at one and the same spot, and some months before I came to the conclusion that there was some kind of a tumor of the brain which would ultimately give him worse trouble. I abandoned the case and advised him to go and consult a gentleman who was one of the most accomplished physicians in Virginia; this he failed to do. When he consulted me on the present occasion, he said the "neuralgia had suddenly left his head and moved to his stomach," and such, indeed, was the case with the pain; the head was perfectly clear of pain, the first time in four years, and all of his trouble was now in the region of his stomach.

On making a most searching examination of his case I discovered a very deep-seated tumor between the navel and pit of the stomach; it was distinctly pulsating, and expansively so, I was quite sure; there was a faint *bruit*, which, on placing him in the genumanual position, became *more distinct*, and left no doubt on my mind but that it was an aneurismal purr. There were some dyspeptic symptoms, which never existed before; there was also a decided jaundiced hue of the eyes, also very great action of the heart, and an aneurismal murmur over the arch of the aorta. I knew his family history very well, and knew that his mother died of angina pectoris, which is but a symptom of degeneration of the coronary arteries; I knew that his sister died of *ramolissement* of the brain, which was doubtless due to thrombosis; in short, I knew that there was an hereditary predisposition to arterial degeneration. In accordance with these facts I made the diagnosis of aneurism of the abdominal aorta, and gave a rather unfavorable opinion as to the result, which shocked him greatly. Being in preparation for a prolonged sojourn in the West, I did not undertake the treatment of his case, but sent him to the distinguished physician alluded to above.

Unfortunately this medical gentleman failed to discern the true nature of the case, but mistook it for neuralgia and prescribed accordingly, and assured the young man that in ten days he would be so far relieved that "he would feel like another man;" and at the end of this period he should return to him, which he did, but alas! only to present himself in a condition growing progressively worse. At this visit the doctor examined him more carefully, but failed to detect the abdominal tumor, but discovered the *bruit* over the arch of the aorta, and construed it as the hygræmic murmur. This was manifestly an error, since the patient was neither, at this time, anæmic nor hygræmic, for he was very well nourished and still weighed nearly two hundred pounds. The doctor adhered to his former opinion, and noticing the jaundiced hue of the eyes and skin, and thinking that some derangement of the liver was protracting the neuralgia, he prescribed active cholagogue cathartics and applied a large blister over the epigastric region, and advised the patient to go to the warm or hot springs of Virginia. The medicine acted very drastically, and by the time he got through with it he was so much worse that he could not leave his house for some time; and he had also lost faith in the doctor, and seemed to be out of faith generally with the profession, since he had consulted two of them in whom he had confidence at least, and they differed so widely that he determined to take his case in his own hands, and did not return to his physician. But to the credit of this physician he admitted to a friend of mine that he had been entirely mistaken in Mr. B.'s case, and that he was then satisfied that the case would terminate fatally.

Just so soon as he had sufficiently rallied from the effects of the drastics, some time towards the last of June, he went to a strong chalybeate spring and remained there for a month or more, but on returning in July he had evidently lost ground. After having been at home for some time, the gastric and other troubles became so annoying that he was forced to call in a doctor from the neighborhood, who, with much promptness, diagnosed a case of *pure "dyspepsy;"* and under the use of remedies directed to the relief of the gastric symptoms he became more comfortable for a few weeks, but he continued to lose weight. Some time in the month of October, and about five months after I had, with very great difficulty, diagnosed aortic aneurism, this doctor was called in the night to relieve some violent symptom in the case, and for the first time discovered the tumor in the patient's abdomen. The patient by this time was reduced to a mere skeleton, and long before this time the tumor must have been as plain as a big apple in an old woman's reticule. After this discovery was made, just like buzzards around carrion, a number of other doctors gathered in to render service in the case, but in spite of their combined skill the poor young man died about the first of the next January. There was no post mortem made. Here was a case of general arterial degeneration; and as a result there were at least three aneurisms, one in the abdomen, one at the arch of the aorta, and a third located somewhere in the brain. I have introduced this case to show the great difficulty in diagnosing diseases in this region, and to show how doctors will differ as to their seat and nature.

I will now close this somewhat rambling and unphilosophical communication, in which I fear that I will be charged with prolixity, as well as tautology; but my apology is, that I am very desirous of convincing the younger members of our profession that affections of the pancreas are *by no means* uncommon, and their diagnosis and cure are by no means impossible in the majority of cases. If I succeed in this I am more than satisfied, even if I should be forced to plead guilty to the charge of inelegance of diction.

INDIANAPOLIS.

# OCCLUSION OF THE ANTERIOR, MIDDLE AND POS-TERIOR COMMUNICATING ARTERIES OF THE LEFT SIDE OF THE BRAIN.

BY C. G. COMEGYS, M. D.

*Lecturer on Clinical Medicine in the Cincinnati Hospital.*

F. K., aged thirty-three years, American, married, railroad clerk, bilio-sanguine temperament, was placed under my charge on the 28th of April. He was semi-conscious only, and could give but little account of himself. I learned that he had not been well for some time, and had manifested unusual irritability for some days. He had not been sleeping well, and had had dreams of a startling character. On the previous night the illness of the baby had kept him awake. On this day he had gone to his office as usual, but soon felt so overcome that he laid down and slept heavily for two hours. His associates thought it best to conduct him home. He could walk with assistance to a carriage, and to his bed on arrival at the hotel, but he was dull and quite unlike himself. He was supposed to be suffering from biliousness only, but his wife soon became alarmed at his stupor.

On my arrival at 3 P. M., he was only semi-conscious, did not answer well, and complained of his head generally. Temperature was not abnormal; respiration twenty-four, regular; pulse ninety, rather feeble; and there was no motor or sensory paralysis. I regarded him as suffering with meningeal congestion of the upper and lateral surfaces of the brain, of a passive character, and due, in the long run, most likely to overwork in an office imperfectly lighted and ventilated. The base of the brain did not seem to be affected.

I directed six ounces of blood to be taken by cups from the nape of the neck, and a hot mustard foot-bath, and ordered a purge of calomel and jalap.

I saw him again at 7½ P. M. His condition was much

worse; besides greater mental hebetude, he was having constant spasms in the fingers of the right hand, and more or less movement of the right humerus, shoulder and leg, but not clearly spasmodic. The eyes, which had presented no abnormal movements on my first visit, were now rolling from side to side. The respiration was twenty-four, temperature one hundred and one, pulse eighty, but not strong; no action of bowels or bladder.

It was now plain, however wide the lesion was spread, that the injury of greatest moment, as shown by the spasms in fingers and movements of right extremities, and deeper mental complications, was in the territory of the left side of the brain supplied by the middle cerebral artery.

I now ordered twelve leeches to the temples, and a stimulating enema; I also injected subcutaneously, in the course of an hour, five grains of ergotin. Ice-bags were to be kept on the forehead and back of the neck during the night. Professor William H. Mussey now came in to see him with me, and concurred in my diagnosis and treatment.

On the next morning he was better, that is the convulsive movements had ceased, the pupils, which had been small, were larger and movable, and much more consciousness existed. His bowels had acted freely, but the urine was detained, and upon using the catheter a stricture was found. He was kept under the fluid extract of ergot during the day, with ice applications as before.

On the following morning we observed a slight hemiplegia of right side and face, but no deviation of the tongue or eyes, and that he was in a slight condition of aphasia. He could speak only a few words, connectedly and with difficulty; it was a great effort to call his wife's name and that of near friends, and his inability to write the name of a person or place was marked, due allowance being made for the paresis of muscles of right hand; the defect was plainly one of the memory to embody his ideas in objective forms. The supervention of the hemiplegia and aphasia left no doubt in our minds of the involvement of the left corpus striatum, the island of Reil, the posterior aspect of the left third frontal convolution, and the superior surface of the anterior portions of the brain.

The question of the nature of the disease was now to be considered, in order to pursue a steady treatment. We had no exact data of his anterior life; his wife had known him less than two years. He had been a confederate officer during the civil war, but no one knew of his having been seriously sick. There was a hint from a friend of some *specific* ailment during his campaigns, but no external signs existed to assure us of the fact. There was no *bruit* connected with the circulation through the heart, nor along the arteries, nor any old articular affection to indicate a point of departure for a clot which could produce the brain lesion; nor could we think, from his age, that atheromatous changes existed in the arteries. There was entire absence of acute inflammatory and of apoplectic symptoms. We determined, therefore, to base our treatment on the theory of syphilitic changes in the brain tissue and vessels of supply of the affected part. He was put upon the use, therefore, of twenty grains iodide of potassium and one-twentieth of a grain of perchloride of mercury, three times a day. Four drops of Fowler's solution were given three times a day also. He was to drink milk mainly for food; beef-tea was also freely given.

Except on the evening of the first day, when his temperature was 101°, it at no time was higher than 99.5°. The pulse also descended to eighty, and the respirations, which were always regular, stood throughout at twenty. It was always necessary to withdraw the urine, and injections or mild cathartics were often given to move his bowels.

The patient seemed to improve under this course; he could get out of bed, stand, and assisted walk to a chair. Moreover his mind was clearer; he could speak more words, and in a coarse way write his name. At the end of two weeks he was taken to Louisville, his wife's home, and was placed under the charge of Dr. J. M. Clemens. I forwarded to that intelligent physician the above narrative of his case, expressing a hope that he might yet recover. Three weeks after his departure, I received a letter from Dr. Clemens, which contains the following remarks:

"LOUISVILLE, May 29, 1876.

"I felt greatly obliged by your history, and I may also say diagnosis, of Mr. K.'s case; for, upon investigating the case, I was fully persuaded of the entire correctness of your diagnosis, and of consequence your treatment. I am of the opinion that your hinted theory of the causation (specific) well grounded, and from a careful study of his case most probably correct. In this opinion, as in fact the opinion entire which you gave, Dr. D. Cummins, of this city, who has visited the case several times with me, fully concurs. I am of opinion that the gummous formation had been going on for some time; that in this way the left middle cerebral artery was gradually encroached upon until nature, in her wisdom, saw fit to make an attempt at establishing collateral circulation, which resulted in the passive congestion under which you found him suffering, and that red softening has followed as a result. I think there can be no question that softening has been going on for more than a fortnight, and for a week or more has been progressing rapidly, as shown by gradual encroachment upon all the voluntary muscles, loss of speech, inability to swallow, immobility of pupils, etc. For three or four days he has been utterly unable to swallow a particle of anything, and has received water and nourishment by the stomach-tube alone. The sphincter ani being paralyzed, administration of nourishment by the bowel has of course been out of the question. He has twice had considerable irritative fever, which I interpreted as an expression of some inflammatory action going on around the periphery of the softening region.

"We have kept him upon your treatment as the only hope of relief to his symptoms. Of course we have occasionally used some additional medication to meet temporary variations in his condition, but our reliance has been upon the iodide of potassium and the mercury.

"I am sorry to say that there is now absolutely nothing on

which to hang the slightest hope, and there is every reason to believe that it is only a question of comparatively brief time with him."

Dr. Clemens subsequently wrote that after the date of his last letter, Mr. K. began to improve; his paralysis, which had been general and almost total for all parts of the body, grew so much better that he had recovered deglutition sufficiently to receive medicine and food by the mouth, could manage both extremities of left side, and regained more or less movement of right arm and leg. This amendment continued for three weeks. Then a hypostatic pneumonia developed, with high fever, rapid pulse and respiration. All of these untoward symptoms yielded, however, to treatment; in a few days, the pulse, respiration and temperature descending to about the normal level. Soon after this a diarrhœa set in, to which he speedily succumbed on the 13th of June.

A post mortem was made by Dr. Clemens, in which he was assisted by Drs. Cummins and Morton, with the following results:

"Unusually firm attachment of the dura mater to the calvaria, in the region of the Pacchionian glands, along the course of the longitudinal sinus. Effusion at base of the brain. Numerous adhesions over both hemispheres of arachnoid to the dura mater, due to arachnitis. The arachnoid, throughout its entire extent, was found intensely congested and thickened. Effusion in the left sylvian fissure, also in the third ventricle. Upon slicing the brain, extensive red softening was found in both hemispheres. The middle lobe of the left hemisphere, evidently the beginning point, almost creamy in consistence. Softening of the anterior portion of the optic thalami. Upon inspection of the vessels of the base of the brain, a plug of fibrine, almost white, was found at the terminus of the left internal carotid, occupying not only the mouth of the left middle cerebral—which we have felt sure was obstructed—but also that of the anterior cerebral and posterior communicating arteries, thus obstructing the entire left side of the circle of Willis. Firm, almost pulverulent coagulæ occupied these arteries. There was no exudation upon the arteries of the base of the brain; but upon the coats of the vessels of the choroid plexus there was found considerable exudation, as also upon the coats of the cerebral arteries forming plexus in fissure of Sylvius, both sides. Cerebellum in normal condition. Heart not examined."

Dr. Clemens goes on to say:

"I am at a loss, considering the entire absence of history of any heart trouble, to account for the presence of the embolon. The most plausible solution, however, seems to me to be that he had, during the war, from exposure contracted a slight rheumatism, resulting in a circumscribed endocarditis, not sufficient to give rise to pronounced symptoms, yet sufficient to produce the fibrinous plug which found its lodgment in the situation above mentioned. I presume the temporary improvement in the paralysis must have been due to the partial absorption of the effused material at the base of the brain and in the ventricle, the presence of which, I have no doubt, did much to paralyze the functions of the already badly crippled brain."

*Remarks.*—Notwithstanding the inability of all parties to detect a point of departure in the heart or vessels for the embolon, yet it is evident that such a place existed; and the occlusion of the arteries began in an imperfect way thereby at the end of the left internal carotid, and grew larger until the anterior, middle and posterior communicating arteries became gradually tightly plugged; for the symptoms seem to indicate the gradual approach of complete embolation, and the maintenance of functions on a low plane afterwards, by supplies through the anastomosis with the posterior cerebral, and branches of the basilar arteries. The field was too large from which the blood supply was cut off—the frontal and most of the middle lobes of the left hemisphere, the corpus striatum, and part of the thalamus opticus of same side being nearly totally deprived of a direct supply of arterial blood—for recovery by the establishment of a collateral circulation. A vast area involving most important physical and psychical centers was doomed to destruction.

Destructive changes involved the right hemisphere also, furnishing well pronounced symptoms in the progress of the case; but no affection of the arteries on that side existed to account for them, and we are left to infer that they were developed *indirectly* by the severity of conditions on the left side.

Another thing seen in the case is the general paralysis that supervened after he reached home, and a subsequent marked improvement of it, which can be accounted for by the functional involvement merely of sound tissues in the environment of the foci of softening, which recovered when the irritation subsided; for no revival of function can ever take place when complete destruction of tissue has occurred. In this way we can account for the improvement so often seen in cases of brain diseases.

It is evident now, that the pathology was not due to syphilitic products in the brain tissue itself, nor in the arterial coats. Thrombi are, it is well known, developed in this way, producing destructive changes of a character with those in this case. In our diagnosis we were mistaken, not in the localization of the malady, but in its nature.

CINCINNATI.

---

## TREATMENT OF PLACENTA PRÆVIA—A VINDICATION.

### BY THEOPHILUS PARVIN, M. D.

In the June number of the American Practitioner was published a paper on the treatment of placenta prævia, which I had read before the State Medical Society of Indiana. In the Transactions of the Society just issued this paper also appears, though greatly to my regret I was not given an opportunity of seeing the *proof*, else typographical errors would have been corrected, some slight alterations and additions would have been made, such as were made in the copy published in the Practitioner. However, the articles are essentially the same. But appended to the article, as it appears in the Transactions, are criticisms made by members of the Society in the discussion of it, a discussion which professional engagements prevented my hearing, and answering the adverse criticisms, so far as answer was demanded, at the time of their utterance. I therefore embrace the earliest opportunity to vindicate the position taken in that paper, and to correct some, as I believe, very erroneous statements that were made.

One of the critics (page 50 of the Transactions) implies my willingness to sacrifice the life of the mother rather than that of the child. And this is gravely said, and with righteous rhetoric condemned, right in the face of my statement (page 38 of Transactions, page 338 of American Practitioner,) "if either life is to be especially imperilled or lost, let it be that of the child rather than of the mother"!

Another thought that after introducing "a Molesworth dilator," an instrument with which he frankly acknowledged himself "not sufficiently familiar," "the dilator allows a dilatation to take place when you are absent, which may be the cause of a fatal hemorrhage." It is presumed that the physician will not leave his patient in labor, especially while he is accomplishing the first stage by a series of dilators.

But passing by minor criticisms and minor critics, I shall restrict myself to the remarks made by Dr. George W. Mears, remarks in condemnation of the practice advocated by me, and those in favor of the tampon. While respecting this gentleman for his many years of active professional life, I can not refrain from a plain but courteous criticism of many of his statements, especially as they are his matured, deliberate utterances since he had the opportunity of revising his remarks prior to their publication. I shall show to every unprejudiced mind that some of his facts are mere opinions, and some others are positively erroneous.

But first let me state the principle I sought to maintain in the paper referred to, and then the practice advised. This principle was that in cases of placenta prævia, when serious hemorrhage occurred after the child was viable, the induction of labor was advisable.   Two eminent obstetricians, one Brit-ish, the other American—Drs. Greenhalgh and Thomas—were quoted as advising this.

In addition to that evidence, let me now present extracts from two recent works on obstetrics, the one the third edition of "Meadows," the other the first of "Playfair."

Dr. Meadows says, "It may be laid down as a rule of gen-eral application, and one, too, which ought to be rigidly ob-served, that, no matter what the period of gestation, any large loss of blood demands the termination of pregnancy; for to leave a patient to be subjected to another attack, coming on as it would do without any warning, is in truth to place her life in imminent danger.   The only justifiable grounds for such temporizing policy is the concurrence of the following conditions: that the discharge is slight, the period of preg-nancy short of six months, the absence of pain, and an undi-lated os."

Dr. Playfair's evidence is quite as strong.   He says, "Not long ago an interesting discussion took place at the London Obstetrical Society, on a paper in which Dr. Greenhalgh ad-vised the immediate induction of labor in all cases of placenta prævia.   No less than six metropolitan teachers of midwifery took part in it; and, although they differed in details, they all agreed as to the unadvisability of allowing pregnancy to pro-gress when the existence of placenta prævia had been dis-tinctly ascertained."

A principle sustained by such evidence can not be thrust aside very readily.

Now as to the practice.   Granted that the induction of labor is advisable in a given case, dilatation of the os by hydrostatic pressure was advocated.   It was claimed that suit-able rubber dilators would not only restrain the hemorrhage, but expand the os so that the first stage of labor could be readily, promptly and safely accomplished.

We will now consider some of the criticisms made by Dr.

Mears. He asserts that in placenta prævia hemorrhage prior to full term is a rare* occurrence; that the induction of premature labor is painful, tedious, dangerous; that "an inflated gum elastic air-bag, even within the internal os," is no "guarantee against fatal hemorrhage."

The first assertion is disproved by statistics. Take those of Johnston and Sinclair, for example, and we find that out of twenty-four cases, nine were in the seventh month, eight in the eighth month, and only seven at the ninth. Trask's† statistics give only forty-six at full term, to one hundred and sixty-nine occurring before.

But this artificial dilatation is painful, tedious, dangerous. The pain probably is frequently not so great in these cases as in natural labor, since the hemorrhage very often promotes relaxation of the tissues concerned, and facilitates the expansion of the os. But even if great, an anæsthetic may blunt it, and at any rate the danger to be avoided far overbalances it.

But it is dangerous. Here is an assertion without proof, an opinion put for a fact. It is contradicted by the experience of Barnes, Thomas, Angus McDonald, and others, who have actually tried, and not merely thought about this practice.

So, too, the "tedious," which, elsewhere in his criticism, Dr. Mears makes mean ten or twelve hours, is contradicted by those who have tried; any one can find conclusive contradictions in Barnes's Obstetric Operations, in an article by Dr. Thomas, in the first volume of the American Journal of Obstetrics, and in the Edinburgh Obstetrical Society's Transactions, Vol. III.

But the "inflated" rubber-bag even within the internal os is no guarantee against fatal hemorrhage. As no reference was made in the article to an inflated rubber-bag, this objection might be passed by as not at all pertinent. But let us

---

* This assertion is such an extraordinary one, so unreasonable and so easily disproved, that I shall give the gentleman's exact words: "The truth is that as such cases," *i. e.*, those of hemorrhage in the last months of gestation, "in comparison with those of the other class, at full term, are exceedingly rare occurrences," etc.

† Transactions of the American Medical Association, 1855.

suppose the writer referred to some of the hydrostatic dilators, there is the testimony of those who have used them, that they do secure against hemorrhage. Dr. J. Matthews Duncan observes that* when "hemorrhage to an alarming extent occurs in placenta prævia, the use of the rubber-bags appears to be the most successful means we can employ."

I think these assertions have been fairly put and completely disproved. It is astonishing that any one familiar with the literature of the subject should have made them.

It might have been well enough to have made such assertions years ago, but they are anachronisms in 1876, and are valueless. After certain things have been accomplished, it is useless to say they can not be. Facts never show their stubbornness better, not in disproving old theories, but in standing their ground in spite of younger theories formed for their overthrow. It is just as useless now to declare that hydrostatic dilators will not, in cases of placenta prævia with hemorrhage demanding interference, accomplish the first stage of labor promptly and safely, as it would be to revive the mathematics of Lardner, proving the impossibility of crossing the Atlantic by steam power, or to awaken the quarrel against Galileo.

It is now proposed briefly to refer to some observations of Dr. Mears in reference to the tampon treatment.

In 1868 he read an exceedingly interesting paper upon placenta prævia before the State Medical Society of Indiana. In it he speaks of resorting to the tampon, "recommended some forty years ago by Professor Wigand, of Hamburg," and states that his own "mode of application differs but little from that advised by the author of the theory." He now states that he claimed then, and claims to-day, "originality in the modus operandi of applying it, and some other circumstances connected with its use." His "modus operandi of applying it" is through a speculum, first introducing "a small piece of sponge thoroughly saturated with the solution of persulphate or pernitrate of iron of one-third or one-fourth its

* Edinburgh Obstetrical Society's Transactions, Vol. III.

ordinary strength," and pressing it upon the bleeding surface, and then thoroughly packing the vagina with charpie or squares of linen or muslin.

His description is excellent, and the method he follows is undoubtedly one of the best ways in which a tampon can be used in such cases. It is cheerfully conceded, too, that Dr. Mears's claims to originality in the "modus operandi of applying" the tampon, are just. At the same time he has been anticipated in almost every essential of his so-called "modus operandi of applying." Frequent instances of plugging the os uteri in placenta prævia prior to this are on record; the use of the speculum* in introducing the tampon will be found mentioned in the London Lancet as early as July 4, 1846; and Depaul, in his Clinical Lectures on Obstetrics, referring to the use of astringents, which others have used or advised, rejects them as generally unnecessary, using himself only when the blood is remarkably fluid a solution of perchloride of iron.

It certainly seems doubtful whether the "small piece of sponge," though saturated with the iron solution, can contribute much, if any, of the fluid to the bleeding uterine surface, for it meets the blood which is being discharged, and it presses more directly upon that portion of the placenta which has been detached, than spreads around the inner surface of the os. But it does make a temporarily efficient uterine tampon, stiffened, too, by the action of the iron, and by the coagulated blood, it probably acts as an excellent irritant, and excites uterine contraction.

Dr. Mears states that when he first considered the suitableness of the tampon, "he could not account for the fact that so plausible and readily applied remedy as that suggested by Leroux, and again urged in a somewhat modified form by Dewees, should have given place to the more hazardous sug-

---

* Dr. E. P. Bennett, American Medical Times, 1863, remarks that in abortion and in placenta prævia the life of many a female is saved only by the judicious use of the tampon; and he points out the facility and the thoroughness with which tamponing can be done by using a glass speculum.

gestions of after times." As the topic of podalic version had just been referred to and the practice condemned, the writer seems to have regarded it as one of the hazardous suggestions of after times. But podalic version in placenta prævia, which probably dates back as far as the time of Ambrose Paré, was never supplanted by the tampon. The latter, from the day of its suggestion by Leroux, has been the subject of much controversy, and so far as its adoption in practice is concerned, Rigby, Dugés, and Dubois did more to promote it than ever Dr. Dewees did. Rigby regarded it as a means to an end, saying, "By means of the plug we enable the patient to go on with perfect security until the pains have produced sufficient dilatation to admit the hand." Davis, in his obstetrical lectures, was accustomed to urge it as "the one thing needful."

Dr. Mears can say nothing more strongly in favor of his method than was said years ago in behalf of the tampon.

If all statistics of results with the tampon were as favorable as those of Dr. Mears,* not a mother or child lost in twenty years' practice, of course nothing could be better; there would not be the least reason for seeking any other treatment.

But as a case of placenta prævia occurs in the proportion of only one in five hundred and seventy-three cases† of pregnancy, the experience of one individual engaged in general practice is but a small contribution to the settlement of the proper method of treating these cases. Valentine Mott stated that he had seen and been engaged in a number of cases of placenta prævia in the course of his long practice. "In every case in which there was interference at a sufficiently early period, the mother has been always saved, and with few exceptions the child also." And yet the method of delivery

---

*Unfortunately for the value of this statement, the number and particulars of cases are not given.

†This is the proportion given by Playfair. Ramsbotham says one in six hundred and thirty five. Dr. Barnes, The Physiology and Treatment of Placenta Prævia, 1857, combining the statistics of Clarke, Collins, and McClintock and Hardy, finds that it occurs only once in fifteen hundred cases.

Dr. Mott resorted to was by the feet. Thus we see how individual experiences come in conflict, and are more than ever impressed with the conviction that the great problems of practice are to be solved by large averages rather than by individual results.

In regard to the security from hemorrhage obtained by the tampon, a security which Dr. Mears regards as so complete, it would be well to read what the first of living British obstetricians, Dr. Robert Barnes, says in his ''Obstetric Operations,'' before adopting such unbounded confidence.

But this subject is a very large one, and much more might be said, especially in reference to the influence of the tampon in inducing* labor, which it is pretty sure to do, an end which can be accomplished more certainly and quickly, and therefore more safely for the child and for the mother, by the dilators referred to.

The question of treatment of placenta prævia will not be settled to-day or this year, not by the voice of one, but by the combined experience and knowledge of many.

For the present I leave the matter, regretting that space will not permit its further consideration; the regret diminished, however, by knowing that our subscribers will soon have the pleasure of reading an article by Prof. T. G. Thomas, on the induction of premature labor in placenta prævia, such article having been promised some months since.

---

* Dugés understood the value of the tampon, not only for the arrest of hemorrhage but also for the induction of labor. In his *Manuel D' Obstetrique*, Paris, 1526, he observes, " If labor has not commenced, the tampon is absolutely neces sary. It is the sole means of preventing the death of the woman. ＊ ＊ ＊ Moreover, the tampon determines labor, which is the best means of cutting the root of the evil."—*Louise Bourgeois.*

And in Smellie's Collection of Preternatural Cases, we find, after the narration of a case of placenta prævia, the following remarks: "At this period of my practice, I did not know that applying styptics in the vagina, and filling it up with dossils of lint, would sometimes restrain the flooding, and assist to bring on labor."

INDIANAPOLIS.

# CÆSARIAN SECTION—DELIVERY OF A LIVING CHILD—DEATH OF THE MOTHER IN THIRTY-TWO HOURS.

BY W. N. M'COY, M. D.

On September 10, 1875, I was called to Scottsburg to meet Dr. Voris in a difficult case of obstetrics, and arrived there at 9 P. M. In addition to Dr. Voris, Dr. H. H. Ferguson, of Henryville, was present upon my arrival, and subsequently Dr. Watson, of Vienna, joined in the consultation.

The patient was forty years of age, five feet and two inches in height, very fleshy, her weight being more than two hundred pounds, and had been two days in her second labor. Her first labor occurred fourteen years previously, and after continuing seventy-two hours was terminated by craniotomy. Severe suppurative inflammation of the vagina and cervix uteri followed, and she did not recover for some months so as to attend to her household affairs. Her husband stated that coition subsequently was imperfect, it being impossible to penetrate more than about one inch.

Upon first visiting the patient, Dr. Voris stated that he found, upon his first examination, the sphincter of the vagina converted into a hard, fibrous ring, and it was with difficulty he could introduce his finger; once introduced he could pass it an inch and a half up a narrow, tense and very sensitive canal, but could not find the os uteri though coming in contact, as he believed, with the cervix.

Labor pains did not become active until the tenth, and by digital examination now made he discovered a constricted opening to the left of the sacrum, semilunar in shape, dilated about three-eighths of an inch; its long diameter being nearly parallel with the transverse diameter of the pelvis; anterior lip was sharp and cord-like, and not to exceed the eighth of an inch in thickness; the posterior lip was continuous with surrounding tissues. Fully satisfied of the desperate nature of the case, he asked that counsel be immediately sent for.

Upon examination, I found at the vaginal orifice a transverse opening, somewhat elliptic in shape, and about an inch in its long diameter. Surrounding this opening was a band of fibrous structure, firm and unyielding to the strongest pressure. Passing the finger through this orifice about an inch and a half, I came to a point of constriction similar in texture to that surrounding the vaginal outlet. The finger was passed with difficulty beyond the stricture, but owing to the extreme tension and firmness of the parts, it was impossible to reach the presenting part of the child.

After consultation, it was the unanimous opinion that the uterus having prolapsed while in a state of suppurative inflammation, following her previous confinement, the vaginal cervix had become adherent within the vagina. The practicability of craniotomy being out of the question, it was decided that hysterotomy was the only measure left us which offered any hope of relief, and this hope seemed small considering the condition of the patient. At this juncture, adding to the difficulties in the case, severe convulsions occurred. She was bled freely from the arm with marked mitigation of the severity of the convulsions. There being no chloroform at hand, a messenger was promptly despatched for it to the town, one mile distant. The nature of the proposed operation, and the arguments for and against it, being particularly stated to the husband and friends, they readily gave their consent.

The patient was removed from her bed and placed upon a straw tick, the tick being well padded with comforts. Taking my position at her right side, assisted by Drs. Voris, Ferguson and Watson, as soon as the patient was sufficiently under the influence of the chloroform, I commenced the operation by making an incision six inches in length through the linea alba from near the umbilicus to the margin of the pubes, the knife passing through about two inches in thickness of adipose tissue. The peritoneum was opened at the upper extremity of the incision sufficiently to pass a grooved director as a guide to the knife. The opening was made large enough to admit the finger, which served as a further guide until the incision was completed. The abdominal viscera being carefully held back, the uterus was brought plainly into view. By rapid strokes, the anterior wall was then divided, beginning at the fundus, and in a line with the external incision, care being taken not to go too deep. A small opening having been made into its cavity, at the upper part of the incision, large enough to admit the finger, this was again used as a guide until the incision was carried four or five inches.

The limbs of the fetus lay open to view; seizing them, I delivered with difficulty, the head being somewhat firmly held in the superior opening of the pelvis. The child being in a state of asphyxia, respiration was established by prompt use of the ordinary measures. The placenta, already detached, immediately followed the delivery of the fetus.

Some blood was lost while incising the uterus, but hardly so much as in ordinary cases of labor. The uterus being cleared of the membranes and its cavity cleansed, the organ contracting held the lips of the incision firmly together; but as a precautionary measure pressure was made on the sides of the uterus, while the peritoneal cavity was sponged, before closing the abdominal incision.

There was no hemorrhage into the peritoneal cavity from the uterine incision after its closure, up to the time of closing the external incision. The latter was closed by five figure of eight sutures, and between each of these was placed a superficial suture, bringing the edges of the skin accurately together. leaving sufficient space below for draining. The dressing was completed by adhesive strips, compress and bandage.

The patient was carefully placed in bed, brandy was freely given, dry friction to the extremities was persevered in, and heat kept constantly applied. Reaction was gradually but completely established, and consciousness soon was fully restored; there was no return of the convulsions after delivery. The operation was performed between the hours of one and two o'clock A. M. Morphiæ sulph., one-eighth of a grain

every four hours, was prescribed, the patient to take no nourishment except rice or barley-water. She was left in the care
of Dr. Voris, who has given me the following history of the
case subsequent to the operation:

"Sept. 11. Called at 12 M.; patient has been comfortable
all morning; complains of headache, also slight after-pains;
pulse 88, skin cool and moist. 5 P. M., pulse 90, skin moist,
after-pains severe, passed urine voluntarily; dose of morphia
increased to one-fourth of a grain. 11 P. M., pulse 94, tympanitis great; on pressure complains mostly of soreness in
left hypogastrium; again passed urine voluntarily; introduced
catheter into rectum, which caused the discharge of a quantity of gas, and rendered her much easier.

"Sept. 12. 4 P. M., patient has rested well since midnight;
vomited this morning; pulse 92, skin very moist; tympanitis
considerable; the catheter was again introduced into rectum,
and gave her great relief.

"Sept. 13. Patient being very comfortable at 7 A. M., I left
promising to return at 11 A. M.; on my arrival at that hour, I
learned that she had commenced vomiting at half past nine,
and died in half an hour. Two women, who were in attendance at the time, stated that the patient, unable to turn herself, was suffocated by the ejected matter, they being incapable of rendering assistance through fright. No autopsy was
obtained."

The house in which the patient resided was a small cabin
with two rooms, standing in the middle of a corn-field. From
the first a favorable result was hardly looked for. Under most
propitious circumstances hysterotomy is one of the gravest of
operations, and the gravity of the prognosis is much increased
when the subject is in such circumstances of comparative des-
titution and without experienced nurses, as was the patient
whose case I have narrated.

JEFFERSONVILLE, IND.

# TRAUMATIC STRICTURE OF THE URETHRA— TREATMENT BY DILATATION—RECOVERY.

BY GEORGE N. MONETTE, M. D.

Isaac P—— called to consult me on account of inability to pass his urine, although an irresistible spasmodic inclination was present.   He had been badly affected with venereal contamination, and at this time, before coming to me, had been deluged for thirty-six hours with all kinds of diuretics and old women's nostrums.

In consideration of his youth I suspected violence of some kind, and upon catechising him ascertained that it was caused while leaping over our street water-plugs, which are about four feet high and boxed about with wood.   One day, in attempting to spring over the plug, he failed and fell astride it, severely contusing the urethral canal, resulting in active hyperæmia of the parts.   I made a gentle attempt to introduce a No. 4 gum catheter, but failed to relieve the bladder, which was greatly distended with urine.   I then directed the patient to go home and take a hot sitz-bath for half an hour. He did so, and on his return the parts were so relaxed that I passed a No. 4 silver catheter without injury, and relieved him of a copious quantity of urine.   I located the obstruction at the prostate gland, and although he suffered greatly from distention of the bladder and strangury, I proceeded leisurely (for fear of making a false passage) to dilate the canal, which gradually yielded.   There was a slight discharge of blood, which I ascribed to transudation.   There was also a tendency to clonic spasms of the canal, which seemed to come on at intervals of fourteen days.   This led me to suspect malaria; so he was treated accordingly, and relieved by antiperiodics.

This case might have recovered ultimately without treatment, if he could have endured the pain of inability to urinate; *au contraire*, it proves the efficiency of gradual dilatation in lesions of the urethral canal.

NEW ORLEANS.

# Reviews.

A Treatise on the Science and Practice of Midwifery. By WILLIAM S.
PLAYFAIR, M. D., etc. With two plates, and one hundred and sixty-six
illustrations on wood. Philadelphia: Henry C. Lea, 1876.

Dr. Playfair, who is the Professor of Obstetrics in King's
College, London, in his preface justly observes that, "Those
who have studied the progress of midwifery know that there
is no department of medicine in which more has been done
of late years, and none in which modern views of practice
differ more widely from, than those prevalent only a short
time ago." Actuated by this view, Dr. Playfair has produced
an admirable book.

We are gratified to find a book on obstetrics not merely
with something new in therapeutics, but with many new
plates, or, at least, if not all new, never associated together
before. The chapters on the female generative organs, and
on ovulation and menstruation, are remarkably good.

In discussing the diseases of pregnancy, the topic of artificial abortion is introduced, and Dr. Playfair advises puncturing the membranes with a uterine sound. This method we
believe is bad, and would much prefer as safer and quicker
the use of tents, and, if necessary, hydrostatic dilators.

Having recently had sent us a case where pregnancy of five
or six months was complicated with cancer of the neck of the
uterus—a case in which able and eminent medical gentlemen
differed as to the expediency of bringing on labor—we turned
with especial interest to the remarks of Dr. Playfair relating
to this subject. He gives the following, as we believe, judicious advice (page 197):

"If we have the opportunity of seeing the patient early in pregnancy, by inducing abortion we may save the mother the dangers of labor at term, possibly of Cæsarian section, if the obstruction is great. Under such circumstances the operation would, no doubt, be justifiable. If the pregnancy has advanced beyond the sixth or seventh month, unless the amount of malignant deposit be very small indeed, it is probable that the risks of labor would be as great to the mother as at term; and it would then be advisable to give her the advantage of the few months delay."

On the subject of anæsthesia in labor, Dr. Playfair speaks of it as "a practice which has become so universal that no argument is required to establish its being a perfectly legitimate means of assuaging the sufferings of child-birth."

As an anæsthetic Dr. Playfair refers favorably to chloral, and gives excellent rules for its administration. In speaking of the inhalation of chloroform he remarks, "If the pains are very materially lessened in force and frequency, it may be necessary to stop the inhalation for a short time, commencing again when the pains get stronger, which effect may be often completely and easily prevented by mixing the chloroform with about one-third of absolute alcohol, which, originally recommended I believe by Dr. Sansom, increases the stimulating effects of the chloroform, and thus diminishes its tendency to produce undue relaxation."

The chapter on puerperal eclampsia is excellent. In speaking of the treatment the author, while not rejecting absolutely venesection, observes that the mortality has been materially diminished since its indiscriminate use has been abandoned. He further remarks: "It does not follow because a remedy, when carried to excess is apt to be hurtful, that it should be discarded altogether; and I have no doubt that, in properly selected cases and judiciously employed, venesection is a valuable aid in the treatment of eclampsia, and that it is specially likely to be useful in mitigating the first violence of the attack, and in giving time for other remedies to come into action. Care should, however, be taken to select the cases properly; and it will be specially indicated when there is marked evidence of great cerebral congestion and vascular tension, such as a livid face, a full bounding pulse, and strong pulsation in the carotids. The general constitution of the patient may also serve as a guide in determining its use, and we shall be more disposed to resort to it if the patient be a strong and healthy woman; while, on the other hand, if she be feeble and weak, we may wisely discard it, and trust entirely to other means. In any case, it must be looked upon as a temporary expedient only, useful in warding off immediate danger to the cerebral tissues, but never as the main agent in treatment. Nor can it be permissible to bleed in the heroic manner frequently recommended; a single bleeding, the amount regulated by the effect produced, is all that is ever likely to be of service."

Few works on obstetrics we have enjoyed the reading of so much as this. We predict for "Playfair" no ordinary success.

***

**A Manual of Midwifery.** By ALFRED MEADOWS, M. D. Second American from the third London edition, revised and enlarged, with one hundred and forty-five illustrations. Philadelphia: Lindsay & Blakiston, 1876.

Let us first heartily commend the form and general appearance of this book.

It is hardly necessary to criticise a book that has been so well received by the profession. The case has been closed, and the verdict rendered, and that verdict is decided approval of the volume. Both for students and practitioners it will prove decidedly useful.

Nevertheless, while finding much to commend, we sometimes find in the work rules of practice that we can not approve; for example, on page 52, the injection of water into the uterus to wash out the ovum in case of abortion. This is a needless risk. We are not surprised to find the author, a sentence or two further on, remarking, "I have seen severe, and in one case fatal, metro-peritonitis result entirely from this simple proceeding." Such an experience ought to more than counterbalance the advice to resort to this treatment.

Nor do we think Dr. Meadows's style incapable of being improved. Such an expression as "we know very little for certain" (page 165) is inelegant, if not incorrect.

Some of the illustrations are bad.

On page 186 we have plate 64, intended to represent the fourth cranial position, but any one who can think it other than the third has sharper optics than ours. Plates 99 and 100 represent the accoucheur attaining the os uteri with the finger passed up over the external surface of the symphysis pubis.

On page 317 we have a description and representation of Dr. Protheroe Smith's apparatus, a sort of harness to be used under certain circumstances by laboring women; and on page 318, we have three female figures nude except as to this Smith device. Some examination has led us to the conclusion, *nothing* could be better.

However the book is a good one, and we hope will continue to have professional favor.

---

On Tracheotomy, especially in relation to Diseases of the Larynx and Trachea. By W. PUGIN THORNTON, Surgeon to the Hospital for Diseases of the Throat, etc. Philadelphia: Lindsay & Blakiston.

Tracheotomy is no longer so dangerous or formidable an operation as it was once regarded, and as indicated by our author is not performed so blindly, as a *dernier ressort*, as formerly; for he says, "since the laryngoscope has come into practical use, any condition of the larynx interfering with respiration can be recognized with certainty and precision, and the desirability of an operation determined."

Dr. Thornton never uses chloroform, but freezes the skin with ether spray; for it is a matter of vital importance that any blood which may run down the trachea be coughed up. He manages children by having them wrapped in a sheet and forcibly held down. He always takes a Faradic battery along to be used in case of suspended respiration. The tube which he prefers to insert after the operation is the Durham or right-angled tube, there being less liability of pressure on the mucous membrane and subsequent ulceration from this, than from the curved tube.

The operation of tracheotomy is treated of very minutely, the author preferring the scalpel to the tracheotome. The dangers during and after tracheotomy are, first, slowness in operating; second, fixing the head too far back; third, passage of blood down into the air passages; fourth, inability to introduce the canula into the trachea; fifth, entrance of air into the veins. The latter part of the book is devoted to diseases and injuries requiring tracheotomy, in which are named eighteen maladies, besides some miscellaneous diseases. The book contains eighteen wood-cuts and three excellent photographs, and is to be recommended as superior to our surgical works for acquiring a knowledge of tracheotomy.    A. M.

---

Micro-Photographs in Histology, Normal and Pathological. By CARL SEILER, M. D. Philadelphia: J. H. Coates & Co. Vol. 1, No. 4. Sixty cents per number.

In the recent International Medical Congress, the discussion of the paper on Microscopy of the Blood raised the old question of the ability of microscopists to distinguish the blood corpuscles of man from those of animals. In this number of the above periodical there is seen, in plate No. XV, a marked difference in size between the blood discs of man and those of the ox. There are also three other plates in this number, namely, hepatic cells from the liver of a fly, leukæmia of the liver, and fat cells from the mesentery of a cat.

**The Student's Guide to Dental Anatomy and Surgery.** By HENRY SEWILL, Member of the Royal College of Surgeons, and Licentiate in Dental Surgery, etc. Philadelphia: Lindsay & Blakiston.

This is a manual, and treats concisely of the anatomy and surgery of the teeth and manipulative dentistry. The cardinal principles of dentistry stand out prominently throughout the work, the author emphasizing the importance of manipulative ability, compared with which theory is easily acquired. In his preface the writer cautiously speaks of the etiology of decay of the teeth, and leaves us to regret that he has not devoted a full chapter to this question. Although a handbook, it treats of dental pathology and therapeutics; and while the student makes it a stepping-stone to more complete works, the practitioner will find in its pages information relative to almost every subject of dental surgery.     J. W. H.

---

**Transactions of the College of Physicians of Philadelphia.** Third Series, Vol. II. Philadelphia, 1876. For sale by Lindsay & Blakiston.

This handsome volume of nearly two hundred pages contains appreciative memoirs of the late Doctors George W. Norris and John S. Parry; a case of empyema, in which cure was effected by Chassaignac's drainage-tube; hepatic abscess, with artificial evacuation and recovery; report on meteorology and epidemics; operative and conservative surgery of the larger joints; excision of the knee in adults; therapeutic uses of compressed and rarefied air; notes on anatomy of the perineum; cases illustrating local injuries of nerves and their trophic consequences; hysterical affections of the eye; gunshot wounds of the thoracic and abdominal cavities; calculous and cystic degeneration of both kidneys; cases of sarcomatous tumor, and case of diabetes insipidus treated by ergot and gallic acid; the authors of these papers, in order, being Doctors Hunt, Ingham, Hutchinson, Hodge, Cleemann, Ashhurst, Hodge, Cohen, Allen, Mitchell, Harlan, Forbes, Morris, Mears and Tyson. This is one of the best of the valuable volumes the Philadel hia Colleɤe has issued.

# Clinic of the Month.

SALICYLIC ACID AS AN ANTISEPTIC.*—These and other experiments, in which proportionally large amounts of ferment were added to fresh grape juice—each fifty cubic centimeters—show, in the most unmistakable way, that the salicylic acid reduced the action of fermentation or prevented it entirely, when a sufficient amount was used; and that when the fermentation had begun, the increase of the salicylic acid slowed it or stopped it entirely according to the proportion. Also that a certain amount of salicylic acid was required to prevent the working of a certain amount of ferment cells. This amount is very small, and is pretty certainly fixed at one hundred grammes of salicylic acid for one thousand liters of grape juice, in active fermentation, to destroy the fermentation entirely and permanently destroy the ferment cells. The salicylic acid works similarly against fungoid vegetation or moulds.

On the 27th of November, fifty cubic centimeters of sweet wine was sowed with the spores of penicilium glaucum; fifty cubic centimeters of the same received 0.0028 grammes of salicylic acid, and in addition the same quantity of the spores; fifty cubic centimeters of the same received the same amount of salicylic acid, but no spores. On the 30th of November, the mould in the first was in full growth, and was seeding on the first of December. In the second there was no growth whatever; the grape juice remained clear, and the mould spores lay poisoned on the surface. The third, which received only salicylic acid, was, on the 15th of December, per-

---

*Continued from the September No. of the American Practitioner, page 184. From the Vierteljahrsschrift für Zahnheilkunde, page 20, 1876. By Prof. H. Humm. Translated from the German by Dr. G. V. Black, Jacksonville, Ill.

fectly clear and pure to the taste, without a trace of fungoid growth of any kind, although it was setting close to a fine growth of mould and uncovered.

The experiments of Newbauer show that as to whether the unfermented wine will ferment sooner or later, or not ferment at all, depends wholly upon the amount of salicylic acid added to it; and that one hundred grammes of the acid to one thousand liters of the wine is sufficient to prevent fermentation entirely, even when ferment is added to it. It is also known that the spores of the ferment are found on the skins of the grapes rather than in the juice, and they may be destroyed there before the grapes are pressed. If we can consider that these propositions are sufficient in the cases mentioned, a very small quantity must be sufficient to prevent any fermentation in the future. Heidenbusch found that new wine, which was in full process of fermentation, was brought to a stand-still by the addition of 8.00 grammes of the acid per one thousand liters. Also that some Trestern wine, which was perfectly clear and one year old, yet on the surface of which flakes of mould continued to form, required four hundred grammes of the acid per one thousand liters, to entirely prevent their formation; two hundred and fifty grammes proved insufficient. From this case Heidenbusch argues that no fixed proportion of the acid can be determined upon with certainty, but that a careful watch is necessary that new additions may be made in case of the reappearance of fermentation or mould. This is on account of the different circumstances, and the different kinds and quantities of ferment or mould spores present, but which can always be controlled by further very slight additions of the acid. The salicylic acid can be depended upon for good results in all the following cases:

First. New wine, in which the fermentation is not quite completed, may be brought to rest at once and be so kept.

Second. In old wine, which has become "sharp" from new fermentation, to again bring it to rest.

Third. In small amounts sent to tropical climates, to prevent renewal of fermentation.

Fourth. In mixtures of different ages and make, to prevent reactions upon each other and consequent refermentation.

Fifth. In small quantities that must stand open or on draught, to prevent mould or souring.

Sixth. In casks which are to be kept in a certain condition, to prevent change and protect them from mould.

Seventh. In old and moulded casks, to render them again fit for service.

In all the foregoing cases a strong alcoholic solution should be used; and as the acid is less soluble in wine, it should be slowly added while the wine is being rapidly stirred.

Newbauer's experiments with wine induced Kolbe to try a series of experiments with beer ferment. He took for this purpose four vessels, each containing five hundred cubic centimeters, of a ten per cent. solution of sugar; in each he placed four grammes of good yeast. To the first he added 0.25 grammes of salicylic acid; to the second, a like quantity of peroxybenzoic acid; to the third, a like quantity of oxybenzoic acid; to the fourth, nothing. These were kept at the temperature of 33° and 35° C. Within six hours fermentation began in all the vessels, except the one containing the salicylic acid, which remained clear, while the others became cloudy and threw off carbonic acid. Again, three vessels in each of which was placed a twelve per cent. solution of grape sugar of one thousand grammes; into each vessel five grammes of good yeast was well stirred. The first received 0.25 grammes of salicylic acid; the second, 0.5 grammes of peroxybenzoic acid; and the third, nothing; and all were covered with paper, and kept at 35° C. In six hours all the solutions were in active fermentation, but the first not so active as the others. The small amount of 0.25 grammes of salicylic acid is, therefore, not sufficient to prevent fermentation being caused by five grammes of yeast in that amount of twelve per cent. solution of sugar. A new quantity was therefore added after six hours, making thirty-five grammes in all. This amount lessened or slowed down the fermentation considerably, but did not stop it entirely; and in four hours more 0.15 grammes were added, after which the fermentation ceased entirely. The next day the liquid was perfectly clear, and the yeast cells lay on the bottom of the vessel; the solution still contained a considerable quantity of sugar, and tasted decidedly sweet.

A. Vögel's experiments with salicylic acid on the germination of seeds are also very interesting. Equal numbers of good cress seeds were placed upon several thicknesses of filter paper. No. 1 was kept wet with distilled water; No. 2, after soaking for half an hour in salicyl water, was placed on the paper and kept wet with distilled water; No. 3 was placed on the paper, and kept wet with salicyl water. In twenty-four hours afterwards No. 1 began to sprout, and the young plants began their development; Nos. 2 and 3 showed no signs whatever of germination, even after a number of days. From this it seems that the salicylic acid hinders the process of germination.

In the use of salicylic acid in medicine, either inwardly or outwardly, there seems no danger of evil results following its use. Kolbe took 1.5 grammes for a number of days together without any evil effect whatever. Fürbinoger, in his experiments in regard to the antiseptic effects of salicylic acid, comes to the conclusion that it has decided power in lowering the temperature, at least when septic fever is present. In his experiments on rabbits, he found it to possess decided antipyrogenic effects. Buss, having found that the salicylic acid had no poisonous effects, even in large doses, although so markedly antiseptic in its qualities, decided to try its antipyrogenic qualities. He states that it proves to be a wonderful antipyrogenic, which, both in its effects and in its relationship with quinia, will in a measure take its place. In doses of from four to eight grammes, according to the intensity of the fever, there are none of the unpleasant effects which are so often occasioned by quinia; collapse and symptoms of intoxication are in no wise to be feared. He has also used it in typhoid fever, erysipelas, acute articular rheumatism, with the best results.

Just here we should say that Firin holds that salicylic acid is the radical of salicin, and that salicin has heretofore been used in intermittent fevers. Especially has Blom made much use of it. (*Medic. Bcobachtungen und Beiträge über die Salicinen ans dem Holländischen. Von Solomon: Potsdam,* 1388.) He used it with good results in intermittents, chronic diarrhœa, consumption, and in the after-treatment of mucus and worm fevers (*Schleim und Wurm Fieber*), and in fevers accompanied with colliquative discharges or excessive sweating. He gave it the preference over quinia, for the reason that it worked no injury to the organs of digestion, nor caused any congestions of the head. In cases of weak stomach, plethoric constitution, etc., he considered it of great value. Wagner and Freiburg say nothing of its antipyrogenic effects in their published reports of their use of it in diphtheria; but we have no reason to suppose that it failed to produce that effect. The epidemic of Frieburg, described by Wagner, was one of great severity, and very many children were lost; many died of common diphtheria, also many from secondary diphtheria of the upper portion of the trachea. (*Kehlkopfdiptheria.*) Wagner at first treated his cases by local and mechanical means, which, according to the investigations of Letzterich, seemed to be indicated. His colleagues employed in part other modes of treatment, but all of them lost a very large per cent. of their cases. The internal use of salicylic acid seems now to have been the best remedy employed, and gave splendid results. For children that could not use a gargle he used 0.15–0.3 grammes, in powder, in water or wine, every two hours; and to those who could use a gargle, he gave the following:

R. Salicylic acid, . . . . 1.5 grammes.
    Alcohol, . . . . . 15.0 "
    Aq. dist., . . . . . 150.0 "

To be used as a gargle every hour. If in this some crystallization should take place, it will be sufficient to shake it before using. In this way Wagner treated fifteen very severe cases without having to regret the loss of a case; also the course of the disease in these cases was very markedly shorter than any of those treated by other means. The lighter cases passed through the course in from three to five days, and very bad cases, in which the local appearances as well as the general symptoms justified an unfavorable prognosis, were generally well in about eight days.

We spoke above of the local use of salicylic acid in water, 1–300. Professor Theirsch has reported a large number of amputations and other large operations (*Sammlung Klinischer Vorträge*, No. 84–85,) which healed readily without fever or swelling, after having been flooded with salicyl water; so that Professor Theirsch feels himself justified in stating that salicylic acid will in the future be very important to the surgeon.

After all this, it is evident that the salicylic acid will become very important to the dental surgeon, for a remedy has long been sought that would perform the office of carbolic acid, thermol acid, etc., without the evil effects, cauterization, bad taste, smell, etc., belonging to them; and now it appears that the salicylic acid will fulfill that office satisfactorily. From my experience it would seem that salicylic acid has an important use in those teeth with dead and decomposing pulps. The decomposing mass in the pulp-chamber and root canals should be removed with suitable instruments, and then the chamber and canals thoroughly washed out with salicyl water. The washing is to be repeated three or four times in as many days, after which the tooth and roots may be filled without any danger of the occurrence of pericementitis. Ostermann uses the salicylic acid in substance in such cases, filling the pulp-chamber with it, and sealing up the cavity temporarily for a few days, afterward removing and filling permanently. Farther experiments by myself have given the best results. Carious teeth, which were exceedingly sensitive but the pulp not yet exposed but nearly so, I washed out thoroughly and repeatedly from two to four days; and then, if the sensitiveness was not abated, I placed salicylic acid in substance in the cavity, sealing it with a temporary filling; at a fixed time this was renewed and the excavating completed, leaving sufficient softened dentine over the pulp to prevent exposure; this part was again covered with salicylic acid and the permanent filling inserted. I have removed fillings, inserted in this manner, after two, three, four and six months, to see what changes had taken place in the condition of the cavity. I found that after two months the softened dentine began to harden, and that after six months this process was so completed that a strong pressure of the plugger could be used over the pulp without evil results. Ostitis, pericemititis, etc., did not occur in any case so treated, although some of the patients were young and very sensitive, and especially liable to inflammatory processes. As fillings I used mostly amalgam, which was afterward partly or wholly replaced by gold. I have now treated about one hundred cases in this manner. We may, therefore, justly say that the salicylic acid is a substance of the utmost importance both to the scientist and the physician, as well as in the arts; and that possibly, through the interest it has awakened in the study of the aromatic combinations, far more important results may yet be arrived at.

Salkowski, of Berlin, is already of the opinion that benzoic acid is a better antiseptic. He has made such a report in the *Berliner Klinische Wochenschrift*, No. 228, 1875. The experiments are mostly with decaying substances containing albumen. These experiments were performed in this wise: eight hundred cubic centimeters of flesh were very finely chopped in water, for the purpose of experiment; half this amount received 0.4 grammes salicylic acid, the other half a like quantity of benzoic acid. They were at first kept at 25° to 30° C. heat, afterward at common room temperature, and the water allowed to evaporate. In one month the portion receiving the salicylic acid was strongly alkaline, smelled badly, was covered with mould, and contained myriads of bacteria; that which received the benzoic acid did not show the same conditions until seventeen days afterward—one month and seventeen days instead of one month: he therefore concludes that benzoic acid possesses far greater power as an antiseptic. Salkowski denies that salicylic acid possesses deodorizing qualities or powers, for the reason that it has no strong chemical affinities, throws down no precipitates, nor has any peculiar smell. When fresh meat, finely chopped or in large pieces, is placed in a strong watery solution of benzoic acid, it will not spoil, and the solution will remain clear and retain the smell of the benzoic acid. For internal administration, as antiseptics or antizymotics, the two acids may be used in like quantities, as they both form salts of soda in the blood. A series of experiments have shown that salicylic acid or the benzoic, either one, will at least entirely stop the motions of bacteria when the solutions containing them are saturated with the acids.

Finally, it must be admitted that the experiments of Professors Salkowski, Lavin and Lhiel, with thymol, salicylic and benzoic acids as disinfectants, are calculated in some slight measure to diminish the hopes first raised by Kolbe's report. But Kolbe's services can never be too highly estimated in that they have given rise to an immense amount of experimenting and study, which have again brought forward and given us a better understanding of thymol and benzoic acid, and the whole series of aromatic combinations.

A New Method of Wound Drainage.—In the Edinburgh Medical Journal for September, John Chiene, F. R. C. S., F. R. S. E., Assistant Surgeon Edinburgh Royal Infirmary, etc., thus speaks on this important subject:

Acknowledging the undoubted advantages of the drainage-tube as regards efficiency, I have long felt its disadvantages; for instance, its interference with rapid healing throughout the whole extent of the wound; the irritation it not unfrequently caused by its presence as a foreign body; the blackening of the protective, showing that irritating compounds were always present in the rubber, however pure; the tendency to regurgitation of air along the elastic tube during the dressing, thereby increasing the danger of mischief passing into the depths of of the wound; the necessity of dressing a case solely in order to shorten the tube; and the impossibility of being able properly to estimate the rate at which this should be done. These are self-evident evils, and their removal has for some time occupied my attention. It may also be observed that a tubular drain is not an essential to efficient drainage. The draining-tube acts when blocked, the discharge passing along the outside of the tube and soaking through the blood-clot or granulations which so frequently fill its cavity. I have myself seen old field-drains when lifted filled with vegetable growths and still acting perfectly, the water making its way through the obstruction or along the outer surface of the hollow tiles. To observe how carelessly drainers lay the hollow tiles, leaving often considerable intervals between each, is further proof, if need be, of the continuity of the tubing not being a necessity. I have lately been informed that, in out-of-the-way places in Scotland where drain-tiles are not easily obtained, branches of trees are laid in their stead, and act efficiently in draining moist lands.

The old method of drainage by bringing the silk ligatures out at the corners of the wound, or at an opening made specially for the purpose, as was Mr. Syme's practice in the ankle-joint amputation, encouraged me to hope that advantage might be taken of the phenomena of capillarity in order to effect a thorough drain. The further advantage of utilizing capillary forces was apparent, that, inasmuch as they act in opposition to gravity, it would not be necessary to have the outlet of the drain dependent.

During last Christmas holidays, Mr. Callender, of St. Bartholomew's Hospital, London, when on a visit to this city, informed me that he had stitched together the ends of the drainage-tubes with a catgut stitch, in order to keep them in position for the first three or four days, when the catgut became absorbed, and then the tubing could be gradually removed. The idea then struck me—Why not make the entire drain of catgut instead of gutta percha? If efficient, its advantages in being absorbable were apparent. This might be done in two ways: either by bringing the catgut ligatures out at the corners of the wound instead of cutting them short; or by passing a skein of catgut through the cavity of the wound before stitching it up. I have made trial of the latter plan.

The first case on which I tried it was Mrs. M., on whom it was necessary to amputate by Carden's method at the knee-joint in consequence of a recurrent sarcoma of the tibia. The operation was performed on the 20th of April, 1876. In this case I carried a skein of thick catgut of eighteen threads through the stump, bringing the ends out at the corners of the wound. I passed two rings of drainage-tubing, each half an inch in length, on to the skein, and placed them in position at the outlets of the catgut drain. My object in doing this was that I did not like, on the first trial, to depend entirely on the skein. This drain acted perfectly. The rings were removed on the third day. On the seventh day, after the greater part of the wound was consolidated, and after the incision had healed by the first intention, except at the corners where the ends of the drain issued, I failed in the antiseptic management of the case, and putrefaction occurred, spreading rapidly along the catgut drain, which soon rotted, and was removed on the tenth day. During the time the drain was in position no tension whatever occurred. This case convinced me that further trial was justifiable, and that capillarity was sufficient to carry off the discharges.

The next case was one of amputation at the ankle-joint. J. B., admitted on the 2t5h of May, a railway truck having run over his right foot, crushing it, and necessitating amputation. In this case I made a counter opening in the posterior and inferior surface of the flap, and, tying at its center a skein of the finest gut of twenty-four threads with a thread of catgut, I divided it into three equal parts and brought one-third out at each corner of the wound, and the remaining third out at the artificial opening. I then placed in position at the inferior outlet a ring of tubing, omitting it at the other two. The object of this triple arrangement was to test the necessity for tubing at the outlets. I found by the staining on the gauze that free drainage was established at all three openings, showing that the tubing was unnecessary, and that in future entire dependence might be placed on the skein. The tubing was removed on the third day. The ends of the skein became loose between the sixth and tenth days. I am not able to fix the exact date, as the deep dressing was not changed between the sixth and tenth days; on the sixth day the ends of the drain were firmly attached; on the tenth day they were lying loose on the dressing. The stump on the tenth day was firmly consolidated, union by first intention occurring throughout the whole extent of the wound.

The next case on which it was used was an excision of the knee. P. F., operated on on the 31st of May for osseous angular anchylosis, the result of a wound of the knee-joint a year previously. In this case a skein of thirty-two threads of medium gut was passed behind the bones, and a skein of sixteen threads in front of the bones, and the ends of both skeins brought out at the corners of the wound. The anterior skein was stitched with a thread of chromic acid gut to the tissues over the femur in order to prevent its displacement. The ends of the drains fell off on the twelfth day. The incision healed by the first intention, except at the corners, from which a slight serous discharge of a yellowish color continued until the twenty-fifth day at the outer corner, until the thirtieth day at the inner corner. Small portions of the gut came away during the period between the twelfth and thirtieth day; and I am of opinion that, in this case, too thick a drain was used, and that, although absorption removed the greater part of the drain, the quantity of gut was in such excess that some came away on the discharge, and prevented the healing of the corners of the wound at a much earlier period. The wound is now firmly healed.

Another case on which I tried the method was one in which it was necessary to remove a small fatty tumor from the subcutaneous tissue of the upper part of the forearm. In this wound, a small one, I laid two threads of catgut along the wound, bringing them out at the corners before stitching up. In the same patient it was necessary also to remove a painful neuroma over the lower end of the ulna. The depth of the wound was considerable, as compared with its superficial extent; in it I stitched with chromic acid gut the drain to the bottom of the wound, bringing the ends out at one corner of the wound. The dressing was reapplied on the second day, and again on the fourth day, when the stitches were removed. The patient was sent home on that day with the drains still in position, and acting efficiently. She returned on the fourteenth day after the operation, when, on removing the dressing, the wounds were healed, the drains having dropped off in the interval. This case illustrates two things: first, the necessity of stitching the drain to the bottom of a deep wound in order to retain it in position; second, that the use of this method materially lessened the number of the dressings, and necessarily the expense; and, further, that the stay of the patient in hospital until the wound was healed was not necessary. These cases are sufficient to illustrate the advantages of this method of drainage by catgut. It is still on its trial, and my thanks are specially due to Mr. Lister, who has kindly put it to further and more extensive test.

The number of threads necessary in each skein will depend on the size and importance of the wound. As I have already said, too large a quantity was used in the case of excision of the knee. In a large wound, as far as I am at present able to judge, eight to sixteen threads should be sufficient in each skein; the number of the skeins depending on the shape and size of the wound. In cases in which very profuse discharge is expected, either in a specially large wound or after a tedious operation, in which the wounded surface is necessarily exposed for a considerable time to the irritation of the carbolic spray, it will be better to increase the number of separate skeins, stitching them to different parts of the wounded surfaces in order to keep them in position, than to depend on one or two thick skeins. I am led to form this opinion from the result in the case of excision of the knee. If it is ever necessary to use a skein of more than sixteen threads, one thread of catgut prepared in chromic acid should be added to act as a drain, if required, during the absorption and molecular disintegration of the drain. Chromic acid gut should also be used to stitch the drain in position when such a procedure is necessary. As regards the thickness of the gut, I have used three thicknesses. The finer the gut the more numerous and the smaller will be the capillary tubes between the threads. The fineness of the gut will not interfere with the capillary action through the threads. For these reasons, I am of opinion that the finest gut should be used; by its use, the better will be the drain for any given thickness of skein. It may be a question how much of the action is due to capillarity through and between the threads, and how much to the drain acting as a lead to the discharges. Capillarity has, I believe, the chief place. I have hitherto used the gut prepared in the usual way by soaking in carbolic oil. Simple soaking of the drain in carbolic lotion for a quarter of an hour before using will be sufficient in cases in which prepared gut is not at hand.

As long as the drain is acting, there will be a current of fluid along and around the threads (as well as in them), separating them from the living tissue, by means of which the process of absorption mainly takes place. When the flow ceases, then absorption of the column of fluid will first take place, the living walls of the canal will then reach the threads, and absorption will then commence. If this is a true explanation of what happens, then it is evident that it will not be necessary to use catgut specially prepared (as Mr. Lister has shown by chromic acid,) in order to delay absorption.

CHLORAL AND TINCTURE OF EUCALYPTUS IN CANCER OF THE UTERUS.—In the *Gazette Obstétricale*, September 5th, chloral and tincture of eucalyptus, dissolved in water, are strongly recommended as an injection in cases of uterine cancer. From a half to one gramme of chloral, and from one to two grammes of the tincture, are dissolved in five hundred grammes of water, and this injection used daily. The results are diminution of pain, of hemorrhage, and of the serous discharge, and improvement in the general condition.

ELEPHANTIASIS OF THE FEMALE GENITALIA.—The following is the report of an unusual form of elephantiasis, the writer remarking that it is the first time in his practice of forty-three years that he has had the opportunity of observing this rare disease:

Johanna S——, aged twenty-nine years, had suffered in her childhood with the general diseases of that age, also from a slight rachitis and from granulations. She menstruated when eleven years old, and gives no history of syphilis. As early as her eighteenth year she gave birth without special fatigue or trouble. In her twenty-third year she gave birth a second time, at which time labor was difficult and had to be terminated with forceps. According to the statement of the patient, the pressure of one of the blades of the forceps must have given rise to her subsequent affliction.* Some time after her confinement, her companion, who lay in a bed next to her, noticed a swelling of her genitalia, on account of which she was brought as a so-called syphilitic to the hospital in Wurzburg, where, from its description, they recognized the true nature of her extensive trouble. There she constantly refused to allow this large tumor, hanging down from the right inner labia, to be removed. In spite of this she visited the clinic several times, the students promising a recompense in case she should give her consent thereto. In the summer of 1875 she lay in the hospital here for many weeks with typhoid fever, but still objected to the operation.

On the 13th of December she again came to our institution, presenting the following condition: She appeared emaciated and broken down in health. The external labia were swollen to a high degree, resembling œdema, and standing apart posteriorly. Beneath them stood out prominently, from the inner labia of both sides, bulbous excrescences which were surrounded with a row of warts; these warts were also upon the buttocks. Just outside of the right inner lip, and from its uppermost part, a tumor projected down over the vulva,

---

* Schroeder, in his treatise on Diseases of Women, page 502, remarks that bruises and thrusts occasionally give rise to elephantiasis.

which was seven and one-fourth centimeters long, four and one-fourth centimeters wide, and three centimeters thick.* Its surface resembled neat's tongue, and in shape was a little like a dog's ear. The speculum could be introduced only with difficulty between the parts and into the vagina. The os uteri stood high and was reddened; the cervical canal was narrow, and the walls of the vagina smooth. In general no anomaly of the internal genitalia was apparent, except some leucorrhœa from the uterus. When near her a badly-smelling chocolate-colored efflux was seen about the nates, and so an examination was made per rectum. The examining finger, about two and a half inches above the anus, pushed against a stricture, through which the end of the finger could be squeezed only with difficulty. By the way, it is to be noted that the patient had had for a long time sluggish movements from her bowels, and passed, with considerable straining, fæces similar to those of a sheep. The walls of the rest of the rectum were smooth. There was not found upon the body any signs of an affliction similar to that upon the external genitals. The inguinal glands were not swollen. The patient had not menstruated for three years.

On the 15th of January, 1876, the swelling projecting over the pudenda was excised with a knife, afterwards the root or pedicle was ligated with a thread. Its weight was sixty-five grammes.† The operation was endured very well. The hemorrhage was insignificant. A microscopical examination confirmed the previous clinical diagnosis, as there was found in the tumor hypertrophied tissue, and the chief characteristics of elephantiasis. The stricture of the rectum was easily distended with the finger, so that in a few days the normal lumen was again pretty well established. The treatment in this case had been somewhat of an experiment. On the 14th of January, the patient was discharged from our institution improved some in general health. (Memorabil., July, 1876.)

* One centimeter is equal to about four lines.

† One gramme is equal to about fifteen grains.

CURE OF STRANGULATED INGUINAL HERNIA.—Dr. Henry Blanc, Surgeon-Major of the Indian Army, Bombay, (Lancet, September 2), gives the following details:

Heerjebhai N——, a Parsee, fifty-two years of age, but looking much older, weak and somewhat emaciated, was admitted into the clinical surgical ward on July 15th for strangulated inguinal hernia of the right side. The patient states that the hernia first made its appearance some five years ago; it was small and reducible, and he always wore a truss. On the morning of July 14th, whilst straining at stool, he felt a sudden sharp pain in the hernia, and, on rising, found that it had somewhat increased in size, and that he was unable to reduce it.

*Condition on Admission.*—11 A. M.: The hernia, situated in the right groin, and extending to the upper part of the scrotum, is elongated, tense, and the seat of pain on pressure; the surrounding tissues are normal. The pulse is small and compressible, the face anxious, the eyes deep set, and the skin somewhat clammy. Temperature in axilla 99°. No motion since yesterday morning. The patient suffered from nausea and eructations yesterday evening, and during the night and to-day vomiting has been frequent; the vomited matters are at present watery and tinged with bile; they are not stercoraceous. Taxis has been tried this morning by a native practitioner, but according to the patient's account much force was not used; the manipulations provoked such excessive pain that he would not allow them to be continued, and was taken to the hospital at his own request. An ice-bag was placed over the tumor, and pieces of ice given him to suck; he was also ordered a belladonna suppository. 3 P. M.: The general and local conditions are very much the same as four hours before. Previous to administering chloroform, the patient was told that should taxis fail, advantage would be taken of the anæsthetic about to be given to proceed at once to operate. The patient positively refused to submit to the operation of herniotomy, and before inhaling the chloroform made me promise that, should taxis fail, I would not perform the other operation. Under chloroform taxis was tried, but a minute of gentle manipulations showed the uselessness of the proceeding in this case. The hernial tumor felt very tense, giving above on percussion a slight resonant sound, and to the hand the feeling of a collection of fluid tightly compressed. Not being allowed to operate, and taking into consideration the character of the strangulated hernia, I decided on puncturing it. I introduced into the hernia the finest trocar of the aspirator, and with this instrument withdrew about an ounce of slightly turbid, amber-yellow serum and a large quantity of gases. On withdrawing the canula, the hernia slipped back into the abdomen with the greatest ease. Ordered half a drachm of tincture of opium, a grain of opium every third hour until its effects were manifest, fomentations to the abdomen, ice to be sucked, and milk and broth diet.

July 16th. The patient passed a good night. The bowels have been moved twice. Complains of no pain in the abdomen; feels well. Temperature in axilla 98.5°; pulse 84, of a fair volume.

The case progressed most favorably; not a single bad symptom showed itself. The opium was discontinued the second day. Liquid diet alone was allowed for a few days, when more substantial food was permitted. On the 24th he was discharged.

FORMATION OF EPIDERMIS BY THE TRANSPLANTING OF HAIRS. Dr. Schweininger, (*Vierteljahr. für die prak. Heilk.*, Erster Band, 1876,) reports successful results in inducing cicatrization by transplanting to granulating surfaces hairs pulled out by the roots. Placed upon ulcers they formed as many centers of new epithelial growth, which spread outwards, coalesced, and produced rapid and complete cicatrization. These islands proceeded without doubt from the cells of the outer root sheath, which is continuous with the epidermal cells of the rete mucosum, so that epithelium is here developed from preëxisting epithelial cells. (Boston Med. and Surg. Jour.)

DIPHTHERIA OF THE VAGINA IN AN INFANT.—M. Orth, *Gazette Obstétricale*, communicated to the Obstetrical Society of Berlin an interesting case of diphtheria, the subject being a year and eleven months old. The labia majóra were swelled, and the whole vaginal mucous membrane covered with a grayish exsudate. Eyes slightly inflamed but not the least diphtheritic covering. On the other hand the kidneys were swelled, and there were hemorrhages in the mesentery and other organs. M. Orth admits that the genital organs were the seat of a mechanical injury, and that this was the point of departure of the diphtheritic process.

SUB-PERIOSTEAL EXTIRPATION OF THE OS CALCIS.—M. Ollier, *Archives Générales*, September, read a paper before the Paris Academy of Medicine upon extirpation of the os calcis by the sub-periosteal method. His conclusion is that by this method in young subjects regeneration of the bone takes place. The form will depend upon the shape of the periosteal sheath preserved. The ossification may continue a long time after the healing of the wound under the influence of pressure or friction in the exercise of the foot. At the same time the functions are established according to the normal type.

EMMENAGOGUE PILL.—An emmenagogue pill (*Union Médicale*) may be made by adding to fifteen grains of aloes seven and a half grains each of rue, saffron and savin, the whole to be divided into ten pills. One of these pills is to be taken morning and evening, commencing two or three days before the supposed menstrual epoch. Warm hip-baths, dry cups to the lumbar region and to the inferior extremities, leeches to the upper and inner portion of the thighs, and exercise in walking. In the menstrual intervals, give iron and quinia.

LINIMENT TO REPRESS THE SECRETION OF MILK.—This liniment, *Ibid*, is made of six parts each of the tinctures of black pepper and of bergamot, and two and a half parts of camphor with eighteen of castor-oil. The breasts are rubbed with it three times a day.

# 𝕹otes and 𝕼ueries.

THE CENTENNIAL MEDICAL CONGRESS.—The First American International Congress, a grand thought more than a year ago of a number of the Philadelphia profession, has been held. The Congress was designed especially to commemorate the advances made in the United States by the various departments of Medicine during the century just closed. Thus the Centennial Commission directed, and one of the shallowest of criticisms we have seen made was that so many of the addresses were restricted to American work.

To say that the Congress was a great success is no extravagance. Commencing its labors on Monday, September 4th, it continued during the week. General meetings, at which addresses were delivered, and other business transacted, were held in the mornings, and then, after an hour for lunch, the various sections met, and spent from three to four hours in good solid work.

Upwards of four hundred and forty delegates were enrolled, and while, of course, the majority were from the United States, yet the foreigners numbered more than one hundred. Such a medical assemblage has never taken place in this country, rarely in the world. You could scarcely occupy a seat anywhere in the hall where the general meetings were held without being near one or more who had done something famous in a professional way, and whose names are familiar to the profession. There was Paul F. Eve, with his giant form, his snow-white hair, past his three-score-and-ten years, but with no tremulousness of age in his clear, ringing voice, and no abatement of kindly feeling in the hearty grasp of his hand. There was Lunsford P. Yandell, with his iron-gray hair, his keen, penetrating eye, and his suave, cordial manners, who was engaged in medical teaching more than half a century ago. There was Henry F. Campbell, of Georgia, rotund of form, of restless activity, and ready of speech in any department of medicine; Chaillé, of New Orleans, whose brilliant address won such general praise; and Richardson, too, so widely known and so greatly honored as surgeon, as writer and as teacher; there was Dunlap, of Ohio, the great ovariotomist, who will die talking of his last extraordinary case, or of ligating the pedicle or of draining the peritoneum; Brodie, of Michigan, a little more silver appearing upon his closely cropped head, but active in mind and body as he was when the American Medical Association last met in Detroit; Skillman, of Lexington, Ky., a whole-souled, noble man; Kinloch, of South Carolina, so well known in the department of surgery; Hunter McGuire, of Virginia, honored son of an honored sire; Hodgen, of St. Louis, with his black eyes and swarthy face. New York sent her Austin Flint, whose black whiskers, sprinkled with gray, look as if some prankish boy had dashed snow on them; her Austin Flint, junior, whose head looks big enough to hold half a dozen more physiologies, and face broad and benevolent enough to establish as many hospitals; she also sent Fordyce Barker, Peaslee, Post, John P. White, Bumstead, John C. Dalton, Sayre, Van Buren, E. M. Moore, Gouley, Lusk, and John P. Gray. New England was represented by Bowditch, William Warren Greene; the famous ovariotomist, Kimball of Lowell; J. B. S. Jackson, Isaac G. Porter, and Edwin M. Snow. Ohio had not only Dunlap, but Williams, Bartholow, Hamilton, Wormley, Pooley, Gordon and others. Indiana had among her representatives those veterans Dr. George W. Mears and Dr. George Sutton. The United States Army had, as two of its representatives, Woodward, whom every one knows, and Billings, whose work in connection with the Surgeon-General's library is placing the profession of this country under such great obligations. Pennsylvania had her Samuel D. Gross, one of the noblest-looking men any profession in any age has produced, presiding over the deliberations of the Congress with the dignity and grace which seem a part of his nature; she also had the Atlees, Drysdale, DaCosta, Traill Green, Hartshorne, Hewson, Keen, Kirkbride, James Aitken Meigs, Pollock, Packard, Albert H. Smith, Francis G. Smith, Wister and Wood. Illinois had that true representative of American Medicine, N. S. Davis. Washington City had Toner and Busey; may their shadows never grow less, though that of the former might without marring its beauty!

But what of our foreign representatives? There was Robert Barnes, not a Beau Brummel in dress, or a Chesterfield in manners, not a bit of austere dignity, but frank, out-spoken, and when he did speak, as in the obstetrical section, over which he presided, speaking plainly, pointedly and most instructively, and apparently caring very little for the manner of utterance. His head is large, quite high, and bald above, while the sides have a profusion of brown hair; his face has the ruddy hue of one who knows the virtues of good beef and porter. Alexander R. Simpson,* the able successor of Sir James in the University of Edinburgh, does not in the least look like his illustrious uncle did, but is tall, slender in form, with long jet-black hair, and his face, with prominent nose, is thin and seems weary with work, or worn with sorrow. He speaks deliberately, plainly and practically. His age is about forty-three. Lister is older, and looks it too, as his hair is quite gray, and his form has more fullness — more fat, in plain English. His complexion is somewhat ruddy, but the ruddiness hidden by a sort of faint white tinge, just like a field of red clay that has been sprinkled with snow. A member of the Society of Friends by birth and early education, his manner is simple, artless, modest, and were one of the society to meet him, and address him as Joseph, it would not surprise you in the least. Brunton, of the London Prac-

---

* Professor Simpson is a man active and earnest in all religious efforts. On the Sabbath before the meeting of the Congress, he addressed a large audience in one of the Philadelphia churches upon medical missions. His address, though not marked by any special oratorical powers, was exceedingly interesting, and was very well received.

titioner, is short, very slight in form, light hair, heavy beard; he is about as tall as Professor Holland of the Louisville University, but more slender, and does not look as old. Adams, of London, with his large bald head, dignified manners, might pass for a college president, or an Episcopalian minister. Joliffe Tufnell,\* of Dublin, was one of the most notable men in the Congress, tall, of large frame, one who would be not less dangerous in a physical struggle than he has been successful in the treatment of aneurism. The handsomest face at the Congress, delicate, perfectly proportioned, as if chiselled in marble, was that of Hingston, of Montreal. But we have no time for further allusions to the *personnel* of the Congress.

Seventy papers were read in the various sections, and of course it would be impossible in the space we have to mention them all, still more to even allude to the discussions many of them elicited. We give the following extract from the Philadelphia Medical Times of September 16th, heartily hoping that every subscriber who was not a member of the Congress, will avail himself of the opportunity indicated in the last sentence: "The addresses were, on the whole, very satisfactory, and many of the papers of much value. These memoirs, with the discussions and conclusions reached, concern some of the most vital practical questions in modern medicine; and, since they in a great measure express the conclusions of the larger proportion of the best medical minds of the country, one would think that almost every physician in the United States would desire to acquire the record. Once in a century is not oftener than once in a lifetime; and certainly most of our readers can afford seven dollars for this bibliographical souvenir of our country's prosperity."†

\* A friend gave me an amusing scene he had witnessed on the corner of Chestnut and Fifth streets, in which Tufnell was the chief speaker. A policeman had ordered a street *gamin* from the curb-stone, Tufnell happening along just at the time, remonstrated, alleging that this was a free country, the boy had a right to his seat, etc.; and kept on some little time "chaffing" the policeman, greatly to the delight of the crowd that had collected.

† Subscriptions should be sent to Dr. Caspar Wister, 1303 Arch street, Philadelphia.

One reason for the marked success of the Congress was the admirably constructed machinery; it worked perfectly. Those gentlemen in Philadelphia who had the devising and arranging of it, deserve the best professional thanks.

Only one thing in the action of the Congress is deserving of adverse and severe criticism, and that was the resolution offered by Dr. Eve forbidding the publication of any of its proceedings, papers, etc., in any medical journal. Dr. Eve's good nature allowed him to be imposed upon in this matter. The resolution, so it was privately whispered in Philadelphia, was offered in the interest of a medical journal whose editor had failed to have any reports prepared, when it was found other journals were having such reports in preparation. Just as soon as the matter was generally understood, there was a feeling that would have secured the reconsideration and repeal of the resolution, only it was thought best simply to let the matter pass in silence, and act as if no such resolution had ever been. The New York Medical Record has shown the absurdity and uselessness of the action, and it is about time such nonsense should be stopped in intelligent medical bodies.

Well, the Congress has become a thing of the past, but the pleasure it afforded those who were members will abide in all their memories; and let us trust that its volume of Transactions will contribute much to medical knowledge, and be an enduring monument to the glory of American medicine.

AMERICAN GYNECOLOGICAL SOCIETY.—This society held its first annual meeting in the Hall of the New York Academy of Medicine, on the 13th, 14th and 15th of September. The attendance was large, including most of the members of the society, and many besides, chiefly from New York City. The papers read were interesting, as well as the discussions elicited by them. Among the most valuable of these papers were those by Drs. Robert Barnes, Emmet and Nœggerath. About twenty papers in all were presented; these, with the admirable inaugural address of the president, Dr. Fordyce Barker, will constitute a most valuable volume.

The society elected as honorary fellows only two Americans, and they were Drs. M. B. Wright, of Cincinnati, and Joseph Eve, of Augusta, Ga. The honor was most worthily bestowed. Dr. Wright is too well known to our readers for us to say a word in reference to him; and Dr. Eve is probably the oldest teacher of obstetrics in the United States, having commenced his work nearly forty years ago.

The next meeting of the society will be held in Boston, the last week of May, 1877.

CHICAGO AND THE AMERICAN MEDICAL ASSOCIATION.—We hope the gentlemen in Chicago having in charge the arrangements for the next meeting of the American Medical Association will take a few hints from the management of the International Congress. Give us a printed list of members, and a programme of each day's work. Give us a building in which both general and sectional meetings can be held, and have only an hour intervening between the former and the latter. And in order for the last, arrange for a lunch at one P. M., so that the members will not be scattered off to their hotels or homes, losing two or three hours, or else their dinners, and returning to their afternoon work late, irregularly, tired or stupid.

THE TRANSACTIONS OF THE STATE MEDICAL SOCIETY OF INDIANA FOR 1876.—We acknowledge the receipt of this handsome volume, and commend the Secretary for its prompt appearance. The book is, comparing it with past volumes, singularly free from typographical errors, though still there are too many. Next month we hope to have a review of it from the pen of one of the ablest of American writers.

INDIANA, ILLINOIS AND KENTUCKY TRI-STATE MEDICAL SOCIETY.—The second annual meeting of this society will be held in the city of Vincennes, Ind., November 21, 1876. Prof. Byford, of Chicago, will deliver the opening address.

G. W. BURTON, Rec. Sec'y.

PHILADELPHIA CORRESPONDENCE OF THE BOSTON MEDICAL AND SURGICAL JOURNAL.—We find in the Boston Medical and Surgical Journal of September 21st, an interesting letter as to the International Congress. We give the concluding portion of this letter:

The social side of the congress included the reception given by the physicians of Philadelphia on Monday evening, the very elegant and hospitable receptions given by Drs. Wilson and Thompson on Tuesday evening, by Dr. George Strawbridge on Wednesday evening, and by H. C. Lea and J. B. Lippincott on Thursday. Besides, scores of private dinners were given. Hospitality was lavishly bestowed.

The grand subscription dinner on Friday night was as enjoyable and as successful as every other feature of the congress had been. Professor Gross sat at the head of the central table; Mr. Lister sat on his right, supported by General Hawley; on his left sat Governor Hartranft, supported by Adams, of London. After the company of two hundred had discussed an excellent dinner, Professor Gross called for responses to several appropriate toasts. The speakers were Lister, Adams, Governor Hartranft, General Hawley, Professors Stillé, Dalton, Chaillé, Dr. Woodward, and Professor Hjort, of Norway. All were eloquent. I wish I might make quotations; suffice it to say that the foreign speakers expressed the warmest satisfaction with the results of the congress, their sense of personal benefit, their surprise at the forwardness of medicine in America, and their gratitude for generous hospitality.

The closing meeting Saturday forenoon was marked by a general expression of fraternal feeling of pleasure in the splendid success of the congress, intermingled with good wishes and cordial farewells.

In boyhood's days, after the wearying, delightful pleasures of a Fourth of July, what one of us but wished the day might be enjoyed all over again? Such, it struck me, was the general feeling at the close of the most memorable medical union in our history.

To the Presidents and Secretaries of Sections, American Medical Association, 1877.—*Gentlemen:* Permit a suggestion—would it not be well for you to see that each of your sections shall have an ample supply of good papers? Do not trust to spontaneous generation for material for the work of sections, but by immediate correspondence with those who are qualified, and whose writings will attract and instruct, secure contributions of suitable variety, length and interest. Efforts of this kind can make the Chicago meeting of the Association as marked a success as was the American International Congress.

An Omission and an Error.—The Clinic, of Cincinnati, September 23d, contained an extract headed "Diseases necessary to human happiness," credited to *The Doctor.* If it will refer to the American Practitioner of June last, it will find that extract as part of a notice of, with extracts from, a manuscript copy of Rush's Lectures, and a quotation from St. George Mivart following the last extract. An omission to read the Practitioner has led it into an error.

An Apology.—We regret exceedingly the tone of Dr. Bartholow's communication in the last number of our journal. He has done himself injury, if not injustice. A printer's error should not cause such denunciation against a writer of the character and integrity of Dr. Wm. Carson. A sufficient study of rhetoric to avoid using the coarse slang "hefty," would be an excellent thing for one of Dr. Bartholow's position and reputation.

# THE AMERICAN PRACTITIONER.

## NOVEMBER, 1876.

Certainly it is excellent discipline for an author to feel that he must say all that he has to say in the fewest possible words, or his reader is sure to skip them; and in the plainest possible words, or his reader will certainly misunderstand them. Generally, also, a downright fact may be told in a plain way; and we want downright facts at present more than any thing else —RUSKIN.

## Original Communications.

## SPECIALISM IN MEDICINE.*

### BY E. D. FORÉE, M. D.

*Professor of Diseases peculiar to Women in the Hospital College of Medicine, Louisville, Ky.*

In the organization of the medical department of Central University, the chair of diseases peculiar to women was established, and he who now addresses you was designated for the place. By this appointment and its acceptance I have become, in fashionable parlance, a specialist. Being so recognized and acknowledged, I shall claim the privilege inherent to the position of using the time allotted to this, our first interview, of offering a few thoughts upon medical specialism, which is now prevalent and rapidly increasing.

You will learn, as you progress in the profession, that *Fashion*, that inexorable tyrant, extends its sway over medicine to a more presumptive limit than over any other science,

* From a lecture delivered by Dr. E. D. Forée, before the class inaugurating his annual course of instructions, September 21, 1876.

excepting, perhaps, the social science alone; and that he who runs counter to it does so at his personal hazard, and may be chargeable with undue temerity. Nevertheless, having become convinced, by ample observation, that the fashion of splitting up the art of medicine into innumerable parts is fraught with mischief to the people, is subversive of the interests of the physician, and retards the progress of the science itself, I shall venture to discuss it in its various bearings.

Specialism in medicine is the outgrowth of the half century just ending. Prior to that there was no division of practice, except into the two great branches of surgery and general practice; and these even were so intimately blended that it was only as a medical man of general and thorough acquirement betrayed the greater aptitude and skill for either branch did he become a devotee to medicine or surgery. For example, our own Physic having made himself a finished anatomist and physiologist, and having learned well the rudiments of all other departments, then by a ripe clinical experience, running through many years, having won distinction in both medicine and surgery, yet excelling in the latter he had surgical practice thrust upon him to such an extent that he had no time to give to other departments of practice. In this way he became a practitioner of surgery alone.

Dr. Gross, who by general consent is styled the Nestor of American surgery, whom we in our city delight to honor, and whose name is familiar to enlightened physicians everywhere, was an assiduous student of general medicine; anatomy, physiology, pathology, therapeutics, histology, indeed all of elementary medicine alike, engaged his earnest attention. Then he sought clinical experience in every department of practice; and not till after he was forty years old, and had accumulated a large experience in the art of recognizing and treating all classes of disease, did he become an exclusive practitioner of surgery.

Simpson, of Edinburgh, having become learned in every branch of medical science and obtained a large clinical experience in both hospital and private practice, was appointed Professor of Obstetrics in the University of Edinburgh. This accident gave the direction of his great mind to the study of the diseases of women. Very soon his achievements in this direction were found to be so grand, and gynecological practice accumulated upon him so largely, that he was compelled to become an exclusive practitioner—a specialist.

In like manner Hewitt, Barnes, Spencer Wells, and others, of Great Britain, Sims, Emmet, Thomas, Peaslee, and many others, of our eastern seaboard, have been driven into specialism. So also did our own lamented Miller, after having acquired a most thorough knowledge of the whole science, and a rich clinical experience in general practice, become a specialist, not by choice but because it was thrust upon him.

Ricord, of Paris, whose education and enlarged observation of diseases qualified him for any and all branches of practice, became a specialist because his saloons were so crowded with subjects of venereal diseases that he had not a moment for any other practice.

Civiale, of Paris, and Sir Henry Thompson, of London, both ripe medical scholars and replete with general experience, became, after they had each reached the zenith of their manhood, the practitioners of their specialty.

Von Gräfe, Bader, Schalber, Stellwag, Politzer, Sichel, Toynbee, Carter and Wilde, of Europe, Agnew, Jeffries, Williams, Loring and Roosa, of our own country—all distinguished for their thoroughness in all departments of medical learning, and having had extensive and enlightened clinical experience, gained deservedly high reputations as ophthalmologists or aurists, or both—devoted themselves especially to diseases of the eye and ear. So I might mention a host of others who are working in special fields, and who are accomplishing great good for medicine and for the public.

Of this class of specialists I can not speak in too high commendation. In them we have many of the most renowned members of our profession, and persons who have contributed most liberally to the progress of our science. They are men who have grown into specialties through great mental training, who have become proficients in all medical learning, and though found in devotion to diseases of a single organ, or of one set of organs, would be fully competent to investigate and treat almost all the diseases to which our frail forms are liable. It is the success of such men which has awakened the ambition of some and aroused the cupidity of others, and thus become the origin of, and the impetus to, the prevalent and increasing fashion of the day to divide the practice of medicine, aye, not merely the practice but unfortunately the study of medicine also, into infinitessimal parts. Men, seeing the reputations made and the large honorariums gained by such distinguished exclusivists, are led into the effort to become specialists also, and that with but little *study*, no personal aptitude, and with scant underlying acquirement. They enter the offices of specialists, with the avowed purpose' of pursuing a single branch of medicine; the private training is with that one object in view, and when in medical institutions this single idea is still dominant. They give but little heed to the instructions of the school save to those which have a direct relation with their chosen field, or at the most strive to obtain only so much knowledge of the general science as will let them through the too lax gates of the colleges, and insure to them an illy-earned doctorate.

This is, in few words, the history of a large number of men who are now in their offices claiming to be endowed with wondrous knowledge, and the highest skill in the art of mending eyes, restoring lost audition, healing rectums, cutting, slashing and burning wombs, giving fecundity to the barren, and instruction to prevent excessive fruition; and of others who claim the power to cure all skin diseases from leprosy down to right up the nasal and laryngeal cavities, whatever their diseases, and so on. They do not publish their claims in newspapers or circulars, as do their cousins, the quacks; but they whisper them in great confidence to the Betsey Malones, Sairey Gamps, and the street tattlers of the male sex, who not merely tell them to all persons whom they meet, and send word to the balance of mankind, but crowd the anterooms and slyly exhibit themselves as living examples of the miraculous cures their favorite specialists can accomplish.

Another and a higher dodge is to get up long papers composed of the opinions and teachings of the able masters in their line, but so grooving and dove-tailing them together as to make a handsome and finished mosaic. These they publish as their own, thus to advertise themselves and bring custom to their doors.

This is the kind of specialism and such the specialists against which and whom I beg, in the interest of true science, to enter my solemn protest, and urge you, gentlemen, to hold in absolute abhorrence. It is this class of specialists which misleads the people and gives extent and permanency to a baneful fashion.

In our larger cities it is now not uncommon for a single individual to have half a dozen doctors, every doctor restricted to his own peculiar sphere. It is Dr. Barnes, I believe, who tells an anecdote to about this effect: A lady, seeking his advice, told him when he was making inquiry about her circulation, that he need not mind that; Dr. A. had her heart; Dr. B. took care of her lungs; Dr. C. looked after her eyes; Dr. D. did her general practice, and she wished to place her genitals only in his charge. The Doctor facetiously adds that he was curious to know to whom her umbilicus would be committed. This picture is no exaggeration; many similar ones are mentioned by the busy practitioner. It is coming to be the very summit of the *ton.*

The result of this fashion is gracefully yet truthfully told in a recent address by Dr. Henry, of New York, to the alumni of the Medical Department of the University of Vermont. He says: "Experience has forced me to the belief that the evils of this subdivision are individually nursed and fostered through lack of proper general qualifications, indolence, and the greater prospect of large fees. Diseases that were skillfully treated in the early part of this century by the general practitioner, are now sent from one 'ologist' to another, until the sufferer, exhausted of patience and means, seeks in utter despair the assistance of the nearest quack."

Such unfortunates as those described by Dr. Henry constitute no small part of the persons who pass into the hands of the homœopathists, or who subject themselves to the torturing processes of the sticking doctors; not unfrequently to be redeemed from their ailments by the do-nothing practice of the one, or conjured into health by the other. Such partitioning of practice, and such sectional study, are debasing our profession, lessening the confidence of the people, and changing the science ·from Athens, the city of light, to Lutetia, the city of mire.

It should, therefore, be the pleasure of every lover of his profession to discountenance superficial, partially-trained, and incompetent specialism. I do not mean by this that we should decline to avail ourselves of the superior skill of all such specialists as have earned their positions by earnest toil, thorough acquaintance with the science of medicine, and careful and extended observation. Such men rarely fail to throw brilliant light upon obscure points in diagnosis, and give valuable hints for treatment. They become, indeed, to the general practitioner what the light-house is to the mariner; they guide him within lines of safety, and save him from hidden rocks and perilous currents; they are in truth towers of strength.

It has been charged that the medical schools of the country are contributing in a large measure to the production and perpetuity of these dangerous forms of specialism. Dr. Henry, in the address already alluded to, says: "For the purpose of leading the mass of the profession and the public into the belief that the schools are progressive, too many of the faculties have yielded to the fashionable spasm of the day and appointed persons to deliver special courses of lectures. With some few exceptions, these special lecturers are scarcely up to the standard which might be fairly asked in so-called specialists."

The proposition made in the first clause of his ·argument, I do not believe is well founded, and must emphatically dissent to it. The schools are not striving to mislead the profession or the public, but are, in my judgment, both honest and wise in their arrangement of the machinery of teaching. They have multiplied chairs and lectureships only as the widening and extending boundaries of the science have imperatively demanded. In the early history of medical teaching, when the science was meager in its principles, and not as now voluminous in detail, but few teachers were required to give instructions in all that was known. The most ancient and renowned school of our continent, the Medical Department of Pennsylvania University, began with but three professors. Those three taught the students who assembled all that was known of medicine at that time, as thoroughly as the most numerously appointed schools can possibly teach it to-day. Thus it will be seen our institutions are merely keeping step with the advancing profession, and striving by a multiplication of lectureships to give to the student, in the most comprehensive yet concise manner, all which constitutes the enlarged science. They do not inculcate, or even propose, the policy of studying for a specialty, but on the contrary insist that every aspirant for the medical doctorate shall faithfully follow the instructions given in every branch, in order to his qualification for general practice or the pursuit of a single department.

I know of no school which is favoring the study of a single branch, none which will accept, in extenuation of imperfect knowledge of the whole science, the plea that the applicant is preparing for a specialty. On the contrary, teachers of specialties themselves insist, in no dubious terms, upon a thorough knowledge of all.

Billroth, in the introduction of his Course on Surgery, says: "The surgeon can only judge safely and correctly of the state of his patient when he is at the same time a physician; moreover, the physician must have surgical knowledge, or he will make the grossest blunders."

Dr. Fordyce Barker, the distinguished teacher of Clinical Midwifery, in the preface to his valuable work on Puerperal Diseases, says: "A man may become eminent as a physician,

and yet know very little of obstetrics; or he may be a successful, even distinguished surgeon, and be quite ignorant of
even the rudiments of obstetrics; but no one can be a really
able obstetrician, unless he be both physician and surgeon."

Sir Henry Thompson says: "No man should become a specialist until he has had a ripe experience engrafted upon a
most liberal professional education, and be forty years old."

Mr. R. Brudenell Carter, in the conclusion of his address
before the International Medical Congress recently sitting in
Philadelphia, said, "It gave him real pleasure to find so many
eminent specialists identified with the great body of the profession. He believed the specialist a man of great utility,
but thought the separation of specialism from general medicine detrimental to the earnest practitioners of both. He
thought the knowledge of the specialist should become the
property of the general practitioner also, and that it is wise in
schools to include in their plan chairs of special branches.
He believed the ranks of useful specialism could only be
reached by the most thorough training in the entire science;
and concluded by saying it is absurd to attempt respectability
in medicine by the study of an exclusive branch." Thus it
becomes apparent that teachers of specialties discourage specialism except of the kind that comes through learning and
observation.

The point made by Dr. Henry, in the second clause of his
argument, is more valid, namely, that "teachers of specialties
are too frequently not up to the standard fairly to be expected;" yet this objection is more apparent than real, for though
a teacher of a specialty may not be a thorough master of it,
his teaching may in the main be correct and useful. Lacking
the necessary store of knowledge, and being deficient in experience, he may nevertheless be a good teacher. He may
draw the instruction which he imparts from the texts of the
most approved authorities, and make it valuable to the student; and though such teaching may not be as complete or
exact as that given by the acknowledged masters, still it will
be vastly better than no teaching. The argument of Dr.

Henry is, therefore, fallacious. The schools do not foster or encourage uneducated and vicious specialism, but are doing all that lies within their power to promote liberal and universal medical education.

I hope I shall not be misunderstood in the positions taken in the course of these remarks. Lest I may be, I beg to reiterate the points taken, and will venture the opinion that the unprejudiced judgment of all intelligent gentlemen of the profession, whether they be general practitioners or specialists, will fully sustain them. They are these: that specialties pursued by men of general and proficient cultivation in the science of medicine, who have had a clinical experience sufficiently enlarged to give them acquaintanceship with the current morbid processes of the body and enable them to distinguish between them, and to trace them to their probable pathological sources, must rarely fail to be productive of good, both to the profession and public, and materially advance the interests of the science, and for the very forcible reason that one field assiduously cultivated by a *wise* laborer yields more abundantly than a number of fields imperfectly tilled. The shortness of time and the limitation of the human intellect render it very evident that a single mind can not reach the perfection in the whole that it can in a part. The second position is, that a person, notwithstanding he may be of gigantic intellect and untiring industry, unless he becomes a general medical scholar and a patient and careful student of diseases generally, can not become a successful and useful specialist, but will retard progress and injure the science by his frequent blunders, and will consequently become the instrument of mischief to the public.

Precisely as it is necessary for the artist to have a familiarity with nature in all its forms, an eye cultivated in the perception of colors, their changes and combinations; the sculptor to have "a knowledge of mathematics, anatomy, physiology and a cultivated imagination;" or the novelist to have a full acquaintance with human nature, a knowledge of history, and be learned in the sciences in order to success—so is it of prime necessity that the specialist in medicine shall combine with a native adaptation a familiarity with the organization of man in health and disease, a profound knowledge of the laws governing both states, and clinical experience sufficient to enable him to recognize disease of whatever form may come before him. Then, and not till then, should he allow himself to enter upon the higher domain of specialism. Even when gentlemen have reached the high standard indicated, and are in all regards useful and distinguished special practitioners, there are difficulties in the way, many of which could be mentioned if time served; but one which is so common to all with whom I have met, I can not pass over in silence. It is that almost every specialist is prone to find in the organs of his peculiar province the morbid change which will account for all the symptoms in every case which is presented to him. He is sincere in this opinion, yet he often finds that it has drifted him into the vortex of error, from which he too frequently does not become extricated until the opportunity of remedying the real malady is lost forever.

In conclusion, gentlemen, allow me to whisper into your ears a little item of information for your personal good. It may seem ignoble to do so in connection with an examination of a subject belonging wholly to the interests of the science of medicine; yet I shall do so for the double purpose of placing you upon your guard, and as an incentive to more diligent study.

It is this: that besides promoting' the science, you will advance your individual interests by so studying every department of medicine as to enable you to manage skillfully all the diseases of your patients, and thus keep them out of the hands of specialists as entirely as possible consistent with their good. For the reason that you will now and then meet with one to whom you entrust your patient for the relief of a special disease, who will retain and treat him and other members of his family for whatever affliction may arise in the course of his connection with the case. He will not be just and liberal as you have been. He will not say to the patient, your physician can treat this new and different disease better than I can, but will hold him as long as possible.

This, I doubt not, is within the personal experience of almost every physician. You will encounter it when you come to practice. Therefore, it will be greatly to your advantage to neglect no branch, but become, as far as the power within you lies, the master of all.

Louisville, Ky.

---

## THREE CASES OF IMPERFORATE HYMEN.*

### BY SAMUEL R. BURROUGHS, M. D.

Case I. In 1868, a negro man consulted me in reference to his infant child, a girl then three days old, whose condition he described as follows: The midwife, an aged negress, stated that the baby had passed no water from the bladder since its birth, but had had free dejections of a watery character from the bowels; that it was extremely restless, and would bend itself backward by sudden jerks and scream as if in great pain, and required almost constant nursing. Thinking there was some mistake in the matter, I gave it as my opinion that the urine probably passed when the bowels were moved, and directed a warm bath and a little spirits of nitre every three hours, and to closely examine the napkins. The next day the father returned, and stated that my directions had been followed, but no urine had been observed to pass; that the child had ceased to nurse, and was having convulsions. I now visited the patient, whom I found with convulsions recurring at intervals of twenty minutes, and between them crying and tossing incessantly. On examining the genitalia, I dis-

* Extracted from a very able paper, entitled *The Hymen: its Anatomy, Malformation, and Treatment of its Imperforate Deformity*, read at the meeting of the Texas State Medical Association, by Dr. S. R. Burroughs, of Guy's Store, Leon County, Texas.—D. W. Y.

covered, slightly protruding between the labia, a thin delicate membrane, containing minute blood-vessels, and somewhat distended by fluid. No meatus urinarius, or opening in the urethra, could be detected. Further examination revealed the membrane to be the hymen attached above to, or rather continuous with, the mucous membrane in front of the meatus urinarius, and completely blocking up the entrance both to the vagina and urethra. On introducing a delicate exploring needle, I discovered the confined fluid to be urine. The adjacent parts were much swollen from infiltration; a distinct and well rounded tumor was observable in the hypogastric region, over the whole of which there was distressing tenderness on pressure. A gentle tap with the finger over either the distended bladder or the protruding hymen revealed that the two contained the same fluid. Being satisfied as to the condition of things, I now enlarged the opening made by the exploring needle with a bistoury, when about a pint and a half of urine came away with a gush. I then proceeded to dissect up the entire membrane. But little hemorrhage occurred. I then introduced a pledget of lint well oiled, ordering it to be renewed as occasion required until the parts healed. The little patient soon after dropped to sleep. In four or five days the cut surfaces had cicatrized, and the case gave no further trouble.

CASE II. Was in the person of a young lady, aged fifteen years, who was well formed and of good constitution. Her tongue was clean, and she had no fever. Yet she was the subject of a severe throbbing pain at the base of the occiput, grinding pains in the uterine region, radiating occasionally to the loins and inside of the thighs, intermittent in character and appearing with a certain degree of regularity, simulating somewhat the advent of a real labor. Examination of the abdomen revealed a pear-shaped tumor, the summit of which reached nearly to the umbilicus. The tumor was firm, though somewhat elastic. When pressed upon, the most excruciating pains were excited in the lower extremity of the tumor, or in that part corresponding to the os uteri.

The most carefully conducted examination failed to discover fluctuation or a placental souffle, or the sound of a fetal heart. The mother said that the patient had never menstruated, and had enjoyed excellent health until six months before, when she complained of dull pains in the head, back and hypogastrium, accompanied by anorexia and slight nausea, a disposition to sleep and an indisposition to either physical or mental exertion. These symptoms, which usually recurred every twenty-five to thirty days, generally reached their height on the third day, and then gradually subsided in about as many more, fair health, or at least comfort, being at first the rule during the interim. But as they were repeated they became more and more severe, until the general health was finally disturbed. No other than domestic remedies had been used in the case. I proposed a digital examination, which was refused. I then gave a dose of chloral-hydrate, which secured a pleasant night's sleep. The pains gradually ceased, and the molimen slowly passed off.

At the end of a month I was called in great haste to see the patient, and found her suffering pains similar to and as great as those of labor; she was in tears, and on the accession of the pains would scream at the top of her voice. There were cramps in the calves of the legs, and sharp transient pains in the mammæ, which were somewhat enlarged and hard. The pulse was a little accelerated, the tongue coated, and the temperature slightly increased. There was frequent desire to micturate, the act being attended by scalding, while only a few drops of urine escaped.

A vaginal examination was now no longer opposed, and led to the discovery of a scarlet red, fluctuating tumor, the size of a goose-egg, lying between the labia majora. The catheter brought away a pint of highly-colored urine. Fluctuation in the tumor was easily detected both in that part of it which lay between the labia and that which occupied the hypogastric region, and a light blow in either situation was communicated to the opposite extremity of the swelling. An examination by the rectum detected the presence of a fluid in the vagina. Being now fully satisfied as to the nature of the case, I plunged a bistoury through the walls of the projecting cyst, when a black, grumous-looking fluid escaped with a force which projected it a distance of five or six feet. The patient experienced almost instantaneous relief. The total amount of fluid discharged at the time was estimated at twenty-five or thirty ounces, but it continued to pass in clots and small quantities for several days longer. As soon as the main flow had ceased, I made a second incision transverse to the first through the entire extent of the membrane, introduced an oiled tent, and enjoined attention to cleanliness. The patient rapidly recovered her health, and had no further trouble.

CASE III. A lady stated that her daughter, who was nearly fourteen years of age, had been in good health until five months before, when she suffered for several days with pain in the head and back, loss of appetite and strength. She furthermore said that these phenomena had, since that time, returned at regular monthly epochs, with some increase in severity at each successive period; that she had never menstruated, and at that time was suffering much from pain in the lower part of the abdomen and back, the former being swollen and rather tender to the touch.

Being unable to visit the patient at the time, and supposing that the symptoms arose from other than a local cause, I directed iron and quinia, warm clothing, out-door exercise, good food, etc. Two months subsequent to this time the girl's mother brought her to my office for examination. An abdominal tumor was as manifest as in Case II. It really simulated a uterus gravid six months. A dense, unyielding, imperforate hymen fluctuating through it, and also through the rectum, and most of the other features noted in Case II, go to complete the picture. The next day I operated at the patient's residence by a crucial incision, giving exit to twenty or thirty ounces of black, decomposed blood, intermingled with purulent matter. After the greater part of this liquid mass had passed, I dissected the four quarters of the disk from their original continuity, and placed an oiled tent in the opening, and directed that with the necessary renewals it should be kept *in situ* until the parts healed. For an hour or two after the operation the girl suffered considerably with uterine pains, which, however, yielded to chloral hydrate, and under proper regimen her health was speedily regained. The membrane removed in this case was about one-eighth of an inch in thickness, very dense in structure, and sufficiently rigid to prevent the pressure of the retained fluid from causing it to bulge or protrude externally.

In conclusion, I may be permitted to remark that Case I is not only interesting from its rare occurrence, but in that it combines both a malformation and a malposition, converting the genito-urinary apparatus into one irregular common canal. I have failed so far to find a record of a similar case in the books and journals to which I have had access.

Cases II and III are important inasmuch as they establish the following facts: First, they show the necessity of carefully examining the genito-urinary organs of all children born under our professional care, and correcting, if possible, such deformity as may be discovered. Second, that great suffering, constitutional disturbance, and much embarrassment both on the part of the patient and medical attendant, may obtain in these cases from a neglect of the above precaution. Finally, it is also worthy of remark that neither of these cases exhibited any symptoms whatever that could be attributed to the results of a regurgitation of the retained liquid through the fallopian tubes, although uterine contractions were excited by its increasing volume and continued presence.

GUY'S STORE, LEON COUNTY, TEXAS.

## MASCULINE METAMORPHOSIS.

BY JAMES D. MAXWELL, M. D.

A case unique in its character, so far as my observation extends, presented itself in April, 1873, which I take the liberty of briefly reporting to you, hoping the researches and experience of some of your readers may give a satisfactory explanation of the phenomenon.

Miss ——, an intelligent young lady in an adjoining county, by profession a music teacher, was suddenly overtaken in March, 1871, by a rain-storm, and thoroughly drenched in the midst of her catamenial period. The immediate result was the cessation of the menses and a severe cold; the remote result, irregular and very painful menstruation for the next twelve months, when amenorrhœa supervened.

About this time, or earlier, the patient complained greatly of pain in the iliac and lumbar regions, and was supposed to be suffering with ulceration of the os uteri; for which she was treated by her physician. The pain was especially severe upon the least exertion; and on one occasion, in attempting to get into a carriage, produced syncope. Intercurrent with these symptoms were chilly sensations and febrile movement, treated at the time as an attack of malarial fever, but with the light subsequently thrown upon the case may have been the accompaniments of ovaritis.

These were the symptoms up to about May 1, 1872, when there were manifested those features in the case which made it so anomalous. The delicate features of the female began to assume a masculine appearance; the voice changed, the throat and neck enlarged, the mammæ shrank away and became like those of a fleshy man, with the heavy circle of dark hair around the nipples; the beard grew luxuriantly, dark and glossy all over the face, unless through shame, as was frequently the case, it was removed with some depilatory ointment or closely cropped with scissors. The hair was thickly set also upon the sternum, extending down the recti muscles of the abdomen and on the legs, as in the male. With all this there was constantly increasing obesity of the whole body, and a corresponding helplessness to such an extent that the patient was confined to an easy chair, made especially for her comfort. From being a delicate girl of slender form, weighing probably in health one hundred and fifteen pounds, she now at the time of my visit, April, 1873, must have weighed two hundred and fifty or three hundred pounds; and such a transformation of features! that no one could realize who had not seen the patient. The case seemed not more hopeless than obscure, and a strong wish was expressed by the physicians present to have a post mortem when the patient died. Upon her death, some two or three months afterward, this privilege was granted.

The autopsy was made, however, "under difficulties" more amusing to relate than instructive. The peculiarities of the case and the sensitiveness of friends, made it necessary to act under the cover of night. The examination was made with reference to a previously formed opinion that there would be found some diseased condition of the ovaries, and was, therefore, confined to the abdominal and pelvic cavities. In making the usual incisions for this purpose, there was nothing remarkable except the depth of adipose tissue penetrated in cutting through the abdominal walls. The omentum and mesentery contained also an unusual amount of fatty matter, and the appendices epiploicæ hung in clusters, like fringes, from the large intestine, much resembling in shape and size very large almonds. The uterus was normal in every particular, except some signs of an eschar upon the os, the result of former treatment for ulceration. The ovaries were very much atrophied, not over one-third the natural size, dusky in hue externally, almost cartilaginous to the touch, and of an ashy, striated appearance when laid open with the knife. The examination might have been carried further, especially to the heart, to ascertain if the immediate cause of death was not dependent on fatty accumulation about this organ; but it was made under stress of circumstances, with limited time and want of opportunity.

The query now presents itself as to the probable cause of this abnormal accumulation of fatty tissue, and the change from the peculiarities of the female to those of the male in the manner specified. Reasoning by analogy and from observation in the animal kingdom, the conclusion would naturally point to the loss of function in the ovaries, by whatever cause produced. The caponed cock and the spayed heifer, and I might add the eunuch, show the proclivity to adipose development.

Our medical literature is not without an example also of the influence of the extirpation of the ovaries, or the impairment of their functions, upon the stimulation of the hair follicles. In the Cyclopedia of Practical Medicine, under the head of Amenorrhœa, occurs the following language: "But there are no protuberant mammæ, no sexual propensities; a slight beard grows on the upper lip, and the general characteristics resemble those of the male. In such a case the probabilities are that the ovaries are either absent or have become so diseased that their functions are entirely lost. A striking instance is related by Mr. Pott, where a precisely similar state was artificially induced by the removal of the ovaries in a young woman in St. Bartholomew's Hospital, although previously to the operation menstruation and all the signs of puberty had regularly existed."

I have thought it unnecessary to refer particularly to the treatment pursued in this case, but may say generally, as I learn from her family physician, that it was adapted first to the dysmenorrhœa, second to the amenorrhœa, and third to amenorrhœa and ulceration of the os uteri. Remedies seeming to prove futile with her family physician, she visited Dr. Byford, of Chicago, under whose advice treatment was still pursued on her return home. It was about this time that the changes began which have been particularly referred to as anomalous, and which continued to increase till her death.

BLOOMINGTON, IND.

# A CLINICAL LECTURE—DIAGNOSTIC VALUE OF ABDOMINAL PALPATION IN PREGNANCY.*

## BY JAMES R. CHADWICK, M. D.

*Fellow of the American Gynecological Society.*

The history of the patient now before you has already suggested to your minds the probability that she is pregnant, but the menstruation has been habitually so irregular that we must all entertain some doubts as to the fact, and must be completely in the dark as to the period to which that state may have advanced. As your text-books give at great length the various signs and symptoms of pregnancy as taught by English, French and American obstetricians, I will devote the short time at our disposal to a minute exposition of the method and advantages of abdominal palpation, which has attained to a prominence and importance in Germany that are unknown and unappreciated in other countries.

The other methods of abdominal examination are *inspection, percussion* and *auscultation;* their objects may be briefly stated as follows:

*Inspection* of the abdomen informs us as to its volume and form; the tension of its walls, the discoloration and scars upon its integument, the changes of the umbilicus, the impediment to respiration, and condition of the ribs; sometimes shows us the movements of the child or of flatus, the twitching of the abdominal muscles, and occasionally a thrill from pulsation of the aorta.

*Percussion* informs us as to the consistence of the contents of the abdomen, giving the size and height of the womb, as well as, imperfectly, the nature of its contents, the presence of ascites, flatus, or a full bladder.

---

* This lecture was published in the Boston Medical and Surgical Journal some time since. But the demand for copies of it being so great that the supply has been exhausted, Dr. Chadwick republishes it, with some important additions and a few alterations, in the American Practitioner.

"The object of *auscultation* is to recognize the fetal heart-sounds, and the maternal vascular murmurs, and to distinguish them from the transmitted heart-sounds of the mother, from the spontaneous movements of the fetus, from the umbilical murmur, from the gurgling of gases and the splashing of fluids in the intestines, and from the aortal pulse." (C. Braun.)

For the purposes of diagnosis, palpation is the determination of the volume, consistence, form and position of the uterus; the size, position, presenting part and spontaneous movements of the fetus; the presence of more than one fetus, or of complicating abdominal or pelvic tumors; the life of the fetus, the transmitted thrill of the aortal pulse, the fullness of the urinary bladder, the presence of ascites, and, in some measure, the question of a previous birth, by the *sense of touch through the abdominal walls.*

*Preliminaries.*—The woman, to be examined, should be flat upon her back on a bed; her legs should be drawn up, and her head supported, in order to relax the abdominal muscles and integuments. Corsets, drawers, and all constricting bands about the abdomen or chest, should be removed. A sheet should cover the lower extremities, and the night-dress or chemise be drawn up under her breasts, thus leaving the abdomen alone exposed. Should modesty require, the sheet, being the cleaner and looser of the two, may be brought up over the abdomen, though this will interfere somewhat with a satisfactory examination. The physician's hands should be warm.

*Manual of Palpation.*—Standing upon the right of the woman, the physician lays his hands upon her abdomen, and proceeds to explore its contents, as revealed to the touch. This is performed by moving the hands, step by step (so to speak) over its surface, while they are rounded over the inequalities, made prominent by pressure, so as to form an idea of the configuration of what is within.. This is best effected by a general "pawing" motion, during which the hands are kept nearly flat upon the abdomen, the pressure being not constant in any one spot, for a rocking motion is imparted to the hands by alternate flexion and extension of the wrist and of the metacarpo-phalangeal articulations. The hands are, during this action, either moved along side by side in the same region of the abdominal surface, or at opposite sides of the abdomen; in the latter case, the one steadies the uterus and fetus, while the other studies their angles and form. This is most useful when the abdominal contents are very movable. When it is wished to test the consistence or mobility (including ballottement) of the underlying parts, the very tips of the fingers of one hand should *first* be placed gently upon the abdominal integument, almost perpendicular to it; and *then*, by a forcible thrust downwards, be brought up against the parts below. As this should be a shove rather than a blow, it may best be executed by an action from the elbow, with stiff but slightly-flexed wrist and hands. In order to examine the presentiug part of the fetus, two other procedures are commonly followed. In the first, the right hand of the investigator, with thumb abducted, is laid, palm downwards, upon the abdomen immediately above the symphysis pubis, the thumb being near the middle of the left Poupart's ligament, and the fingers at the same point on the other side; the ring and middle finger come chiefly into play. The thumb and fingers are then thrust downwards into the abdomen, and approximated, until they grasp between them the presenting part of the fetus. The distinguishing characteristics of a presenting head or breech may best be brought out by giving the part a sort of shake in this way, by which it is tossed to and fro between the thumb and fingers.

The second method of palpating the presenting part is by laying the two hands flat upon the opposite sides of the abdomen, the points of the fingers being directed toward and lying just above the middle of Poupart's ligaments on each side; they are then thrust downward and inward towards the cavity of the pelvis, until they come upon and hold between them the presenting part. This method is rarely resorted to, unless the previous one yields an ambiguous or negative result. It is slightly painful, but the examiner is by it enabled to explore deeper in the pelvis, and thus often reach a deep-seated head, which would not be accessible to the former procedure. No force sufficient to cause the woman any real pain need ever be employed during these manipulations.

Attention to the minutiæ enumerated above is of importance, for a promiscuous punching will not only subject the woman to much discomfort and pain, but will also excite reflex contractions of the abdominal or uterine muscles, and thus defeat the object in view.

*At the Bedside.*—While facing the woman, the obstetrician lays his hands, with the fingers directed toward her head, upon the opposite sides of her abdomen, to make sure that the long axis of the fetus corresponds to the longitudinal axis of the uterus; in other words, that he has a longitudinal position before him. This proved, he proceeds to estimate the period of the pregnancy by defining the height to which the fundus uteri rises. This may be done by depressing, as far as possible, the ulnar border of the left hand above the fundus, and measuring, while it is closely applied to the latter and in a perpendicular position, its distance from certain fixed points. The right hand may be required to support the body of the uterus, should it incline to fall away from the median line of the body.

*The Period of the Pregnancy* is determined chiefly from the height of the fundus, which depends in the later months almost entirely upon the size of the fetus. The measurement of the abdominal circumference gives no data, as proved by Hecker, Spiegelberg and Richelot, who, for example, found for the tenth month of pregnancy variations of 34½–45½ inches (H.), 33–42½ inches (S.), and 32¼–44½ inches (R.)

In transverse and twin pregnancies, this manner of diagnosticating the period gives untrustworthy results, for then the long axis of the uterus will be the transverse, and in consequence the fundus will not attain to the same altitude. The general size of the child or children, the size and hardness of the head or heads, and the testimony derivable from the vaginal examination, and from the statements of the mother, must then be relied upon.

The following are the rules to be observed in making the calculation: The line connecting the symphysis pubis to the ensiform cartilage is supposed to be crossed, at right angles, by six equidistant transverse lines; two intersecting each of the spaces from the pubes to the umbilicus, and from the umbilicus to the tip of the ensiform cartilage, and one passing through each of the last two points.

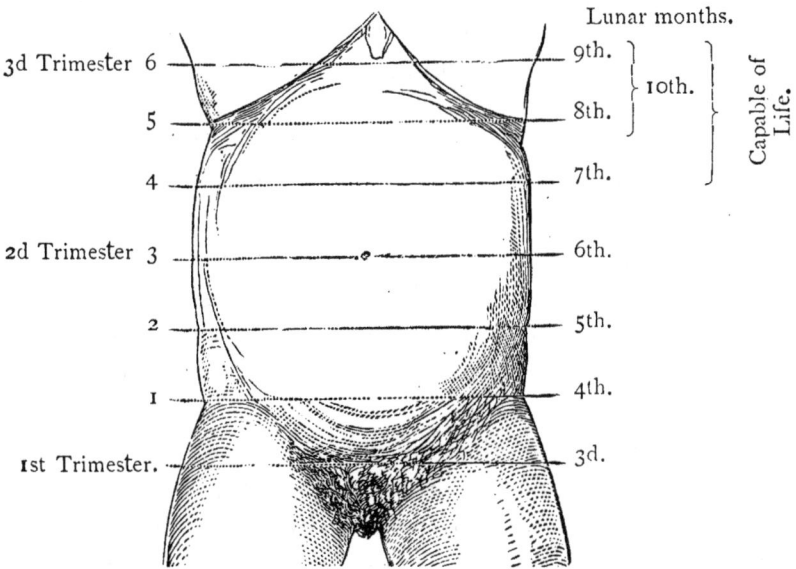

The normal term of gestation—two hundred and eighty days, reckoned from the commencement of the last menstruation—is then divided into ten lunar months; these, exclusive of the tenth month, are arranged in trimesters. During the first trimester the fundus uteri is rising to the level of the pelvic brim, and is not accessible to palpation; at the end of the second trimester it has reached the height of the umbilicus, and at the end of the third that of the ensiform cartilage. The altitude attained by the fundus at the end of the several months of each trimester corresponds to the other lines of the scale.

The distance between each of these lines is about equal to the breadth of two fingers, whence the common saying that the fundus stands "two fingers above the symphysis pubis, or two fingers below the navel," etc., indicating the end of the fourth and fifth lunar months respectively, and so on.

During the tenth lunar month, the uterus is generally supposed to be settling into the pelvis; therefore, although it has been increasing in size, the fundus has really been sinking from its position at the end of the ninth month. This descent is, however, far from constant, and should not be allowed for, until further abdominal and vaginal examination has confirmed the supposition. A complete descent of the uterus would, consequently, carry the fundus, in the course of the tenth lunar month, through the various altitudes through which it had passed in its ascent during the ninth, and bring it finally, at the end of the tenth, to the level at which it stood at the end of the eighth. This is exceptional, so that it is more correct to place the normal height of the fundus, at the end of the tenth month, somewhere *between* the lines corresponding to the end of the eighth and ninth months, with the proviso that the fundus will not infrequently be found as high as the line of the ninth month.

In estimating the period of pregnancy, no mention has thus far been made of the other less reliable, but not unimportant, data to be obtained from palpation. These will be more fully described in other connections later, and will here be only mentioned as they successively appear in the several months.

*Fourth lunar month.*—The uterus is felt as a rounded, elastic tumor, above the symphysis pubis, and continued into the pelvis; its consistency is soft, and in multiparæ often uneven. It may be a little harder in several places adjoining the fetal parts, but the latter are not distinctly felt. Ballottement through the abdominal walls is very rare.

*Fifth lunar month.*—Uterus a little to one side of the median line, generally to the right. Spontaneous movement of the fetus, and abdominal ballottement rarely felt. (Fetal heart-sounds, in rare cases, heard on auscultation.)

*Sixth lunar month.*—Fetal parts, and consequently the presentation, can commonly be made out.  Spontaneous movements felt.  (Fetal heart-sounds heard.)

*Seventh and eighth lunar months.*—All the parts of the fetus gradually become more manifest to palpation.  Fetus gradually loses its extreme mobility.  Head increasing in hardness, as well as in size.

*Ninth lunar month.*—The fetus, constantly gaining in size in proportion to the uterus, obliges the latter to conform more and more to its shape.  Ballottement of the head commonly felt.

*Tenth lunar month.*—Uterus generally descends into the pelvis, by which the presenting part of the fetus becomes more or less immovable, and the fundus is caused to fall more forward, by which a flattening of the epigastric region may ensue.

All these signs are to be earlier and more easily obtained in multiparæ than in primiparæ, owing to the greater tension of the abdominal walls in the latter.  The fetus is, of course, supposed to be alive.

This method of determining the period of the pregnancy will be found in general satisfactory, despite its manifest imperfections.  Three points are important in applying it, however: that the fetus should not be in a transverse position; that the fundus should be in the middle line of the body, and that the bladder should be empty, it being evident that a dilatation of the uterus in a transverse direction would shorten its vertical axis; that any deflection of the womb from the median line of the body would lessen its apparent height, and that a full bladder might prevent the uterus from sinking to its proper level in the pelvis.

Fullness of the rectum is said to affect, in some measure, the height of the fundus uteri, but is rarely taken into account.  The thickness of the abdominal walls is also to be considered and allowed for; it is determined by taking up a fold between the thumb and fingers.  This gives another indication, for it has been proved that the amount of adipose tissue in the walls decreases with each successive pregnancy.

Deformity of the pelvis, of the vertical column, or of the thorax, an unusual amount of amniotic fluid, and the presence of complicating tumors, may lead us astray, unless such conditions are discovered and due allowance made.

Having thus settled, preliminarily, the duration of the pregnancy, subject, however, to modification or correction after the vaginal examination, the physician proceeds to diagnosticate the position and presenting part of the fetus, and to detect any abnormal condition that may exist. If the urinary bladder is full, it will be felt as a more or less prominent, elastic tumor, immediately above the symphysis pubis, and must be evacuated.

The consistence of the abdomen varies with the nature of its walls, and more especially of its contents. The walls, when fat, will be soft to the feel, even when somewhat distended; yet in primiparæ they are apt to be very tense toward the end of the pregnancy, owing to the unusual dilatation.

The uterus is felt as an elastic, more or less firm bladder, rounded above and prolonged downwards into the pelvis. Toward the end of gestation it assumes more nearly the ovoid form of the fetus; it never, however, quite loses a slight antero-posterior groove in its fundus, the last trace of its formation by the union of Muller's ducts; this is more marked during a contraction. Its shape when pregnant (and contracting) or dilated from other cause, is acknowledged to be chiefly dependent upon its contents. Up to the seventh or eighth lunar month the uterus is so distended by the proportionately great amount of liquor amnii, that the fetus floats free of its walls, and does not mar the symmetry of its rounded outline. After that time, however, the relation of the fetus to the fluid is gradually reversed, and the uterus assumes, in a measure, the form given it by the fetus.

*Peculiarities of the Fetal Parts.*—The two great extremities of the fetus, as it lies doubled up in the uterus, are the head and the breech; they are recognized by their individual peculiarities, and by the rounded terminal character common to both.

The *head* is felt as a round, hard body, entirely free from angles or even prominences, more movable than the breech, and more or less isolated (because of the hollow at the neck) from the neighboring resistant points. When the head is freely movable, one of its chief distinctive features is its *ballottement*, or quick rebound upon the exploring fingers, after a sudden push. The sensation imparted to the hand, in this case, is peculiar and characteristic, being such as is caused by a hard ball floating in a liquid. Its rebound is quicker and more bouncing than that of the breech, which alone could resemble it, because it swings from the body by the flexible neck, and thus describes the arc of a small circle only; whereas the breech, when thus propelled, describes an arc of greater radius, and is restrained by the inflexibility and greater inertia of the body, as well as the more extended surface which it exposes to the resistant action of the fluid; for these reasons the rebound of the breech is slower and less sudden than that of the head. This peculiar feel is enhanced by the different consistence of the two parts, the head being hard and bony, whereas the breech is soft and fleshy. As the size of the head increases, this ballottement is less marked, but as its bones gradually become more ossified, with the increase in size of the fetus, what is lost in mobility is gained in hardness.

The *breech* is known by its being directly continuous with the back, by not being symmetrically round, but somewhat pointed (the tuberosities of the ischia), by not being hard, and by not rebounding suddenly upon the fingers after a blow (ballottement).

The *back* is recognized by the long, uninterrupted resistant surface it presents to palpation. It is said that the spinous processes of the vertebræ can, in some instances, be felt; if so, the occurrence must be of extreme rarity.

The *small extremities*—the legs and arms—are generally detected as small, irregularly-shaped bodies, easily pushed about by the hands, often spontaneously changing their positions, and frequently dealing blows to the hand of the observer.

The momentary application of cold to the abdomen is said to increase these spontaneous movements of the fetus; it is inconceivable that the cold itself should penetrate to the fetus and excite the unwonted activity, especially if we are to believe Hebra's statement, made in my hearing, that a thermometer placed between the teeth and cheek is not sensibly affected by the continued application of ice to the cheek externally. It is more probable that the reflex nervous current excited in the woman in such a case, has an effect upon her uterus, and thus indirectly produces an impression upon the fetus.

BOSTON, MASS.                                  (To be continued )

---

## SUCCESSFUL CASE OF OVARIOTOMY.*

BY DRS. A. J. SMITH AND R. F. BLOUNT.

The subject of the above operation was Mrs. C. Latchen, residing six miles north of this city, aged fifty-one years, small and delicate in stature, native-born, and the mother of twelve large, healthy children, the youngest of whom is fourteen years. In November, 1874, she detected an enlargement in the left iliac region, which continued to increase in size, until in April, 1875, she presented herself to us for examination and treatment.

After a careful and thorough examination, we diagnosed an ovarian tumor. At this time it appeared to be solid, and about the size of a fetal head at full term of gestation. We gave treatment for the improvement of her general health. The tumor continued to grow rapidly, soon so encroaching upon the abdominal viscera that digestion and assimilation were imperfectly performed, and so embarrassing respiration that to lie down was impossible, even to sleep.

* Read before the Wabash County Medical Society, February, 1876.

June 22.—Fluctuation now being apparent, as a measure of palliation we introduced No. 3 needle, Dieulafoy's aspirator, two inches below the umbilicus, in the mesial line, and succeeded in removing six ounces of a thick, glairy fluid, highly albuminous.

August 30.—Our patient still rapidly declining, and the tumor enlarging; aspirated with the same needle as before, and in same locality, but with no results. Thinking the caliber of the needle too small to admit the flow of so tenacious a fluid, it was followed with a medium-sized trocar; still a dry tap. This being unsatisfactory, and confident we could detect fluctuation, the No. 3 needle was again inserted at a point about two inches above the anterior superior spinous process of the ilium, with the satisfaction of securing about four ounces of a similar fluid to that of the first operation. The needle was cautiously passed in different directions, with the hope of emptying other cysts, but with only slight results. Now knowing we had to do with a polycystic tumor, which could not be reduced by tapping, and our patient presenting marked signs of decline, we advised extirpation as the only means of relief, to which full consent was given.

December 2, 10 A. M.—Time appointed for the operation. The patient was put upon preparatory treatment some weeks previous, such as tinct. of chloride of iron, strychnia, good nourishment, sponging, etc. On the day preceding the operation she took quinia and a cathartic of castor oil. Promptly at the hour appointed we were joined by our friends, Drs. Dicken, Donaldson, J. and J. H. Ford, of this city, and Drs. Kidd and Murphy, of Roann, to all of whom we owe much for very efficient assistance.

We found the patient prepared as previously directed. The temperature of the apartment was raised to 85° F., and all avenues to external air closed. Squibbs's sulphuric ether was administered, complete anæsthesia induced, and the patient placed upon a table provided for the occasion and catheterized. An exploratory incision was now made, two and a half inches long, through the linea alba, beginning at a point two and a half inches below the umbilicus; here we found rather firm adhesions, which were with some difficulty broken up. A No. 10 male sound was introduced, and swept around the tumor in search of other adhesions; none were found, except that to the left at a point where we had previously aspirated, which was easily broken up.

The incision was now enlarged to the extent of seven inches, downward to within one inch of the symphysis pubis, and upward to the umbilicus. A Spencer Wells' trocar was introduced into the sac, and passed from cyst to cyst, until the tumor was so diminished that it could be turned out through the incision. During the emptying of the cysts, the walls of same were firmly clasped with a Sims' double-toothed forceps and gradually withdrawn, a Wells' clamp firmly adjusted to the pedicle, and the tumor, weighing about twenty pounds, severed therefrom. The pedicle was transfixed with a double-plaited silk ligature, and tied firmly in two halves, the clamp removed, stump nicely trimmed, and, all oozing of blood arrested, was dropped back, the ligatures left hanging from the lower angle of the incision for drainage.

The opposite ovary and uterus were examined and found to be healthy. Next the abdominal cavity was carefully and thoroughly cleansed, and the wound closed by seven interrupted sutures passed from within, including the peritoneum. A few adhesive straps, lint saturated with carbolated oil applied to the wound, and a compress of raw cotton, secured by a double flannel bandage, completed the dressing, and the patient then placed in bed. Fresh air was now admitted, and the temperature lowered to 65° F. The patient soon rallied from the effects of the anæsthetic, also from the shock of the operation. A single dose of brandy and carbonate of ammonia, and one hour later two grains of opium, was given.

At 5 P. M. the patient had slight vomiting; 8 P. M. vomiting more frequent and continued. At the end of the third day removed one half of the stitches.

Fifth day.—Vomiting still persisting; removed the remaining stitches, wound entirely united.

Sixth day.—Vomiting stercoraceous matter; patient feeble; gave essence of beef, milk, quinia and brandy, per rectum; gave repeated enemata of flaxseed tea, until a thorough evacuation of the bowels was obtained, after which the patient was more comfortable and tolerated nourishment by the stomach.

Eighth day.—Patient much improved; rested well during the past night.

Eleventh day.—Pulse small and frequent, skin dry and hot, tongue dry and red, urine highly ammoniacal; gave five grains of quinia, beef tea, milk and brandy, per rectum, every four hours.

Twelfth and thirteenth days.—General appearance better; so much improved that light food was allowed by the stomach.

Fourteenth day.—Doing well; ligatures removed and wound dressed.

Seventeenth day.—Wound entirely healed, and the case dismissed cured.

The wound was thoroughly cleansed daily, and dressed with carbolated oil. The vomiting was excessive, some days almost constant, every attempt to arrest it failing. The hypodermic injections of morphia afforded greater relief than any other remedy tried.

Mrs. L. has been a great sufferer from indigestion for many years, and subject to severe paroxysms of vomiting, which will in part account for the great gastric irritability during the entire treatment incident to the operation.

WABASH, IND.

---

# A CASE OF HEPATIC ABSCESS.

### BY GEORGE N. MONETTE, M. D.

David B——, aged nineteen, general jobber, always temperate, came to me to be treated for a "swelling," as he termed it, in the right hypochondrium. After a thorough physical examination, I diagnosed hepatic abscess. The engorged and hypertrophied liver extended from the crest of the ilium on one side to the crest of the ilium on the other; the largest abdominal circumference being thirty-six inches, the smallest, or lumbo-sacral, measuring thirty-four inches. The antero-lateral portion of the liver corresponding to the right lobe was the most prominent part, over which there was some tenderness on pressure. There was uniform distension of the abdominal parietes until within a few weeks of his death, at which time the left iliac region assumed a concave aspect. He had had intermittent fever the preceding spring, which yielded to quinia and iron. About two months prior to his visit to me he had a return of the paroxysms, which culminated in acute engorgement of the liver, the organ attaining great dimensions in a very short time. In addition to the above symptoms, there was general circulatory impairment with emaciation. The conjunctiva had a slight tinge of an icteroid hue, and the complexion was sallow and cachectic. There was no diarrhœa, dysentery, or other intestinal derangement. There was anorexia, dyspnœa, and podœdema. The urine was comparatively normal, straw-colored, but occasionally a dark red, and of muddy consistence.

The prognosis was unfavorable from the first, and the treatment I suggested was to puncture; but I informed the family that death was inevitable, and so concluded to do nothing. Treatment was superfluous almost, save to ameliorate his suffering; however, I ordered quinia, tinct. ferri chlor. and acidi nitro mur. dil., which only served to intensify his appetite. There was no autopsy, but the local hypostasis and the prominence and thinning of the parietal walls, pointed to the formation of pus and confirmed the diagnosis.

New Orleans, La.

# Reviews.

Transactions of the Indiana State Medical Society, 1876. Twenty-
Sixth Annual Session.

The circling months bring to us another volume of our
State Society Transactions, and it is again our duty to examine it and render to its contents such praise or censure as to
our judgment they may seem to demand. The task is not
one of our choice, yet in undertaking it we feel assured of a
spirit of impartiality, and trust that we shall execute it with
justice.

We are presented, in this volume, with two papers on the
Use of Tobacco, the first by Dr. S. S. Boyd, of Dublin, the
second by Dr. William F. Harvey, of Plainfield. Both are
counterblasts of the extreme kind, such as would have delighted the heart of old King James, and probably would
have won from him the honor of knighthood for their writers.
We are not going to write an anti-blast, for we are neither a
user nor an admirer of the weed. But we must say that we
do not think its use will be diminished by such writing as
this; and say farther, with regret, that we do not think these
papers are worthy a place in the Transactions. The sweeping
assertions, the unmeasured denunciation even to tirade, with
the entire lack of accurate and detailed personal experience,
of both papers, must sustain our judgment.

The second paper does, it is true, make a general statement
of personal experience with tobacco as a remedy, but it is
only general and not presented so as to be of any value, while
what little force it has is destroyed on the same page by the
statement that "it is a remedy too dangerous to use except
where every other known remedy has failed to relieve a given

case." Passing beyond the consideration of personal cleanliness, which is "next to godliness," the greatest objection to the use of tobacco is that it creates or increases the appetite for strong drinks. Both authors call attention to this fact; both mention, but do not urge as they might, the next great objection, its destruction of energy and ambition, its production of a mental state of dreamy lethargy and content, not compatible with the activity and exertion of the battle-field of life. Neither of them lays any particular stress upon its effect in producing irregular action of the great central organ of the circulation, or in causing dyspepsia, cases of which come so frequently under the observation of every physician, and of which we are sure every member of the Society sees a score to one of the dire and terrible effects set forth as of daily occurrence.

One point in the first paper we are glad to see urged, the ever positive and multiform injury resulting from the use of this powerful article by the young; and we wish the author had said a word in regard to another article, less potent but more generally used. We allude to coffee, so frequently in the west given to children, even to infants, as a daily beverage, a custom which is certainly not only unnecessary but very injurious.

We can not pass these papers without calling attention to some most extraordinary statements contained in the second one. One of them is that delirium tremens does not occur in persons who do not use both tobacco and alcoholic stimulants. This may be so, we can not gainsay it; but had the author established it he would have given a very considerahle value to his paper. As to some other statements, such as tobacco producing malignant disease, causing "aching pains in every part of the body, pains in every organ and joiut" (l), causing "a large percentage of the sudden deaths daily reported in the papers," with all the dire catalogue of evils on page 91; of these we will say that they should not appear in a scientific paper without proof or reference to the authority upon which they are based. These are of a piece, however, with the logic which appears at the end. The tobacco tax of France, from 1812 to 1842, is compared with the number of lunatics, and the tax of to-day compared with the lunatics now, whereby it is shown "that the increase of lunacy has kept pace with the increase of the tobacco revenue!" Now, suppose the author had compared the number of miles of railroad in France before 1842 with the number of-insane, and made the same comparison for 1876, would it not have shown beyond a question that the increase of lunatics has kept pace with improved modes of locomotion!

The subject of State Medicine is presented in two papers. The first is the address of the President, Dr. Helm, of Peru, in which the subject is very briefly but ably presented. The greater portion is taken up in urging better provisions for the care of the insane, and from the figures given there is certainly need for our state to act in this matter. The Doctor warmly advocates the treatment of the insane practiced at Gheel, in Belgium.

The second paper is by Dr. Hervey, of Indianapolis, and is an earnest plea for the establishment of a State Asylum for Inebriates, in regard to which we think the tax-payers of the state will have something to say. In this paper the author regrets that the legislature has failed "to recognize some standard of medical qualification."

And this brings us to the paper on Medical Education, by Dr. J. S. Gregg, of Fort Wayne. The subject is one upon which it would be difficult to say anything new, so frequently has it been treated and maltreated. The author is, we are glad to see, a warm advocate of the graded system of instruction, in which the student passes through, and is examined in, the more elementary branches of medical science before passing to the higher and more practical ones; and also advocates a better preliminary education. The means by which an elevation in medical education is to be attained are, the enlightenment of the people, and the efforts of the profession itself. The latter is the only reliable and effectual means; and the sooner the profession sees it and recognizes it, the better. Im provement of the people is a slow process, while legislative interference presents, in our opinion, no hope whatever. We express this opinion the more freely because we started in life a warm advocate of it. In one of our neighboring states the thing has been fairly tried through all its phases, and finally a law requiring only graduation from any legally constituted medical college remains a dead letter on the statute books. It is an open question whether enactments of this kind are not foreign to the spirit of our institutions; they certainly are at present to the spirit of popular opinion.

Finally, we have some exceptions to take to this paper, written by a gentleman evidently warmly interested in the welfare of the profession. We think all the colleges which have adopted the graded system should have been equally mentioned, and not one alone selected for praise, however high its standing. Again, while devoting so much attention to that which really is the greatest curse to the advance of the profession—the multiplication of medical colleges—why not say a few words upon the influence of the general practitioner? Are there no sins at his door? If young men, known to be without proper preliminary education, are permitted, even induced, to enter the office of a practitioner, merely to gratify the miserable vanity of having students, how can the colleges turn out worthy graduates? We propose to begin at the beginning in this matter, and advocate in our State Society a plan we have always pursued, the requirement of a pledge from every member to receive no person into his office who has not already shown himself a student by acquiring a fair amount of general education, and then exacting from him a pledge that he complete his course and graduate before going into practice. After a while the Society will, perhaps, be able to turn its attention to the colleges.

The paper by Dr. George Sutton, of Aurora, upon Reduction of Dislocation of the Hip-Joint by means of a Fulcrum, a subject which has been heretofore presented to our readers, is excellent, indeed of the highest order, because of its practical character. We have had no opportunity to test this method since it was published. It is an addition to our resources, to be borne in mind when others fail us, if it does not supercede them; and we believe that when the head of the femur rests in the ischiatic notch, it will prove a decided improvement. As an original contribution to a practical subject, this paper takes high rank.

Another practical subject of great importance is well presented in the paper on Reflex Morbid Conditions arising from Disease of the Uterus, by Dr. W. H. Bell, of Logansport. It treats of a class of cases of which no practitioner can see many unless placed in unusually favorable circumstances, and they are never plain or apparent; reports of cases are therefore always of interest, and only good can result from awakened attention to the subject. We, therefore, think the Society indebted to Dr. Bell for his able paper; and his remarks upon the local treatment of uterine disease are judicious, practical, and evidently the result of observation and study. In so good a paper, however, it surprises us to find such a glaring instance of *non sequitur* as the first case reported. We are told that "a critical post mortem examination proved beyond doubt that the initial cause of the knee affection was located in some of the generative organs;" yet there is not a word of any pathological change found in these organs at the post mortem, nor does the report of the case contain a syllable as to any symptoms on the part of these organs during the patient's life !

The Treatment of Puerperal Convulsions is considered in a paper by Dr. G. W. Mears, of Indianapolis. The title should have been, "A Plea for Blood-Letting as a Remedy" in this disease. It is a strong protest against the abandonment of venesection, and a strong presentation of its claims to our confidence. So far we are in entire sympathy with the author; we believe that a rapid abstraction of blood is one of the most useful measures of treatment in this frightful accident of parturition, one that is very generally demanded, and one which often can not be omitted with proper regard for the safety of our patient. Beyond this we can not go. Yet the author seems to wish to lead us further. But because venesection is a good remedy, it is no reason that chloroform and chloral, as well as opiates, may not be also good remedies. Because we advocate one, and have confidence in it, we are not compelled to abandon the others. It is a plain fact that no exclusive plan of treatment can be followed, and warmly as we would advocate blood-letting, we have seen cases with such a condition of the pulse that we are sure no physician would have bled the patient, unless he bled rather for the name of the disease than for the condition of the patient. The author advocates too exclusive a pathology, as well as plan of treatment. If the proximate cause of the convulsions be congestion of the nervous centers, a congestion which can be relieved by venesection, then the problem is an easy one—bleed again and again—*coup sur coup*, following Bouillaud. But there are able advocates of cerebral anæmia being the immediate preceding condition of convulsion. According to the theory of Traube and Rosenstein, which seems at present in the ascendant, there is cerebral serous effusion arising from the hydræmic condition of the blood. The good effect of early blood-letting can be understood if this theory be correct; but at the same time it is clear that too much or too frequently repeated, it can not but prove injurious by increasing the conditions upon which the disease depends. Singularly enough the objection urged by the author against chloroform is that it only removes temporarily the signs and manifestations of the disease. There is, unfortunately, a good deal that we don't know about the pathology of puerperal convulsions, and until the pathology is clear we can not base treatment upon it. In the light of clinical experience, we believe venesection to be one of the best of remedies, but, as before said, think the author too exclusive in his advocacy of it.

Another practical and very important subject is presented in the paper on the Treatment of Placenta Prævia, by Dr. Parvin, of Indianapolis, an able and scholarly paper, as we believe are all emanating from his facile pen. The subject elicited a discussion equal in interest to the paper, and both demand from us a brief notice. We have here the same difficulty as with puerperal convulsions; cases are not all alike. Not only are they not alike as to symptoms and pathological conditions, but we are prepared to maintain that a choice of treatment may be forced on a physician by the circumstances under which he is placed, as to such matters as the distance he is from the patient, and the time required to reach her, a thing which can be said of few, if any, other cases. The essential difference in cases was fully recognized and very plainly stated by the last speaker; yet we have again, unfortunately, the betrayal of a partisanship which would seem to rigidly advocate one plan of treatment, and to unduly depreciate others, a spirit into which all are likely to fall, especially during a discussion; yet one that is incompatible with scientific investigation.

We fully believe that the induction of premature labor in placenta prævia, when the child is viable, to be an advance and an improvement in obstetrics. It was the object of the paper, it seems to us, to present and advocate this plan. Yet we do not suppose that upon being called to a case the author would proceed at once to so important a measure under all circumstances and conditions. The paper fails to state as explicitly as it should have done, the class of cases, and just when and why, a resort should be had to a mode of treatment not yet generally accepted. Nor do we think it places a just estimate upon some other measures of relief, and instance puncture of the membranes, which is advised by the highest authorities, and which we can by no means believe to be as dangerous to the child as ergot. The danger of concealed hemorrhage after this, as well as after the tampon, we believe to be overestimated by the Doctor, and by some who took part in the debate; it is a possible, by no means a probable occurrence.

Now as to the tampon. The practitioner who has found it always reliable has been fortunate indeed, and we congratulate him, as well as those who find the hemorrhage, before eight and a half months, yield to rest and moderate remedies; but when he expresses entire and abiding confidence in this remedy—that in all cases at full term the safety of both mother and child is assured by it—we are very certain that he is misled by limited experience, (for all individual experience is limited), and trust he may never be awakened from his fancied security by disaster. That any particular form of tampon affords perfect security is likewise fallacious; and as to the application of solution of iron as a hemostatic, one of the latest and highest authorities says that astringents have been tried in every possible way in these cases, and "their action is not even in the slightest degree to be depended upon; a result which will not excite wonder if the purely mechanical cause of the hemorrhage be kept in mind." (Leishman.) We have equally strong testimony from equally competent clinical observers that a dilator introduced into the cervix acts as an "efficient plug." (Playfair.) Yet we find in this debate the value of dilators openly called in question, if not denied.

So it is again; the "old, old story" told once more. He who sees the white side of the shield swears it is silver; he who is on the other side, will fight to maintain that it is gold! Still, nothing but good results from these intellectual jousts; comparison of experience, enlarged views, increased knowledge; therefore, we welcome such papers as this on placenta prævia, and mark them as among the best in the annals of our Society.

There are several other papers in the volume, but we must conclude. The remarks upon the preventive treatment of apoplexy, appended to the Report of the Final Illness of Dr. James S. Athon, by Dr. I. C. Walker, of Indianapolis, are well worthy of consideration, and should have been presented in a separate paper.

The paper upon Hysteria, by Dr. F. J. Van Vorhis, of Indianapolis, deserves a notice which we can not give it.

The appearance of the volume is creditable to the Society; binding, paper and type are excellent; but as to proof-reading, we should characterize it as execrable, did the pages bear evidence that there had been any at all.           *

**A Practical Treatise on Materia Medica and Therapeutics.** By Roberts
Bartholow, M. A., M. D.   New York:   D. Appleton & Co.   1876.

Medical bookmakers are not greatly given to originality of
matter or novelty of style, and it is refreshing to encounter a
volume like the one under review, in which the author has
departed from the beaten path.   The plan of Dr. Bartholow's
work differs from that of any with which we are acquainted.
His classification is physiological, but in its scheme is unlike
anything published in the English language.

Remedies used to promote constructive metamorphosis.
Remedies used to promote destructive metamorphosis.
Remedies used to modify the functions of the nervous system.
Remedies used to cause some evacuation from the body.
Topical remedies.

These are the five orders into which he divides therapeutical
agents.   To our mind no better classification has been suggested; indeed, it impresses us as decidedly the most convenient yet offered to the student of therapy.   But, while
expressing delight with this classification because of its convenience, we frankly confess our inability to coincide with the
author in his cordial faith in physiological therapeutics.   Physiology, doubtless, has a magnificent future.   Its possibilities
are immense.   But, at present, it can not claim, with justice,
to be more than a promising young science; and so far as
practical medicine is concerned, it is certainly not yet developed beyond the *pupa* state.   The author's manner of writing
is clear and exceedingly concise, and if fault was found with
it, dogmatism would most likely be the sin alleged against it.
His excessive positivism, doubtless, arises from a naturally
ardent nature, and an unbounded confidence in the puissance
of drugs.

Avoiding tedious discourse on natural history and pharma-
cology, a condensed, but at the same time full account is given
of the physical and therapeutical properties of remedies.

Instead of quoting the views of authors, Dr. Bartholow
publishes his own opinions, educed from reading and clinical

observation; and at the end of each article a list of the authorities to whom he is indebted is given. This is a saving
of time to the reader, while it is a proper acknowledgment to
the authors.

In his descriptions of drugs, when it is practicable, he gives
the properties and applications, and doses of some medicine
representative of a class, and simply enumerates the names
and doses of the other substances having similar powers.
Thus, much space is saved. Too much time is given to the
mineral springs of America and Europe; and the chapter on
alimentation, though elaborately prepared and exceedingly
voluminous, does not, in our judgment, add anything to the
practical usefulness of the book. It is founded on physiological facts, or more truthfully speaking, on physiological experiments; and after a careful study of the diet tables and instructions as to food, we remain unshaken in the belief that the
instinctive appetite of the patient is the safest of all guides in
the selection of aliment for the invalid. The enthusiasts who
offer the results of experiments made on cats and dogs and
guinea-pigs, as indicating the correct method of feeding sick
people, will not be accepted in this day as true prophets. On
this point, however, the profession is by no means of one
mind.

Both to the medical student and practitioner, Dr. Bartholow's book commends itself by its originality and modernness,
and by its condensed form and the practical character of its
contents.

The following extracts may prove of interest. Some of
the statements are confirmatory of the teachings of previous
writers. Others are the result of the author's personal observation. We give them without comment:

" Arsenic may cure epithelioma; is useful in scirrhus, and palliative in uterine
cases."

"Eucalyptus, though an unequalled remedy in catarrh of the bladder, is a
very inferior antiperiodic."

" Hydrastia stands next to quinia as an antiperiodic; is useful in all the conditions in which quinia is used, and is an excellent injection for gonorrhœa."

" Quinia performs its offices by means of its antiseptic powers; is an anti-ferment. It may produce permanent deafness. It arrests inflammation in its forming stage, and is excellent in scarlatina, variola, and rubeola."

" Alkalies, in the treatment of rheumatism, are losing ground; and quinia, blisters and cold baths give better results."

" A solution of common soda, freely applied, will often remove bromidrosis from the feet and axillary glands.' '

" The sulphites, vaunted by Polli, are of no avail."

" Blue Lick water (of Kentucky) is useful in abdominal plethora and obesity. Hemorrhoids and engorgement of the pelvic viscera are relieved by it, and excellent results are obtained from its prolonged use in glandular affections, hepatic, splenetic, uterine and prostatic."

" Numerous cases of spina bifida have been cured by injection of tincture of iodine."

" Mercury increases the flow of bile, not by augmenting its secretion, but by producing reflex constriction of the gall-bladder, mechanically forcing out the bile."

" Scheffer's (Louisville) pepsin is the best of all pepsins."

" Spare women, by warm baths and inunctions of oil, may acquire flesh and roundness of form."

" Phosphorus is the best remedy for impotence. Oleum phosphoratum consists of twelve grains of phosphorus, and one ounce of olive oil. Dose, five to ten drops."

" Fowler's solution, in drop doses before meals, arrests the vomiting of pregnancy, and also the vomiting of chronic gastric catarrh from alcohol. Lienteric diarrhœa is cured by arsenic."

" Permanganate of potash relieves the condition in which lumbar pain, frequent micturition, and urine with profuse brick-dust sediment and intestinal indigestion, are associated symptoms."

" Chloride of gold and sodium in 1-20 grain doses, thrice daily, will relieve nervous dyspepsia; prevents decline of sexual power, cures sterility, and likewise weak and ineffectual erections and diurnal seminal emissions."

" Chloride of gold, in 1-20 to 1-30 grain doses, produces remarkable improvement in chronic Bright's disease."

" Seminal troubles that are relieved by gold, are aggravated by bromide of potash, and *vice versa.*"

" Alum is the best cure for lead colic, and relieves the pain and nausea more certainly than any other remedy."

" Digitalis possesses great utility in scarlet fever. It lowers the temperature, and maintains the action of the kidneys."

" Belladonna has real curative power in erysipelas, and without doubt has power to arrest lacteal secretion."

" Opium is the most important agent we possess in the treatment of various inflammations."

" Aconite is of the highest value in the eruptive fevers, especially in scarlatina. It lowers the temperature, promotes diuresis and diaphoresis, and checks

nasal, faucial and aural inflammations. In measles it arrests the catarrhal pneumonia. In idiopathic erysipelas we have no better remedy; and in cerebral and
spinal meningitis, prior to effusion, aconite is as serviceable as in other inflammations."

" Salicylic acid in typhoid, erysipelas, acute rheumatism, pneumonia, phthisis,
etc., is only second to quinia as an antipyretic. For intermittents it seems nearly,
if not quite equal to quinia."

" Aqua puncture is so decided in its relief of pain, that some physicians con-
tend that the anodyne effects of hypodermic injections of morphia are due to the
water, and not to the opiate. The injection of water, to be efficacious, must be
near to the seat of pain. In facial neuralgia, sciatica, lumbo-abdominal neuralgia, lumbago, uterine colic, and irritability of the bladder, aqua puncture possesses extraordinary power. In paralyzed and wasting muscles, it promotes
nutrition of the muscles and contributes to the regeneration of muscular power.
Thirty to sixty minims of water should be injected at the painful points; and if
no relief occurs in two minutes, repeat the remedy."

" An ingenious use of bicarbonate of sodium to produce emesis, applicable in
narcotic poisoning: Sufficient soda is first swallowed, and immediately after a
suitable proportion of tartaric acid is taken. Brisk effervescence ensues, thoroughly emptying the stomach."

---

**Blood-Letting in Puerperal Eclampsia.** By HENRY FRASER CAMPBELL,
M. D., Corresponding Member of the Imperial Academy of Medicine at St.
Petersburgh, Russia, Professor of Surgery in the University of Georgia, etc.

This little treatise is the production of one of the first medical scholars of the South. Dr. Campbell, years ago, excited
great interest in the profession by his researches in respect to
the excito-secretory system of nerves in its relations to physiology and pathology. An essay which he wrote on the subject was awarded, in 1857, a prize by the American Medical
Association. In the dark period that has intervened but little
was heard of this promising writer, and it was, therefore, with
no common feelings of pleasure that we received this pamphlet, reprinted from the American Journal of Obstetrics, and
showing that the author is pursuing his old line of investigations. In the work before us he traces puerperal eclampsia
to inordinate polarity of the receptive nerve centers. Those
centers, in that excited or irritable condition, receiving an

impression from the irritated womb, give rise to convulsive movements in the muscles. Urea in the blood may act as an irritant, and congestion of those centers may lead to the same convulsions; but whatever the exciting cause, the pathological condition out of which the phenomena arise is undue polarity, or irritability of the cerebral surface, or the motor tract of the cord.

Dr. Campbell has written this treatise not so much in defense of the lancet as to show that its former use in puerperal eclampsia was justifiable on true principles of pathology, and that blood-letting was salutary. Other remedies have been substituted which, he believes, are preferable as being less exhausting, but he finds that the number of recoveries under their administration has not been largely increased. Sixty-five per cent. was the average of cures when blood-letting was the practice, and under our improved methods it has only risen to eighty-nine per cent. But if anæmia of the brain causes the convulsions, as some modern writers hold, how, asks Dr. Campbell, are we to explain the fact that any recovered under the old plan? Chloroform, chloral, the bromides, have certainly increased our success; but then these agents, it is known, diminish the quantity of blood in the brain, and their mode of action is a justification of blood-letting.

The cause of these convulsions, as in fact of all convulsions, being "centric and peripheral irritation, or exaggeration of reflex excitability," the indication of cure is "to quiet and to subdue irritation." For this purpose we possess no remedy equal to opium, which in some form is readily applied either under the skin or by the rectum. The lancet, in Dr. Campbell's judgment, comes next, and in some cases is "utterly indispensable—the most reliable of all our reliances." The *modus operandi* of our new remedies—chloral, the bromides, etc.—is in the same direction; they are sedatives, "the subduers of nervous irritation."

The argument of the author is clear and convincing. He shows that the cause of this disease is not anæmia nor uræmia, though a toxic element in the blood may sometimes give rise to it. The reader would catch the meaning of his sentences a little sooner, perhaps, if they were not quite so long; but the style of the pamphlet is not only vigorous but elevated and eloquent. It will be followed soon, we hope, by papers on other subjects, which will add to his fame as well as enrich medical science.

---

**Clinical Studies of Disease in Children.** By EUSTACE SMITH, M. D., London, Fellow of the Royal College of Physicians, etc. Philadelphia: Lindsay and Blakiston. 1876.

This book is attractive in form. Its binding, typography, paper, etc., give it a remarkably neat appearance, and its size is such that it is as convenient for the doctor to hold after a weary day's work, as one of the volumes of Daniel Deronda, and—may "George Eliot" in her great mercy forgive us if we have sinned—quite as interesting in the perusal.

We need in diseases of children more just such books as Dr. Smith has given us—not just now any other great volumes like the encyclopædic collection of Bouchut, of Meigs and Pepper, that sometimes prove exhaustive in an additional sense, but books devoted to the study of particular diseases; books that are portable, and that we can have with us when we are going our daily rounds, or in longer travel, or off on our recreations, dipping into a volume in casual minutes and feeding our knowledge by the way with new truths and experiences, making the most of the hours that hurry away so fast and of the days that die so soon. Large books have their uses, and we can not give them up; but, oh! publishers, let not your presses be groaning forever under "Ziemssen," "Gross," "Holmes," "Aitken," and many others of the great big volumes, without which no physician's library is said to be complete; but let them throw off now and again such a gem—not less admirable in its setting than in itself— as "Eustace Smith."

These "Studies" occupy nearly three hundred pages, and

are included in ten chapters. The first of the chapters is devoted to some of the peculiarities of disease in children, and to general remarks on diagnosis, prognosis and treatment. In taking the temperature of the patient, Dr. Smith prefers the rectum to the axilla, as more convenient, and more reliable in the result. He also remarks: "Very slight causes will, in infants, produce a remarkable increase of heat; and during natural dentition, just before the passage of the tooth through the gum, a temperature of 104° or 105° F., even in the morning, is not at all an uncommon circumstance. Besides, the normal temperature of young children is rather higher than that of the adult. In a perfectly healthy child of three or four years old the thermometer will often register a temperature of 99½°."

In speaking of treatment, he well observes that this "does not consist entirely, or even principally, in the administration of medicines." He refers to the alkalies as of singular value in the treatment of diseases of young children; this remark applying to many of the acute, and also especially to the chronic maladies. The second chapter is devoted to collapse of the lung, four cases being narrated.

The succeeding chapters are occupied with the consideration of croupous pneumonia, pleurisy, acute catarrhal pneumonia, chronic catarrhal pneumonia, and unabsorbed pneumonic deposits; pneumonic phthisis, cirrhosis of the lung, acute general tuberculosis, tubercular meningitis, and tubercular peritonitis.

Finally, an excellent index is appended, the completeness of which is indicated by the fact that it occupies eleven pages.

---

**Micro-Photographs in Histology, Normal and Pathological.** By CARL SEILER, M. D. Philadelphia: J. H. Coates & Co. August, 1876. No. V. Price 60 cents per number; $6.00 per annum.

In this number, in the first plate, No. XVII, is seen the injected kidney of a mouse, magnified thirty diameters. The general shape is similar to the human kidney, and the malpighian corpuscles are seen as black spots in the cortex. The tubes and vessels from the cortical portion are seen converging at the pelvis. Plate XVIII is a pathological specimen of chronic nephritis. The tubules are filled with albuminoid substance, and the granular mass exhibited on cross section has in places undergone fatty degeneration, and the same process is seen to have occurred in the adjacent connective tissue. Plate XIX, showing the glomeruli, is good so far as it goes, the afferent vessels only being seen. Plate XX exhibits crystals of urea as well as one would wish to see them.

The three plates relating to the kidney are not perfect, but will be an aid in obtaining a knowledge of the minute anatomy and diseases of the kidney, and a serviceable review for those versed in histology.

---

The Theory and Practice of Medicine. By FREDERICK T. ROBERTS, M. D., etc. Second edition from the last London edition, revised and enlarged. Philadelphia: Lindsay and Blakiston, 1876.

The first edition of this book has been most favorably received by the profession in Great Britain and in this country, and similar success undoubtedly awaits this second edition, for it is an excellent work, excellent for the student and for the practitioner.

Were we disposed to be critical, we should dispute the *implied* statement (page 82) that the *corpus luteum* results from a blood-clot; we should object to the omission of cinchonidia as a remedy in intermittent and remittent fever, of salicylic acid in rheumatism, of quinia in cerebro-spinal meningitis; and we should express a doubt as to whether western and southern physicians would agree with the author in his statement that "remittent fever usually lasts from five to fourteen days;" or whether they, in the treatment of this disease, would do as he directs, wait for a remission, and then give fifteen or twenty grains of quinia every two hours.

# Clinic of the Month.

---

TREATMENT OF ECZEMA.—The following is an extract from one of Dr. L. P. Yandell's excellent clinical lectures on Diseases of the Skin, in the Louisville Medical News:

The crustæ are the skin troubles characterized by crusts. Under this head we might discuss the vaccine and small-pox and rupia and itch crusts, but only the latter is a skin disease proper, and it will be treated of in a subsequent discourse.

Eczema in its various forms is the sole dermatitis I ask your attention to in this connection. Eczema means literally a boiling up or a boiling over. It is a moist eruption in its earlier stages, but becomes finally, in certain situations and under certain conditions, a dry eruption. The drying of the moist exudation of eczema produces the crusts; observe they are crusts, not scales. They are met with on all parts of the body, and the various eczemas obtain their names from their location, color, or some other feature. Under the moisture and crusts you find a red, raw surface; itching is usually decided and often tormenting. Smarting pain exists in some cases. The eczema you see in the leg pictured in the Sydenham plate is called E. rubrum, or red eczema, from its color. It is also called weeping sore-leg, because in some cases you have a serous exudation trickling down the leg like tears. E. rubrum is probably always associated with varicose veins. You notice them in the picture. An astringent and anodyne ointment on the leg, and a well-applied roller bandage, together with such constitutional treatment as may be indicated by deranged organs and functions, will heal this eczema, though often it is most obstinate.

Eczema capitis and faciei you see on the face and head in the picture, and in these two little children. In one of them you notice eczema on the neck also. You have in both these cases crusts, moisture, redness, itching. The children are rosy and vigorous-looking; but on inquiry of the mother we learn that the little ones are teething; and furthermore, that in one the itching is most intense about four o'clock P. M., and in the other the pruritus is most vexatious at night. In these patients there probably existed latent malaria and the irritation of dentition to erupt as an eczema. Cold, indigestible food, or lice, might have produced the same result, the malaria being present. Quinia is the remedy for acute eczema in a vast majority of cases. Arsenic and other antiperiodics may substitute it. Iron is always needed. Calomel in cathartic doses promotes recovery. Local treatment is not without benefit. These children will get the following prescriptions:

R̥ Tannin, . . . . . . . . . . gr. x;
  Morphia, . . . . . . . . gr. ij;
  Carbolic acid, . . . . . . . . gr. ij;
  Benzoated oxide-of-zinc ointment (any
    other unirritating ointment might do as
    well), . . . . . . . . . . . ℥ i.

Mix thoroughly and apply to the eruption. No soap must be used, and washing even with simple water should be done as seldom as possible.

R̥ Calomel, . . . . . . . . . . gr. x;
  Bicarb. soda, . . . . . . . . gr. l.

Mix and make ten powders. Give one thrice a week at bedtime.

R̥ Sulphate of quinia, . . . . . . ʒ i;
  Tannin, . . . . . . . . . . gr. xv;
  Syrup of tolu, . . . . . . . . ℥ iij.

Mix carefully. Direct to shake well before administering, and give each child four teaspoonfuls daily, the last to be taken two hours before the period of severe itching is expected to commence. The first dose is to be given four to six hours preceding the last. Properly compounded, this is a tasteless mixture, and therefore excellent for children. It is readily absorbed. It seldom nauseates. One of these children is two and a half years old; the other is a year younger. Children bear and ·require larger doses of quinia in proportion than adults. The antiperiodic treatment will be followed by the ferruginous and bitter tonics. As to diet, the children should have whatever they will eat. Meat and fruits are especially good for them. Never put on low diet any of your patients with skin diseases, and encourage all to use fats.

Chronic eczema may be mistaken by the careless observer for psoriasis. Psoriasis has silvery scales; eczema has crusts. Psoriasis·is always dry; eczema is always moist in its earliest stages. Psoriasis is worst in winter; eczema is often worst in summer. Psoriasis almost invariably exists on the knees when the disease affects the lower limbs, and on the elbows when the trunk is affected; eczema does not especially affect the knees and elbows. Eczema, as a rule, tends to recovery; psoriasis remains stationary or increases. Eczema is generally associated with some functional or systemic disturbance; psoriasis is often found in persons apparently otherwise in perfect health. Eczema is peculiar to no diathesis; psoriasis is a scrofulide, and evidences of the strumous diathesis may always be discovered by careful examination. The spots of psoriasis are smooth-edged, clean-cut in their roundish and ovoid shapes; the spots of eczema are irregular, rough-edged, unsymmetrical, and always rough on top. The psoriasis scales are often smooth to the touch. Remembering these distinctions, diagnosis is without difficulty.

TREATMENT OF FRACTURED PATELLA BY SANBORN'S METHOD. Dr. M. A. Morris, Boston Medical and Surgical Journal, October 5th, gives this valuable report:

The following case occurred in the service of Dr. D. W. Cheever, at the City Hospital, while the reporter was serving under him as house surgeon: On the 30th of November, 1872, C. F., aged forty-five years, a stout, muscular laborer, fell on the street while intoxicated, and fractured his left patella. The bone was broken transversely through its middle, and the lower fragment longitudinally, making a T-shaped fracture. The interval between the upper and lower pieces was three-quarters of an inch, and that between the two lower fragments was very slight indeed. The amount of swelling about the joint was moderate. The limb was put on an inclined plane, with the heel well raised, in a long fracture-box, which extended two-thirds of the way up the thigh, and an evaporating lotion and a figure of eight bandage were applied. On the tenth day Sanborn's method was adopted. (This consists in sticking a long strip of plaster to the anterior surface of the thigh and leg, and securing it by a neatly-adjusted bandage; a loop is left over the knee-joint; under this loop and above the upper fragment is placed a pad or a roller bandage, and another in the same manner below the lower fragment. A piece of stick is inserted into the loop, and by twisting the loop by means of the stick the rollers are forced towards each other and drag the fragments of the patella with them.) By this means the fragments were kept in almost perfect apposition, there being only a tendency of the broken ends to tilt upwards; this was overcome by the pressure of a bandage passed around the joint. On the forty-fourth day a dextrine bandage was applied, and the patient, a few days later, was allowed to go about the ward on crutches, and, two weeks afterwards, to his home, the fracture having apparently united by bone. There was anchylosis of the knee-joint, but he refused to have passive motion practiced. Not long since this man stopped the writer on the street, and pulled up the leg of his pantaloons to show how perfect his knee-pan was. The utmost care was required to discover that ligamentous and not bony union had taken place. At first the attempt to obtain motion between the fragments failed, it was so limited. It is now nearly four years since the accident occurred, and the patient declares that the limb is as strong and perfect in every way as it ever was.

About ten months ago the writer saw a young lady, twenty-four years old, who, in stepping from a train, slipped and fell, striking the left patella against the platform, while the limb was flexed, causing a fracture of the knee-pan through its lower third transversely. Sanborn's method was adopted in this case, and when the apparatus was removed at the end of seven weeks the space between the fragments was probably less than a tenth of an inch. The patient was advised to keep the limb in a straight position, and two weeks later an elastic knee-cap was adjusted.

Regarding the time when passive motion should be commenced, Sir Astley Cooper and others say that it should be carefully employed at the end of five weeks in adults, and a week later in elderly subjects.

Bryant says: "To allow the patient to flex the limb under three months is a hazardous proceeding, for the uniting ligament is sure to be stretched and elongated, and the limb weakened." Erichsen is of the same opinion.

THE USE OF THE OPHTHALMOSCOPE IN INSANITY.—The Dublin Journal of Medical Science, from the *Annales Medico-Psychologiques*, for March, has the following:

Dr. Jehu, of Leigburg, has recently published a series of ophthalmoscopic observations made on 153 cases of different forms of mental alienation, with the following results: 40 cases of melancholia, 17 of mania, 14 of monomania, 19 of dementia, and 16 epileptics were examined, and the anomalies discovered were quite independent of the brain lesion, and included myopia, floccular opacity of the vitreous, alteration in visual accommodation, etc. The ophthalmoscope did not reveal any lesion characteristic of any one or other form of mental derangement; but in a small number of cases a common lesion, affecting the circulation of the papilla and retina, was found concomitantly with a congestive state of the head. Thus, in four cases of melancholia, with intermittent congestion of the head, the posterior plane of the eye participated in the congestion; it was red, the vessels engorged, the veins sinuous and more dilated than the arteries. In these cases the pupils were dilated. The same appearances were found in a maniac and two monomaniacs during a period of intense congestion of the head. The examination was entirely negative in dements and epileptics, except in the case of one dement who presented atrophy of the optic nerve, contrary to what has been asserted by Kostl and Kiemetschek. Whenever inequality of the pupil existed it did not indicate any pathological condition of the fundus oculi. In forty-seven general paralytics examined, M. Jehu has found atrophy of the optic nerve four times at both sides, and three times at one side; eight times the atrophy showed itself by a white coloration, with diminution and contraction of the vessels. In all the cases, with the exception of four, the examination showed that the atrophy comes on early in the disease, but not sufficiently so, however, to aid in the diagnosis at the period before there is any appreciable anomaly of the faculties. The optic atrophy and the cerebral *ramollissement* are not developed coequally. The inequality of the pupils observed in the generality of cases does not count as a point in the march of the atrophy. Amongst the forty-seven paralytics observed, the state of the pupils did not corroborate the assertion of Allbutt, that after the contraction of the pupils the development of the atrophy and dilatation was slower.

SALICYLIC ACID.—Professor H. Köhler, of Halle, states that all the remote therapeutic effects of this remedy may be obtained by administering its salt, the salicylate of soda. The latter is not an antiseptic, and where such is desired, the acid itself must be used. To prevent zymotic action in the blood it is of little or no use, as the acid enters the circulation only in the form of salicylate of soda, which latter has no anti-zymotic virtues. The salt is a most powerful febrifuge, and is by him regarded as even better than quinia in this respect. It will reduce the temperature in fevers with remarkable uniformity, and is very much more convenient to administer than the acid. In rheumatic fever it acts admirably, but is not so good an antiperiodic as quinia in malarial diseases. (Medical and Surgical Reporter.)

# 𝔑otes and 𝔔ueries.

---

Shippen's Lectures on Midwifery.—In this Centennial year of American independence, and especially after our great International Medical Congress, it is natural to revert to the work of the Fathers of American Medicine. On our own part this feeling is just now receiving a fresh stimulus in having before us a manuscript copy of Professor William Shippen's lectures on midwifery.

Dr. Shippen returned to Philadelphia from London, where John Hunter had taught him anatomy and surgery, and William Hunter and Mackenzie had been his obstetric teachers; and from Edinburgh, where he had been under the teaching of Cullen and the elder Monro, and where he was graduated; and just one hundred and fourteen years ago inaugurated medical teaching in this country. At that time and for many years afterward, he taught anatomy, surgery and midwifery.

The copy of his lectures on midwifery, to which we have referred, was made in 1781. The number of lectures is twenty-four.

The introductory is chiefly devoted to "the different authors on midwifery." Hippocrates is declared "the first man midwife." After reference to him and his teaching, we next have Celsus brought forward. Then by long transition we are brought to Paré, "who wrote a short treatise, but scarce worth purchasing." Mauriceau is commended, so are Chamberlen, La Motte, Deventer, Portal, Chapman, Maubray, Burton, Gifford, and Ould, and their special contributions to obstetrics referred to. He speaks of the best British obstetric teacher of the eighteenth century thus: "Smellie* is a good practical writer, and his observations are in general to be depended upon. His directions for using the forceps are judicious, though not perspicuous. However, he is not always to be followed, since he recommends using the forceps where the head is high up, at which time they should never be used." Then follows an account of the improvement in the instrument made by him. Both in the warning given as to the use of the forceps, and in various other passages in these lectures, we see how thoroughly indoctrinated Dr. Shippen was with the teachings of William Hunter, whom Tyler Smith has so commended as the founder of the *physiological* school of obstetrics, and who for a while in practice pushed his worship and waiting upon nature to such an extreme in reference to the delivery† of the placenta.

In connection with his description of the external organs of generation, Dr. Shippen gives the following direction as to the introduction of the catheter: "Place the instrument in the groove between the nymphæ, then pass the end down a little way till you meet with some obstruction, which is no other than the protuberant surface of the meatus, and if you humor it a little, it will easily slip into the passage," etc. "Humor it a little!" Just the word—just the way, as every doctor who has tried knows.

Not much can be said in favor of Dr. Shippen's theory of

* In Hutchinson's *Biographia Medica*, London, 1799, this curious fact—probably little known to-day—is mentioned: "Smellie was at one time seriously endeavoring to substitute wooden forceps in the place of the steel ones, and actually made several experiments with them, and, as he says, with success."

But Smellie's big blunder was calling Lithopædus Senonenis an obstetric author, when lithopædii senonensis icon was simply the representation of a petrified substance; a blunder which Dr. Burton, of York, so severely criticized; a blunder, too, which Sterne has perpetuated, as readers of Tristram Shandy will remember.

† "Teaching that nature, unassisted, was adequate to the expulsion of the placenta in every case, he never interfered; but experience, says Dr. Hamilton, soon taught him the error of this position; for by suffering the placenta to remain too long, he lost five patients of rank in one year." (James's Burns.)

impregnation as thus given: "It is probable in the act of coition the more volatile parts of the semen, after being received into the fallopian tubes, are conveyed by the vessels lining their inner surface into the ovaria, whereby an ovum becomes impregnated, which being enlarged by a proper nutriment, breaks through the external coat of the ovarium."

In speaking of Labor and its Management, after stating that "the old have generally hard labor," etc., he adds, "and hence their labors may go some days without having recourse to art, which must be avoided as much as possible."

Further on he remarks, "timorous women must be soothed, and the hump-backed kept in a chair, as they breathe with difficulty in a horizontal posture." "All weak, delicate women are subject to floodings, and, therefore, should be delivered naked in bed, with proper cloths under them, to avoid any disturbance in undressing them."

In reference to the delivery of the placenta, his teaching was decidedly Hunterian; he says that "there are instances where the placenta was retained in the uterus seven days or more, and then expelled without danger."

The Third Class of Preternatural Labors, in Shippen's order, includes presentations of the back, belly, and shoulders. Podalic version is the treatment he advises, and he explicitly states that if there be difficulty in performing it, "the woman may be placed upon her knees, which will greatly relax the abdominal muscles."

Do the younger obstetricians of to-day all know what "a sheath case" is? Dr. Shippen remarks, in speaking of transverse presentations, "If the waters have been gone a long time, and the uterus contracted like a sheath around the body of the child, it is then called a *sheath case.*"

In regard to the management of women after delivery, he remarks, that "formerly it was customary to swathe the abdomen, but now the petticoat with the broad band is thought to be preferable;" "the breasts should be covered with flannel or rabbit skins;" "a bladder of warm water, or a galbanum plaister applied to the abdomen for after pains;" "wine caudle, given for the first three or four days, if the woman is not liable to inflammation," etc.

But we must terminate our notice. In reading the old authors in medicine we are sometimes tempted to smile at some of their queer faiths and practices, and pride ourselves upon our greater knowledge. But let us repress our mirth and humble our pride with the truth recently so well uttered by Dr. Maudsley: * "No doubt in the future, as in the past, the knowledge of one period will sometimes appear foolishness at a more advanced period of human evolution—the truth of one age become the laughing-stock of the next; but we may profitably reflect that decaying doctrine had its use in its day, and it may teach us modesty to consider that much which has its place in our mental organization now, and is serving its proper end in the development theory, will one day probably be put aside as obsolete belief. Let it be our prayer that when that day comes, and this generation comes up for critical judgment as a historical study before the tribunal of posterity, it may be justly said of it that it has done as much for the progress of mankind as some of the generations upon which the wisest of us look back perhaps with indulgent compassion, and the unwise among us with foolish scorn."

FOREIGN APPRECIATION OF THE LABORS OF DR. J. S. BILLINGS.—In the British and Foreign Medico-Chirurgical Review, October, there is a very favorable notice of the Specimen Fasciculus of a Catalogue of the National Medical Library. In the course of the notice it is stated that "by the energy and unflagging perseverance of Dr. Billings, a comparatively small and little known library at the Surgeon-General's office has rapidly developed into a magnificent collection of medical works of all nations, well deserving the recently assumed title of 'The National Medical Library,' though essentially the medical section of the Library of Congress."

In concluding, the writer observes: "We heartily wish Dr. Billings health and success in carrying out this vast

---

* This is an extract from the very able and admirable introductory lecture delivered at University College, October 2, 1876.

amount of labor in the interests of his professional colleagues; and we feel we can do him no better service than by calling the attention of our readers to his desire to further enrich his library both by independent treatises and by the more ephemeral literature of the present and past days, to his readiness to receive donations of works, and to his courtesy in acknowledging them."

This just tribute will be heartily endorsed, and these kindly wishes promptly echoed by every physician who knows the worth and work of Dr. Billings. The duty of American physicians in regard to this work is plain and positive. Let them see to it by personal appeal to individual members of the United States Congress, if necessary, that sufficient appropriations are made for its completion.

DOUBLE MONSTER.—An interesting teratological specimen was recently observed in the practice of Dr. J. D. O'Brien, of Pembroke, Ky., and the doctor has promised the Practitioner a description of it. It probably belonged to the class of double monsters, and to that particular kind which has been described by Vrolik under the title of *anterior duplicity*. Vrolik observes "that the most complete examples of duplicity yet known are found in this class, whose distinctive characters are, that two bodies, in a state of nearly equal development, are placed exactly opposite to one another, with their sterna connected together, and with their abdominal cavities either partially or completely coalesced. Here, however, as in all the other classes, examples are found of gradations towards a state of singleness."

DEATH OF DR. A. G. WALTERS.—Dr. Walters, of Pittsburgh, died of pneumonia on the 14th of last month. He was a native of Prussia, a graduate of the University of Berlin, and had been residing in Pittsburgh since 1841. Dr. Walters, sixty-five years old at his death, was a man of no ordinary abilities and attainments, and achieved great eminence as a surgeon, not only by brilliant operations, but also by his many contributions to surgical literature.

DR. CARSON IN REPLY TO DR. BARTHOLOW.—We hoped this discussion was over, but Dr. Carson has sent the following, requesting its insertion:

*Editors Practitioner:* It is scarcely necessary for me to notice Dr. Bartholow's last communication in your September number, as you have called attention to the typographical error which afforded Dr. Bartholow the slenderest possible foundation for the toppling mass of epithet behind which he endeavors to hide his palpable contradictions. But as Dr. Bartholow desires a correction, I shall gratify him. The typographical error was doubtless evident to every one who read my article. It consisted in putting *depuration* for *deposition* in the paragraph quoted from Dr. Bartholow's recent work on Therapeutics.

Dr. Bartholow chose the action of digitalis as an illustration of the principle of "physiological antagonism" in the treatment of "pneumonia," and presented their opposition in the following form:

| DIGITALIS. | PNEUMONIA. |
|---|---|
| Exudation checked or prevented by the heightened tonicity of the vessels. | Exudation of fibrinous material. Migration of white blood corpuscles. |

The reading of this is that digitalis checks or prevents exudation by heightening the tonicity of the vessels. In pneumonia there are exudation of fibrinous material and migration of white blood corpuscles; therefore digitalis antagonizes these conditions in pneumonia. Then let us add what, on page 14 of the Seguin lecture, follows the Doctor's tabular statement, in precisely his own language:

"There are two periods, speaking from the point of view of my personal experience, in which digitalis renders the most important service in pneumonia, viz., during the stage of hyperæmia and *exudation*, to limit the area of the inflammatory action, and at the period of crisis to maintain the power of the heart."

This means, if it means anything, that digitalis limits "the area of inflammatory action" in pneumonia, by controlling hyperæmia and *exudation* (of fibrin and white blood corpuscles; see the Doctor's table of opposites above).

We now add the quotation from Dr. Bartholow's work on Therapeutics, page 275. Both the lecture and the book were published in 1876:

"That digitalis has any power to prevent the *deposition* of fibrinous material, to *prevent* or check *the migration of the white blood corpuscles,* or to arrest the multiplication of the cellular elements of inflamed parts, seems to the author highly improbable."

Now no amount of personal abuse of me, or substitution of irrelevant topics, can reconcile this contradiction. Is this antagonism of statement pathological? or is this the physiological play of a many-sided and flexible intellect?

The profession have a right to ask as to the exponent of medical doctrines, Is he honest? Manifest and intentional avoidance of the true and fair issues of criticism, and the substitution of epithet for argument, do not constitute elements of honesty or courage. The profession have also a right to ask, Is he capable? Imperfect knowledge of general and special pathology; hasty adoption of crude theories; investing remedies with preconceived qualities, with wonderful facility for finding the occasion for the precise adjustments required; misunderstanding and misstatements of the certainties of medicine, and thereby misleading the untrained or unsuspecting minds of the profession; and failure, in proper clinical basis, for statements that can not be accepted without something more than doubtful assertion, constitute capacity for mischief only. Practical and honest medicine is unduly weighted every day by such obstructions.

*Cincinnati.* WILLIAM CARSON.

BILLINGS, CLAPP & CO.—Visitors to the Centennial, especially those of the medical profession, could not fail to be struck with the handsome display made by this celebrated Boston firm of manufacturing chemists, the successors of James R. Nichols & Co.

OPIUM ANTIDOTES EXPOSED.—We copy from the Boston Medical and Surgical Journal, of October 26th, the following, and urge the especial attention of our Indiana subscribers:

In the month of August last, Dr. George F. French, of Portland, Maine, was applied to by an opium-eater who asked his advice about a preparation advertised as a sure cure for the opium-habit. Naturally being suspicious of such an article, he sent to the manufacturer, Mrs. J. A. Drollinger, of La Porte, Ind., for a sample bottle. This was furnished, but, as we understand, the proprietress declined to give any information as to its composition, saying, however, that it "is harmless when taken as directed," and "does not contain opium in any form." Failing to be satisfied with this assertion, the doctor applied such chemical tests as he conveniently could and got the reactions of morphia. But to make assurance doubly sure, and to supplement and confirm the chemical test by a physiological one, he secretly administered a small dose of the antidote to a person who had a peculiar idiosyncrasy with reference to opium. The speedy result was, as had been anticipated, a manifestation of the symptoms which in this individual had always followed the exhibition of opium, namely, suffusion of the eyes, loss of voice, pain in the head, and insomnia. Dr. French then reported these facts to the Cumberland County Medical Society, which, at his suggestion, at once appointed a committee to further investigate the matter, and voted to bear the expense of whatever analyses might be necessary. At the regular meeting of the society in September the committee presented the following report:

The committee to whom was assigned the duty of investigating the so-called "opium antidote" prepared by Mrs. J. A. Drollinger, of La Porte, Indiana, beg leave to report that a sample bottle of the article, which was obtained directly from the manufacturer, was sent to Dr. Edward R. Squibb, of Brooklyn, N. Y., for quantitative analysis. His onerous engagements rendered it impossible for him to conduct the investigation in person, but he sent the specimen to Messrs. Walz and Stillwell, chemists, New York, a firm which he thoroughly confides in and endorses. So deeply interested did he become in the project that he insisted upon bearing the expense of the analysis, in spite of the committee's expressed unwillingness to have him assume such a tax.

Walz and Stillwell report that "this sample is glycerine colored with aniline red, and containing in solution crystallized sulphate of morphia, 1.383 per cent. by weight"—about seven grains to the ounce.

While this investigation was progressing, the committee found another alleged "opium antidote," prepared by "Dr. S. B. Collins, the Great Narcologist of the Age," likewise of La Porte, Indiana. A specimen of this was submitted to Dr. Henry Carmichael, Professor of Chemistry in Bowdoin College and Assayer of the State of Maine, who arrived at the following conclusions:

"1. The opium antidote contains morphine.

"2. The morphine is combined with sulphuric acid.

"3. The sulphate of morphine amounts to 3.2 per cent., or fourteen grains to the ounce."

Dr. Walz says that he made an analysis of Collins's "antidote" in 1871, and found that it contained morphia, though he did not ascertain the quantity.

In conclusion, your committee respectfully suggest that the society take some action which will result in the wide dissemination of the information which has been acquired concerning these dangerous preparations.

Frederick Henry Gerrish, George F. French, and Thomas A. Foster, committee.

The society instructed the committee to present their report to some prominent medical journal, and, if it seemed to them advisable, to give the public warning of the danger to which it is exposed through the newspapers of the state. A vote of thanks was passed to Dr. Squibb for his generous assistance.

The importance of this exposure is too obvious to require any extensive comment on our part. Physicians now have something better than general reasons to offer their patients when warning them to shun such nostrums. The profession will not be insensible to the valuable service which the Cumberland County Medical Society has rendered it and the community, and it is to be hoped that other similar bodies will be encouraged to display equal enterprise and spirit. There is a great opportunity for our brethren in the region of La Porte to distinguish themselves as guardians of the health of the people, and we trust that they will not be slow to follow up the track so well opened by their fellows in Maine.

PROFESSOR THOMAS G. PRIOLEAU.—The Charleston Medical Journal announces the death of this venerable physician. Doctor Prioleau was a graduate* of the University of Pennsylvania, and one of the founders of the Medical College of South Carolina, in which school he held the chair of obstetrics until a few years ago. He was nearly ninety years of age, but retained full possession of his faculties to the last.

WARNER'S SUGAR-COATED PILLS.—Wm. R. Warner & Co. have received the Centennial award for their soluble sugar-coated pills. This is the third World's Fair prize attesting the superiority over both home and foreign competition, of these preparations.

TO CONTRIBUTORS.—Papers have been received from Dr. Robert Battey and from Professors Pooley and Thompson, which will appear in our next number.

TYPOGRAPHICAL ERROR.—In the foot-note, page 219 of the last number of this journal, the date 1526 should be 1826.

*In looking over the Medical and Philosophical Register, Vol. V, 1808, we find that Dr. Prioleau was graduated that year, and among his associates were W. P. C. Barton, Samuel Jackson, Isaac Heister, and Thomas Worthington.

# THE AMERICAN PRACTITIONER.

### DECEMBER, 1876.

## Original Communications.

## A CLINICAL LECTURE—DIAGNOSTIC VALUE OF ABDOMINAL PALPATION IN PREGNANCY.

BY JAMES R. CHADWICK, M. D.

*Fellow of the American Gynecological Society.*

(Continued from page 284.)

*At the Bedside.*—Having first established the longitudinal or transverse position of the fetus, and the period of the pregnancy, the next step is to decide upon the presentation which we may have before us.

*Longitudinal Positions.*—The *head* is first to be sought for, and will commonly be found, by suitable palpation, over the symphysis pubis; not unfrequently, it lies somewhat to one side, especially in the earlier months of pregnancy, when it is less crowded down into the pelvis by the pressure of the fundus uteri upon the breech. If not discovered over the symphysis pubis, the head must be located in the vicinity of the fundus.

One extremity of the ovoid having been found, the other, the *breech*, is to be sought. It must lie in the opposite verti-cal half to that in which the head lies.

The presenting part, whether head or breech, may be above the brim of the pelvis, where it will be freely movable, and easily accessible to palpation; or it may have descended into the pelvis, and become more or less fixed, in proportion to the depth to which it has sunk, and its size relatively to that of the pelvis. In the latter case, the presenting head *may* still be reached by palpation, or often the neck only, which can be recognized by its appearing, when grasped, too small to be either the head or the breech. The bimanual method of examining the presenting part may, in cases of "deep-seated head," be resorted to with success. When the breech has descended into the pelvis, the part seized by the hand is not small, but consisting as it does of the body and perhaps the legs, it is as large and may even be larger than the breech itself.

The remaining regions of the abdomen are then to be explored to determine in which direction the *back* is turned, and in which quarter the small extremities lie. The *back* is commonly directed either to the right or left side of the mother, and may be recognized rather by the greater resistance, imparted by it to the lateral half of the abdomen in which it is located, than by its long, resistant surface being absolutely felt, though this last may often happen. In the opposite lateral half of the abdomen, the limbs are to be sought for, both by deep pressure and by gentle manipulation.

*Transverse Positions.*—In these the *head* and *breech* are first to be distinguished from each other as they lie in the opposite lateral segments of the abdomen.

The *back* and *limbs* are then felt for, with a view to determining whether the former is turned more to the front or more to the back of the mother. No presenting parts will be detected, an arm or a leg being too small to be appreciable by palpation. All these signs of the position of the fetus may not be elucidated in every case, but enough will almost invariably be made out to enable us to decide upon the presentations and positions, recognized in the classification adopted. The examiner should not, however, be satisfied until he has tried at least to obtain each of the data given above.

Before giving the classification, I must apologize for substituting the English term "presentation" for the exact translation of the German word "lage," which would be "position." This is all the more to be deplored, for "position" (lage) seems to have been specially chosen, because of the importance accorded in Germany to external examination, in which the presenting part plays but a subordinate *role*. The danger of being misunderstood, from the use of the term "position" in a more restricted sense in English and American treatises, seems to justify this change. As no two schools in Germany have the same classification, that used in Vienna will be given, because it is the simplest and best.

The third and fourth occipital presentations, of English and American authors, are designated as abnormal "rotations" of the other two occipital presentations.

After the vaginal examination, in breech presentations, more exactitude is sometimes gained by accepting knee and foot presentations, as subdivisions of the first; very little stress is, however, laid upon this point, as it is devoid of all practical worth. The German names are added, to aid such as may occasionally refer to German text-books.

## *Classification of Presentations and Positions of the Vienna School.*

### I.—LONGITUDINAL PRESENTATIONS.

#### (Längenlage.)

HEAD.—(Kopflage.)

Breech.
(Steisslage.)

Occipital.
(Schadellage.)

Face.
(Gesichtslage.)

2d. (Rücken nach rechts.) Back toward right side.

1st. (Rücken nach links.) Back toward left side.

2d. (Rücken nach rechts.) Back toward right side.

1st. (Rücken nach links.) Back toward left side.

2d. (Rücken nach rechts.) Back toward right side.

1st. (Rücken nach links.) Back toward left side.

Oblique presentations (schieflage) always change into longitudinal or transverse.

## II.—TRANSVERSE PRESENTATIONS.

### (Querlage.)

| First.<br>Head in left side.<br>(Kopf links.) | | Second.<br>Head in right side.<br>(Kopf rechts.) | |
| --- | --- | --- | --- |
| 2d. Position.<br>(Stellung.)<br>Back backwards.<br>(Rücken nach hinten.) | 1st. Position.<br>(Stellung.)<br>Back forwards.<br>(Rücken nach vorne.) | 2d. Position.<br>(Stellung.)<br>Back backwards.<br>(Rücken nach hinten.) | 1st. Position.<br>(Stellung.)<br>Back forwards.<br>(Rücken nach vorne.) |

It will be observed that this classification and nomenclature are the direct result of the prominence given, in Germany, to the external examination, as all the different presentations and positions can be determined, *exclusively*, from the data thus furnished. From this are the diagnoses made, and then later confirmed, made doubtful, or, in rare cases, refuted by the vaginal examination. The division is extremely simple, and has been proved to give all the indications of real importance in practice. Before reviewing the signs yielded by palpation, in each of the presentations and positions, I must briefly refer to the assistance furnished in this respect by another mode of examination.

*Auscultation of the Fetal Heart.*—This may be performed, with the ear applied to the integument of the abdomen, through the medium of a sheet, or better still by means of a stethoscope, because this instrument may be applied to any

part of the abdomen, without necessitating a constrained posture or a congested head, on the part of the auscultator; it is
open to only one objection, that the woman's abdomen must
be laid bare. It has been proved that the fetal heart-sounds
are, almost invariably, best heard through the back of the
fetus, hence at that part of the abdominal surface of the
woman beneath which the back lies. This is based upon the
fact that the back is generally forced, by the motions of the
fetal extremities, into immediate apposition with the uterine
walls, hence the distance through the back to the auscultator's
ear is less than through the breast; moreover, a considerable
layer of fluid is apt to intervene between the breast and the
uterine walls, a condition peculiarly unfavorable to the transmission of sound. This rule has but one recognized exception, though, of course, unusual circumstances may render it
unreliable. In face presentations, from the unnatural position
of the head, the occiput being pushed back upon the vertebral column, the dorsum of the fetus is separated from the
uterine walls on that side, and the breast is thrust forward
against them on the other, thus reversing the ordinary condition of things. Here the heart-sounds will best be heard in
that region of the abdomen nearest to the breast of the fetus.
In all other presentations, the spot at which the fetal heart-
sounds are heard with the greatest distinctness will always
guide us to the position of the back. If the back of the fetus
is directed toward the back of the mother, the heart-sounds
will be but faintly audible, if at all. During contractions of
the uterus, the fetal heart-sounds are never heard. It will now
be seen how auscultation of the fetal heart-sounds will confirm
or refute the data, furnished by palpation, as to the lay of the
back.

*Signs obtained in each of the Presentations and Positions
through Palpation and Auscultation.*

*First Occipital.*—Head over the pubes. Breech in fundus
uteri. Back in left side of abdomen; small extremities in
right. Fetal heart-sounds in left lower segment of abdomen.

*Second Occipital.*—Head and breech as above. Back and fetal heart-sounds in right side; small extremities in left.

*First Face.*—Head over pubes, somewhat to left. Breech in fundus somewhat to left. Small extremities in right side, also fetal heart-sounds.

*Second Face.*—Head over pubes, and somewhat to right. Breech in fundus, somewhat to right. Small extremities and fetal heart-sounds in left side.

*Oblique* are merely divergencies from one or another of the occipital or transverse presentation; hence the signs will be but modifications of those found in these presentations.

*First Breech.*—Breech over pubes. Head in fundus uteri. Back in left side of abdomen; small extremities in right.

*Second Breech.*—Breech and head as above. Back in right side; small extremities in left.

*First Transverse.*—Head in left side; breech in right.

*First Position.*—Back forwards. Small extremities backwards. Heart-sounds heard.

*Second Position.*—Back backwards. Small extremities forwards. Heart-sounds not heard, or but very faintly.

*Second Transverse.*—Head in right side; breech in left.

*First Position* as in first transverse.

*Second Position* as in first transverse.

*The Diagnosis of Twins* is, in general, very uncertain, and in primiparæ rarely successful. A depression running across the abdomen is rather the exception than the rule, and even if present is not conclusive. Up to the tenth lunar month, the two fetuses are so movable that they yield but few data on which to base a diagnosis. During the tenth lunar month the following signs, if satisfactorily made out, will justify us in pronouncing in favor of twins; yet there is no condition in midwifery which so frequently baffles the skill of the most experienced obstetricians as this:

First. The recognition, by palpation, of several similar large fetal parts (head or breech). Perhaps, while one is deep in the pelvis, two others may be felt through the abdomen.

Second. The recognition, by palpation, of numerous,

small, movable, fetal parts (legs and arms), or their spontaneous motions in several regions of the abdomen. ·

Third. The exact diagnosis, by palpation, of position of each fetus.

Fourth. The immobility of the presenting part (as revealed by palpation and vaginal examination), especially after evacuation of the liquor amnii, while the parts felt through the abdominal walls are very movable.

Fifth. The perception, by auscultation, of the fetal heart-sounds at two opposite sides of the abdomen, while they are inaudible in the intervening space.

Sixth. A striking want of accord between the presenting part (as revealed by palpation and vaginal examination) and the place of the heart-sounds.

In general, an unusual size of the abdomen, a lateral distention of the uterus, the sensation by the mother of fetal motions in many regions, are signs of subordinate value, but should at least raise suspicions of a multiple pregnancy.

*The Signs of Extra-Uterine Pregnancy,* revealed to palpation, vary so greatly in different cases that scarcely any rule can be given for them. The chief peculiarity is the presence of two abdominal tumors; one being the fetus with its inclosing cyst, in which, early in the pregnancy, movable, resistant parts may be felt, and later even the position, etc., of the fetus be determined; the second tumor is the uterus, somewhat enlarged, but not so much so as the supposed duration of the pregnancy would require. Until the fetal parts or their motions can be made out, or the fetal heart-sounds can be heard, extra-uterine pregnancy can not be diagnosticated, by external examination, from any other cystic tumor.

*Complications of Pregnancy revealed by Palpation.*

*The Death of the Fetus* during pregnancy can never be recognized with certainty, but may be suspected from the following signs: The general flabbiness and want of fixed shape of an abdomen, which had previously been firm and resistant, as well as difficulty in defining the outline of the uterus; the impossibility of feeling the spontaneous movements of the fetus (very unreliable); the softness and non-resistance of the fetal parts, and their remaining passively in any spot into which they are pushed; the non-ballottement and soft feel of the head. Confirmatory evidence is derived from the fact that the fetal heart-sound, which had been audible to a skilled auscultator, can no longer be detected in any region of the abdomen.

*The Size of the Fetal Head* relatively to that of the pelves. This, in all cases of narrow or deformed pelvis, is of the utmost importance, as determining whether the delivery should be left to the course of nature, or whether manual or instrumental interference is called for. The size and hardness of the head may be presumed from the general size of the fetus, and estimated directly by palpation. The head can seldom be fairly grasped, and its dimensions arrived at, except when over the pubes, and even then it requires long and constant practice to enable its size to be calculated with any degree of accuracy.

*Hydrocephalus* is diagnosticated from the large size, and the absence of the usual hardness of the head, as well as from its remaining above the pelvic brim, in spite of strong uterine contractions, when previous easy births, or an exact measurement, has established the normal dimensions of the pelvis.

*Contractions of the Uterus* are plainly detected through the abdominal walls, and their character determined. The different conditions of inertia, atony, exhaustion, paralysis, either general or partial, and tetanus of the uterus, during delivery, are thus recognized and appropriately treated. Colicky pains, from contractions of the uterus before the full term, may be distinguished from other similar pains, and proper means be taken to avert a threatening abortion or miscarriage.

*Retroversion* of the pregnant uterus is commonly first indicated by retention of urine and colicky abdominal pains; on palpation the bladder will be detected, extending often as high as the umbilicus. The uterus will be out of reach.

*Rupture of the Uterus,* during natural delivery, occurs, according to C. Braun, from the violence of the contractions, and is located transversely at the junction of neck and body. It can only be certainly diagnosticated from the vaginal examination, but may be suspected from the sudden cessation of pains, previously severe; from the great change in the position of the fetus, and the retreat of the presenting part; from the recognition of the contracted uterus as a hard tumor upon one side; and from the greater distinctness with which the fetus, having escaped into the peritoneal cavity, is felt. When the fetus does not thus escape, the fundus uteri commonly falls to the opposite side to that in which the rupture has taken place, owing to the local paralysis of the latter. The abdomen becomes large, and fluids collect in its deep parts.

*Tumors,* such as fibroids, ovarian cysts, etc. The former will often mar the symmetry of the uterine contour, and may then be carelessly taken for the small extremities, or even a second fetus; their persistence in one spot, in spite of manipulation, and their possible want of accord with the position of the fetus, will dispel the illusion. Ovarian cysts can generally be made out as distinct elastic tumors, separated from the uterus by a well-marked furrow.

## Hindrances and Expedients.

*Tension of the abdominal walls,* when due simply to the unusual dilatation as often happens with primiparæ, may generally be overcome by attention to the details of examination, given in the early pages of this paper. Yet this condition will occasionally prove so obstinate as to render palpation fruitless. Percussion may then be resorted to.

*Muscular contractions* of the abdominal and uterine walls. The latter are involuntary and unavoidable, unless through the delicacy of the explorer's touch. The intervals between the spasms must then be made the most of. The abdominal muscles are, for the most part, under the influence of the will, and should but rarely prove an obstacle to their examination. The woman's attention may often have to be distracted by conversation, or better still she should be required to hold her mouth open, or to count in order to prevent her straining.

*Hydramnios* may cause such distension of the uterus as to interfere seriously with palpation. The uterus will then be large and symmetrical, even yielding fluctuation in extreme cases. The fetus is freely movable, and ballottement easy. The fetal heart-sounds are weak or unheard. Too small an amount of liquor amnii, on the other hand, will allow the uterus to cling to the fetus before the contractions, and enable a long and tedious first stage of labor to be foreseen.

*Tenderness of the abdomen* is rarely so great as to interfere seriously with careful palpation, though a circumscribed spot may be rendered so sensitive from the continual kicking of a lively child, especially if it be against the ribs, as not to bear the least touch. Cases, of which I have seen one, occur occasionally, in which, at any time during the early months of pregnancy, an hyperæsthesia of the peritoneum is excited by spasms of the uterus; many of the local symptoms of a subacute peritonitis, such as pain, extreme tenderness on pressure, etc., are present, with entire absence of the constitutional disturbance, effusion, and other diagnostic symptoms of such a condition. The true nature of the affection has never been satisfactorily shown, so far as I can learn. It is pleasant, however, to feel that this state will improve with time and treatment, and have no prejudicial effect upon the regular course of the pregnancy, provided abortion is at the time guarded against. Such a complication would evidently prevent all palpation, as might also a true circumscribed peritonitis, such as is caused by the bursting of the cyst in extrauterine pregnancy.

*Adipose tissue*, when deposited in great amount in the abdominal walls, adds greatly to their thickness, and may thus form a serious hindrance to abdominal examination. No change occurs in the uterine walls from successive pregnancies, except a little unevenness of surface in some instances.

*Ascites and Flatus* may occur during pregnancy and prevent all access to the uterus through the abdomen. They are distinguished from each other by percussion and fluctuation. Graviditas nervosa is a form of the latter, which is often met with at the time of the grand climacteric, and may then give rise to much doubt and distress.

You have seen, gentlemen, that while describing the various steps to be taken, I have illustrated my words by a manual demonstration. I have in this way discovered that the fundus of my patient's uterus rises to a point two inches above the navel. I have recognized the head over the pubes a little to the right of the median line ; in the left side I am able to trace a continuous resistant surface which I assume to be the back, especially as I find some small, fleeting objects in the right side of the abdomen. If this assumption is correct, I shall hear the fetal heart-sounds most plainly—though but faintly at this early period of pregnancy—at about this spot, which corresponds with the back of the child's thorax. It is audible, but could scarcely be caught by an untrained ear.

The abdominal wall is so thin and lax in this patient that I should not hesitate, with this examination alone, to assert that the woman has reached the seventh lunar month of her pregnancy, and that the child is in the first occipital presentation.

I shall continue this subject, on the next opportunity, by describing the combination of the internal and external examination, and subsequently the application of palpation to the treatment of malpresentation.

Boston, Mass.

---

## CASE OF MAMMARY CANCER.

### BY ROBERT BATTEY, M. D.

It is always interesting to be able to follow up surgical cases after they have passed from under our hands, and to note their progress towards the final results. At page 751 of Beard and

Rockwell's treatise on the Medical and Surgical Uses of Electricity, 1875, will be found a partial history of the case of Mrs. H. As this case, in many of its features, is one of more than ordinary interest, it may not be unacceptable to the readers of the Practitioner to learn more of it; and I am, fortunately, in a position to add to the history, having had the case under my observation both before and subsequent to the operative procedures detailed in the work cited.

In the early spring of 1873, Mrs. H., whilst visiting relatives in this place, consulted me in regard to a tumor in her left breast, which was hard and painful, and gave her some mental disquietude. The tumor was as large as a hen's egg, very hard, nodular, the nipple retracted, and a distinct cord passing from it to the tumor. There was an enlarged lymphatic in the left axilla. The diagnosis was scirrhus tumor of the breast, and she was advised to have it removed at the earliest moment. Upon her return to Virginia she applied at once to Professor Cabell, and was referred by him to Drs. Beard and Rockwell, who detail the operative history in their work before referred to.

In consequence of the unfavorable prognosis of the electricians, the patient put herself afterwards in the hands of a cancer quack, who applied caustics quite extensively and perseveringly to the breast, and sloughed off the tissues freely, including much of the pectoral muscles. Under this treatment, her general health and strength gave way greatly; and finding herself in a sad plight she came south, hoping a more congenial climate might recuperate her.

In May, 1875, she came under the care of my business copartner, Dr. Holmes. Her condition was at this time a sad one; her flesh and strength wasted; her appetite gone; her nervous system racked with constant and intolerable pain. A large open ulcer upon the thorax, which could scarcely be covered by a man's hand, and discharging a thin, ichorous pus, was a burden too grievous to be borne. What with sleepless nights and long, wearisome days, life seemed verging to a longed-for close.

She was at first put upon morphia, and the nervous system tranquilized and good refreshing sleep obtained, which, in two weeks' time, presented the case in a much more favorable aspect. Dr. Holmes now prescribed an alterative course of the potassic iodide with corrosive sublimate, allowing sufficient morphia to secure comfortable rest at night. The ulcer soon began to heal, and went steadily on to a full and perfect cicatrization. She rapidly gained strength and flesh, until she now presents the semblance of robust health. All appearance of cachexia is gone; her complexion is clear and ruddy. The appetite is excellent, the digestion good, the bowels regular, and indeed all of her functions are regular and healthy. She is able to do, and does do, household work in all departments. There is now no enlargement of the axillary glands, but beneath the skin upon the chest, and in the subclavicular region, there are scattered about a number of small nodules, varying in size from that of a pea to the dimensions of a small hazel-nut. These are not painful, nor do they progress, rather diminishing in size and number than increasing.

Under this treatment she has become addicted to the use of morphia; but with this allowance she enjoys excellent health and spirits. How long this may continue, the future alone can disclose.

ROME, GEORGIA.

---

## CASE OF PELIOSIS RHEUMATICA.

BY W. T. TAYLOR, M. D.

Mrs. J. C.; aged forty-eight. Her health has been poor for several years. Some ten or twelve years ago she had a severe attack of acute gastritis—I was told—since which time she has had occasional attacks of pain in the stomach, sometimes so severe as to render her incapable of taking anything into the stomach, except articles of the blandest character. She has borne several children; the youngest being twelve or fourteen years of age.   About one year ago I treated her for leucorrhœa, which readily yielded to treatment.

In January last I was called to see her, and found her suffering the most acute pain.   On examination, the characteristic eruption of herpes zoster was found extending from the middle of the spine obliquely round the body, and terminating in the left groin, near the inner side of the thigh.   The vesicles were distinct, in irregular patches, and passed through the regular course of increase, maturation, decline and termination, in about fourteen days; so that there could be no doubt about the nature of the disease.

The pain, as she described it, began in the spine, and, following the general course of the eruption, terminated in the groin.   As already said, the herpes ran the usual course, and terminated in about two weeks; but unfortunately the pain continued, becoming if anything more severe after the cessation of the eruption.   She described it as deep-seated, burning, continuous, and so severe as to be almost unbearable. Not one moment of rest could be secured, except as she took opiates.   This continued for three or four weeks, and in the meantime everything was tried that would, in any degree, seem to promise relief.

About this time the pain shifted its location, or rather the pain in the track of the eruption became less, while the thigh and leg now became affected, the pain following the course of the great ischiatic and posterior tibial nerves and terminating in the foot.   Its intensity was in no wise lessened by its change of location.   This continued for, perhaps, three or four days, when the foot and ankle began to swell, and in a few hours were immensely puffed up, pitting on pressure, and very painful to the touch, particularly in the neighborhood of the joint.

The next morning, covering the anterior portion of the foot and lower half of the leg, were dark red, livid or purple spots, more numerous immediately about the ankle-joint, from the size of a shot to that of a silver dime.   They did not rise above the surface, the skin preserving its uniform appearance, and remained unaltered under the pressure of the fingers.

They retained this color for two days, became darker, then reddish brown, and finally passed into yellow, and gradually faded out without any desquamation; the whole time of their appearance being eight or ten days.

On the appearance of the eruption the pain and swelling became very much lessened, but did not cease entirely. Indeed, throughout the whole course of the affection, covering a period of six or seven months, was there ever a moment when she was entirely free from pain, or that the swelling entirely left the leg; but from the date of the eruption, the pain left its original seat and localized itself in the foot and leg.

Two weeks passed of comparative freedom from pain, the swelling much reduced. At this time her appetite was better than at any time since the attack, and we were beginning to hope that she had worn the disease out, for nothing she had taken seemed to have done her a particle of good. But we were doomed to disappointment. The limb again began to swell and become painful. The next day the swelling had increased, and the pain was great as ever. In a few hours the same kind of eruption made its appearance. It ran about the same course; its duration corresponding with that of the first.

A third and fourth attack followed; the same interval of comparative ease between; the same set of symptoms following each other with clock-like regularity, so that the patient herself stated she could always foretell an eruption by the pain and swelling. Only one difference was noticed; the swelling, followed by the eruption, gradually extended higher until the fourth or fifth eruption, when the entire limb was implicated.

This continued for months with no cessation, or even modification, of any of the symptoms; the successive attacks and crops of petechiæ following each other every two weeks or thereabouts; sometimes a day or two sooner, and more rarely a day or two later. Toward the last the spots would not entirely fade out before a new crop would take their place. During all this time the patient was gradually losing ground, in spite of iron, bark and stimulants, together with the most nourishing diet, worn down by continued suffering. Finally, on the approach of the cool autumn weather, seven months after the first attack, a change for the better was noticed. The eruption ceased to make its periodical appearance, the swelling gradually went down, and she began to get strength.

One other symptom I failed to mention. Some weeks before improvement began, the joints of one hand became stiff and much swollen, so that for several days she could not use that hand. In a few days, however, this passed away, and did not return.

On examining the heart, a loud systolic murmur was detected, heard with the greatest intensity at the apex. The irregular pulse, accompanying the heart-sounds, led me to conclude that there was regurgitation through a diseased mitral valve, together with thickening and possibly warty vegetations. Could it be possible, as claimed by not a few distinguished medical writers, that these morbid conditions are the result of small fibrinous masses becoming detached from the valves of the heart, and passing into the small arteries, and even into the capillaries, by which congestion is set up followed by stagnation and coagulation of the blood, and all the consequent changes such coagulated blood is liable to undergo in the living body? Or, again, could such conditions be the result of softening and breaking up of fibrinous masses into a finely granulated material, by which the blood would be poisoned? But if these symptoms be the result of either of the above pathological causes, why the periodicity that was present throughout? And if this periodicity was the result of malaria, why should it not yield to quinia and arsenic, which were pushed to the utmost limit of safety?

While believing that the whole series of symptoms were in some way dependent on the morbid changes in the heart, I will leave the above questions to be answered by some gentleman better able to solve them. One or two more questions: Was the first eruption shingles? And if so, were the subsequent eruptions in any way connected with, or dependent on the first? Were the last eruptions purpura rheumatica? And if so, can it be that this disease is dependent on heart disease?

FISHERVILLE, KY.

# CASE OF DISLOCATION OF THE HIP REDUCED BY THE USE OF THE FULCRUM.

BY J. H. POOLEY, M. D.

*Professor of Surgery in Starling Medical College, Columbus, Ohio.*

In the April and September numbers of the American Practitioner for the present year, I was very much interested in two short communications by Dr. George Sutton, Aurora, Ind., on the use of the fulcrum in the reduction of dislocations of the hip. The principle there advocated struck me as being sound and rational, as well as exceedingly simple, and the illustrative cases seemed very convincing. I determined upon the first opportunity that should occur to put it to the test of actual trial, and having done so I am more than ever convinced that it is a most valuable addition to our resources in dealing with this sometimes very troublesome class of injuries. And as every actual trial of a new expedient in surgery is of value in settling the usefulness of the proposed improvement, and as I feel it to be due both to the profession and to Dr. Sutton, that, for a time at least, all the cases in which his method is employed should be recorded, I publish the following account of my case:

October 19, 1876, I was requested by Dr. A. Dunlap, of Springfield, Ohio, to see, in consultation with him, a case of dislocation of the hip, in which he had failed to effect reduction after a fair and repeated trial of the ordinary method of manipulation. The patient, the wife of a farmer residing near Catawba, Clarke county, Ohio, about fifteen miles from Springfield, had been thrown from a wagon the day before—October 18th—about four o'clock in the afternoon, and sustained a dislocation of the left hip. She had been first seen by Dr. John Clark, of Mechanicsburg, who had been unsuccessful in his attempts at reduction. Dr. Dunlap had then been sent for, and had made repeated attempts to reduce the hip, but

also without success.    All these attempts had been by manipulation; pulleys had not been used.

I arrived at the house early on the morning of the 20th,
about three o'clock.    I found the patient—a spare, nervous
woman of thirty-three—in bed, suffering considerably from
pain, and severely from nausea, the result of chloroform which
had been administered on several occasions.

The left limb was an inch and a half shorter than its fellow,
the foot very slightly everted, and the head of the bone could
be plainly felt in front of the ilium, just above the acetabulum.
Dr. Dunlap informed me that the dislocation had been primarily on to the dorsum ilii, and the present position of the head
of the femur was the result of the last manipulation.    It had
been found, on manipulating it, to be extraordinarily movable,
and had been carried once or twice into the thyroid foramen,
and also up on the ilium just above the acetabulum, in which
situation I found it.    In fact it would go almost anywhere
except into the right place.    Dr. Dunlap said that he had
carried it right across the acetabulum on two occasions, and
as he did so, he felt a distinct crushing crepitus, but it went
over, and not in.    His belief, which I presume was correct,
was that a portion of the lip of the acetabulum was broken
off, and as the head of the thigh-bone was brought up against
this broken portion, it was forced before it, and partially filling
up the acetabular depression, prevented it from going in, and
guided it over on to the other side instead.

I directed, according to Dr. Sutton's plan, a firm cylinder
to be made, by tightly and evenly rolling two sheets, which
was three inches in diameter, and about two feet in length; it
was firmly tied round with narrow strips of bandage to prevent
it unrolling.    The patient was now anæsthetized with a mixture of alcohol, chloroform, and ether, and laid upon a firm,
narrow mattress, laid upon the floor.    The cylinder, prepared
as described, was now placed across the upper part of the
thigh in the groin, and firmly held at each end by an assistant;
over this, as a fulcrum, Dr. Dunlap made the manipulations,
while I attempted to follow the excursions of the bone with

my fingers. Drs. Clark and Newcomb, of Mechanicsburg, Drs. Beach and Hunter, of Catawba, and Dr. C. W. Dunlap, were also present and assisting. The first two attempts failed, as I very plainly saw, from not fully carrying out the principle involved in the use of the fulcrum; that is by abducting the knee before complete flexion of the thigh over the cylinder had been accomplished. The first time the head of the femur lodged in the thyroid foramen; the second time at the top of the ilium, where it was when we began; it had skirted round the base of the acetabulum, without rising to its level, much less going into it.

The third trial, in which the principle of the fulcrum was deliberately and thoroughly carried out, was perfectly and speedily successful. The thigh was slowly and fully flexed on to the abdomen over the fulcrum, the head of the bone was lifted up to a level with the acetabulum, and when the knee was abducted, and the motion of bringing the thigh down barely commenced, it slipped in with a distinct snap; the limb was found to be restored in length and position, and the dislocation was reduced. A broad, firm, pelvic bandage was applied, and the patient returned to bed.

This may almost be looked upon as a test case for the new method. Ordinary manipulation had been tried by skillful hands, in which it had never before failed; and I think that there can be little doubt that Dr. Dunlap's explanation of his failure was the correct one. What was wanted then was some means by which the head of the femur could be carried up to a level with the top of the acetabulum, and thus prevented from pushing the broken acetabular rim before it; this was found in Dr. Sutton's method, the obstacle was overcome, and the reduction accomplished.

It seems to me, therefore, that we are indebted to Dr. Sutton for a valuable improvement; and I do not know a more beautiful and philosophical piece of practical surgery, than the reduction of a dislocated hip by Reid's manipulation performed over Sutton's fulcrum.

COLUMBUS, OHIO.

# DANGEROUS SYRINGES.*

BY JOSEPH R. BECK, M. D.

Perhaps there exists no better way to point out the danger that lurks in the use of some of the common appliances of surgery than to illustrate the risks we run in their employment by the relation of typical cases of injury resulting therefrom. It has frequently been noticed and stated by shrewd observers that the ordinary female syringe is occasionally, and, I may safely add on my own account, semi-occasionally demonstrated to be a perfect magazine of mishaps and danger.

It has several times occurred to me in practice that uterine colic has followed the use of the female syringe so commonly and universally employed; and I have been accustomed for the last three years, when ordering syringes for patients, to have the instruments brought to me for inspection before using. When so submitted to my hands, I have invariably, with a splinter of wood, plugged the aperture in the end of the barrel, if it were an ordinary piston syringe, or the opening in the end of the female tube, if a Davidson or other bulb instrument. Since taking this precaution, my case-book has not recorded a single accident to any of my patients from the use of a syringe.

I conclude, therefore, that cutlers and instrument-makers generally would confer a great and lasting favor upon physicians, if they would manufacture their female syringes without a perforation in the distal extremity. To remedy any impediment to the flow of the fluid which might possibly arise from the closure of the end aperture, the manufacturer could easily perforate the side of the tube or barrel at one or more additional points.

That accidents arising from this source are more common than is generally believed, I am sure; and I only expect in

* Read before the Allen County (Ind.) Medical Society, October 3, 1876.

this relation to continue to further sound the alarm, and call the attention of the profession again to a danger of which it has frequently been reminded, by the relation of a case which recently came under my notice.

On the 9th of last July, I was telegraphed to come to Lancaster, Ohio, to see, in consultation with Dr. G. W. Boerstler, of that place, Mrs. M. E. E——, a resident ordinarily of Cincinnati, but at this time, in accordance with her usual habit, spending her summer at the former place. I reached Lancaster on Monday morning, July 10th, at ten o'clock, and immediately saw the patient. She was suffering from general peritonitis, involving the endometrium and the cystic mucous membrane, and, in the face of the most profuse exhibition of opiates, was suffering the most atrocious pain that can be imagined. A vaginal examination revealed, in addition to the ordinary symptoms of peritonitis, a laceration of the cervix uteri, and, deeming this to have been the *fons et origo mali*, directed my inquiries so as to ascertain its manner of production.

It seems that the patient was yet in the puerperal state, her baby, which was her second one, being only three months old. Her first labor, which had occurred nearly four years prior to the last, had been very protracted; but by the advice of her accoucheur, whom I shall call W——, nature was allowed to take her own good time, and the process was concluded without injury to mother or child. This accouchement was followed by a good "getting up." In her last labor, owing to the absence of her regular medical attendant, the services of another individual, whom I shall call Z——, were obtained. The latter party was duly informed of the protracted nature of the first labor, but he probably found some degree of dilatation present, and very improperly, in my opinion, gave ergot, while the labor pains had suffered not the slightest diminution. Of course the uterine spasm was reinforced to an intense degree, and the fetal head was driven through the cervical canal with such celerity that the cervix was lacerated from the internal to the external os as completely as if the operation of "discission after Sims" had been done.

Here a hiatus occurs in the history of the case, which may be bridged over by the remark that the "getting up" this time was not at all good, and the patient, not convalescing as rapidly as was anticipated, went out of the city earlier in the season than usual, feeling quite badly. At this point we can again resume the history of the case.

For a number of weeks after her arrival in Lancaster, Mrs. E—— noticed that she was subject to a constant but slight sanguinous discharge from the vagina, which occasioned her more annoyance and inconvenience than positive alarm. On the occasion of a visit from her husband, only a short time before her last attack, she mentioned this state of affairs to him, and requested him on his return to Cincinnati to see her regular physician, and have some medicine sent her to check the discharge. This errand Mr. E—— did, and a solution, presumably a weak one, of sulphate of zinc was sent up, with directions to use it as a vaginal injection. The directions were followed but once by the patient, when a sharp uterine pain admonished her to desist. The application had been made with a Davidson bulb syringe, and in less than two hours thereafter she had a rigor and a hemorrhage, small in amount it is true, but *from the urethra.* The day following she was the subject of a *second urethral hemorrhage,* amounting to perhaps three or four ounces, which was closely followed by a second rigor.

She now consulted Dr. Boerstler, who placed her upon the tincture of the chloride of iron, and no more hemorrhages occurred. This description carries the case up to July 11th, on which day the general peritonitis, which had been gathering intensity for several days, became almost unmanageable and absolutely terrific, and immense amounts of morphia were exhibited to hold the pain in check. Poultices were applied to the abdomen, and the other necessary treatment was had.

After I saw and examined the case on Monday, as the inflammation was still running riot, light cloths wrung out in almost boiling water were substituted for the heavy poultices, chloral hydrate for the morphia, and a large vaginal douche of very hot water ordered. This douche was applied several times for all of a full hour at each time, with the same Davidson syringe, but with the central orifice plugged up. It was productive of a great amount of good. She also had ten grains of sulphate of quinia each evening, and received large amounts of nutritious food, mostly nitrogenous.

I left the patient on the following Thursday morning on the high road to convalescence; but I have since then been advised by Dr. Boerstler that her recovery has been very much retarded by an intense pain in the abdomen, which recurred each evening with great persistency, and which he was disposed to attribute to the forming of a pelvic abscess. In this I dissented, and advised the free use of the iodide of potassium internally. I have since learned from a brother of the patient, under date of August 23d, that she was fully recovered, and had returned to her home in Cincinnati the day before.

There exists not the slightest doubt in my mind that all this trouble arose from the injection matter being sent, by reason of the lacerated cervix, directly from the tube of the syringe into the uterine cavity; and it is even possible that some of the fluid penetrated one or both of the fallopian tubes, and thus reached the cavity of the peritoneum. Patients have no idea of the propelling force which they employ when using these bulb syringes; and with the central vent open, a lacerated cervix, and patulous fallopian tubes present, it is necessarily quite easy to inflict untold damage ignorantly.

I relate this case, as I have before said, only to put others on their guard against using a stream directly against the os from a syringe with a central orifice, and to ask that manufacturers will so amend this abomination as that their instruments shall become perfectly safe, even in the hands of the most ignorant.

Fort Wayne, Ind

# SUCCESSFUL EXCISION OF THE KNEE-JOINT UNDER UNFAVORABLE CIRCUMSTANCES.

BY JOSEPH EASTMAN, M. D.

Thomas Collins, aged eleven years, was admitted to the Indianapolis City Hospital, March 25th, 1876. As consulting surgeon of the institution I saw him in less than thirty minutes afterwards, and found him in the following condition, caused by a fall between the wheels and belts of a rolling-mill: Dislocation of the femur on dorsum of the ilium, and deep contused wound over inner condyle of femur and head of the tibia of the left leg. The right thigh presented an immense laceration of the quadriceps extensor, sartorius, and abductor muscles, their lower two-thirds having been entirely carried away. The femoral artery protruded from the flesh and fascia some three inches, it having been severed near the apex of Scarpa's triangle. There was very little hemorrhage; the pulsations of the artery were very weak, reaction not having taken place sufficient to wash out the clots.

Previous to my arrival, Dr. Smith, one of the superintendents of the hospital, had given the patient an unusual amount of stimulants, and continued their use internally and externally. As reaction was brought on, the internal clots began to escape from the proximal end of the lacerated vessel, necessitating the immediate application of compression over the the ramus of the pubis.

There was no question as to what was to be done. Accordingly as soon as the temperature in the axilla came up to 97° F., he was brought under the influence of chloroform, and I reduced the dislocated femur by manipulation, and amputated the lacerated limb by the circular method at the junction of the upper with the middle third of the thigh.

We had no further trouble with the stump of the right leg or the dislocation; but in spite of our early and constant preventive treatment, the contused wound on the inner side of the left knee set up acute suppurative arthritis, with all its accompanying evils, reducing the patient very much.

On the twenty-first day after the amputation a consultation of the hospital staff, Dr. Walker, and others of the city, was had, and all agreed that life with no legs would be very undesirable, and that excision of the knee-joint offered a faint hope. I expressed my willingness to undertake what seemed to all present the nearly hopeless task of saving the limb by the operation referred to. The patient was again brought under the influence of chloroform. I excised the joint by the transverse incision, carefully removing the patella and all fragments of ligamentous structure. I avoided going beyond the epiphyseal junction on both femur and tibia, that the subsequent growth of the limb should not be interfered with. The leg was put up in a plaster-of-paris gutter, the boy placed in bed, and given every chance of life afforded by egg-nog, milk-punch, beef-tea, quinia, strychnia, iron, etc., for two months, at the end of which time his limb was firmly united, straight, and healed completely. He soon began to walk with the aid of crutches, and withal seemed to enjoy life quite well.

I report this case simply to place on record one more case of excision of the knee-joint in a case that promised very little, believing that very many limbs are removed which could be saved by timely and careful excision. I do not believe many cases occur where the powers of life are lower at the time of operating, or where the result is ultimately more satisfactory. Dr. Ashhurst, in a very able and complete article in the transactions of the College of Physicians of Philadelphia, for July, 1876, reports ten successful cases of excision of the knee, and not one failed. Dr. Hodge, in the same volume, reports two in which the result was most satisfactory. For a complete description as to the best mode of operating, I would refer to the reports of Drs. Ashhurst and Hodge.

INDIANAPOLIS.

Michael N——, of Terre Haute, a young machinist, had the palm of his hand slightly lacerated between the thumb and forefinger by a piece of railroad iron. The wound healed completely in six days. Fifteen days after the injury he was seized with trismus and tetanic spasms. When I first saw him his tongue had been wounded; he lay upon his back with jaws firmly fixed; the cervical muscles rigid, pulse 112 and small. He was comfortable in the absence of spasms, which came on every twenty to forty minutes. Opisthotonos was constant, but increased during a convulsion. These symptoms gradually increased, except the pulse-rate, which ranged from 100 to 110. The disease reached its height about the nineteenth day, the patient suffering with pain between the shoulders, in the neck and spine, loins and scrobiculus cordis, having a most painful expression of countenance. In this condition he remained without fever for thirty days, when the convulsions gradually ceased and the muscles relaxed. During all this time his family declared he had no sleep: this statement should be received *cum grano salis*. The treatment consisted in the administration of three grains of calomel in one grain doses daily, and five grains of quinia four times a day for five days, the quinia being directed more to the malarial influence, as he had had several chills before the tetanus supervened. I gave hydrate of chloral for three days, which lessened the frequency of the spasms; but fearing the cumulative tendency I substituted whisky instead, of which he drank three pints daily; he called for it constantly, and was really drunk from day to day. During all his illness I gave him animal broth, beef-tea, and corn-meal gruel. He is now well, but very stiff in the hips and back. I am now fully persuaded that the whisky brought about the cure, and think that tetanus is not a mortal and incurable disease.

Terre Haute, Ind.

* Part of a paper read before the Tri-State Medical Society, October 22, 1876.

# Reviews.

---

Practical Treatise on Diseases of the Eye. By ROBERT BRUDENELL
CARTER, F. R. C. S., Ophthalmic Surgeon to St. George's Hospital, etc.

This book is from the pen of an able scholar and teacher,
"whose aim"—see author's preface—"in the preparation of
its pages, has been to place before the profession, in a concise
and readable form, a general view of the present state of
knowledge with regard to the nature and treatment of the
more important diseases of the eye." He further states: "I
have not thought it necessary to dwell minutely upon maladies
of rare occurrence, or upon details which are interesting only
to specialists; neither have I attempted to achieve that kind
of completeness which is produced by undigested compilation.
. . . . The book contains but slight reference to modes
of practice of which I am unable to speak from experience."

Every page bears evidence of a sound judgment, a large
experience, and an unusual practicality on the part of the
author. In support of the above view, we will quote a few
sentences from the fifth chapter: "Surgical mechanicians have
provided us with instruments in almost infinite variety, but
the hands take precedence of them all, and deserve our earliest
and most careful consideration. It was said by many that an
ophthalmic operator must spoil a hatful of eyes before he cures
one. As the instruments of any period are a fixed quantity,
and as adequate knowledge concerning when and·why to
operate, may be obtained by attentively observing the practice
of others, it is manifest that the hatful of eyes must be a sacrifice offered up to the training of the hands. A familiar
maxim of political economy is that all learners spoil a portion
of raw material. This maxim expresses one of the verities

of life; and a surgeon who learns to operate by using the eyes of human beings to begin with, and by thus in time gaining manual dexterity at hap-hazard—gaining by sheer practice the power to do things well which he at first did badly—although he may eventually become skillful, obtains his skillfulness at an unwarrantable cost. Instead of seeking such dearly bought experience, it is better first to consider carefully the nature of the mechanical acts which are to be undertaken, and then to see how far, and by what means, the hands can be trained to the possession of the qualities required of them."

The author advocates the operating frequently on the eyes of the inferior animals, until one has acquired a large degree of ambidexterity before a human eye is operated on; this "will render the accidents which may result from awkwardness unlikely, if not impossible."

The qualities of hand which are combined in an accomplished eye operator may be summed up under the following heads, each of which will demand a brief consideration:

"First. A high development of what is called by physiologists 'muscular sense;' the faculty by which we feel and estimate the degree of force we are exerting, either in pressure or traction. Second, the power of uniting two hands in consentaneous movement, and of directing the intelligence to them simultaneously; so that they may work smoothly and harmoniously together as a single organ for the attainment of a common object, and may both at once be equally under the control and governance of the will. Third, the power to employ the left hand, indifferently with the right, for the guidance and use of cutting or other instruments. Fourth, steadiness."

On the subject of instruments, after speaking about the many useless ones which have been produced, and "which are the representatives of inventive awkwardness," he says:

" But in all ages and countries the bad workman has complained of his tools, and the good workman has produced the most varied results by the most simple means. A man who is very awkward, and whose awkwardness is perpetually bringing him to grief, hits upon a contrivance by which he hopes that this natural result may be in some degree obviated. He calls his contrivance an invention; and, like those persons of whom it is said that their glory is in their shame, he is often somewhat proud of it. Many surgeons of great and deserved repute have invented each but a single instrument, such as a Beers's knife or a Tyrrel's hook, chiefly because they have struck out some new procedure for which new appliances were indispensable. . . . . The, safest man is he who never invented an instrument in his life, but whose daily practice affords evidence that he can use those which have been invented for him by others."

We would like to quote further from this chapter, which is a long one, and which is full of practical suggestions, but space will not permit.

Chapter VII is also full of useful hints and suggestions, and would well repay the superintendents and medical officers of our charitable institutions for its perusal. A few words from this valuable chapter are as follows:

"The history of contagious ophthalmia in a charity school is usually, that the disease has been introduced in some accidental manner, probably by a new inmate, whose conjunctivitis escaped observation and quarantine. It would find a large portion of the children with follicular granulations, the result of insanitary conditions, some of which were perhaps unavoidable. . . . . The surgeon to the school may not at first fully appreciate the gravity of the crisis with which he has to deal, or he may not have enjoyed sufficient opportunities of studying diseases of the eye to be perfectly conversant with all the conditions which should guide his treatment. One child after another goes into the infirmary with 'bad eyes;' and the cases increase in number and severity week by week. At first it has often happened that some undiscriminating plan of treatment has been adopted, and that its application has been intrusted to some careless or incompetent person. Under such circumstances the bad cases go wrong, and the mild cases are discharged from the infirmary half cured, with mischief still lurking in their palpebral folds, to spread contagion among the playmates and themselves to undergo relapse. Matters proceed from bad to worse; the whole establishment becomes saturated with contagium, nurses and helpers suffer, many eyes are lost, and a public scandal is created. Then, at last, a specialist is called in; and is too often asked to banish the epidemic, notwithstanding the continued existence of all the causes which have fostered and perpetuated it."

The author then goes on to speak of the segregation of the affected ones, and the thorough and systematic disinfection of the building and its contents, and urges upon officers the importance of examining the palpebral folds of the conjunctivæ before discharging a patient as cured. Had such an examination been made during our late war many recruits would have been rejected, hundreds of eyes would have been saved, and hundreds of thousands of dollars would thereby have been saved which are now used on pensioners; and one might further add that fewer cases would have been scattered over our land as nuclei for the dissemination and propagation of granular ophthalmia; which disease, as all are aware, has vastly increased since the commencement of our internecine war.

On page 306, while speaking of the diagnostic symptoms of cataract, the author relates an incident which ought to convince those who lay so much stress on, or who attach so much weight to the fact of one's having been *abroad*, that the fools are not all confined within the limits of the United States, but that the metropolis of the world has its full share of asses. He says: "As far as I know, there are only two conditions which could by any possibility be mistaken for cataract in early life; and these are, first, glioma of the retina; and secondly, a deposit of lymph behind the lens. Some years ago a child was brought to the Kent County Ophthalmic Hospital (of which I was in temporary charge), who presented a whiteness of the pupil; the child had been taken to another hospital a day or two previously, and there the mother had been told that there was cataract, and that, it being then December, a needle operation must be performed in the ensuing spring.

On close examination I found that there was no perception of light; that there was increase of tension; that the iris was pushed forward into contact with the cornea, and that the almost primrose-colored, opaque, homogeneous surface seen through the pupil was manifestly behind a clear lens. These conditions indicated the presence of a morbid growth within the eye, and enucleation was performed without delay, the tumor proving to be a glioma."

On page 469, while speaking concerning the diagnosis of various anomalies of refraction with the ophthalmoscope alone, he says: "For my own part, I not only claim no such power, but am certain that I do not possess it; and I greatly doubt whether some of those who claim it, do not deceive themselves."

It is the opinion of the writer that not only do some deceive themselves, but that many others publish gross fabrications concerning their powers in the above named direction. And of the certainty of the correctness of this opinion, I have frequently proved by subsequent examinations of patients, under atropia, after they have been examined by others claiming to be experts in the use of said instrument.

On page 480, in his remarks upon muscular asthenopia, he mentions a case, that of a young man brought to him by his father for an examination ophthalmoscopically, in order to throw light on an obscure and intractable brain disease. He was suddenly attacked while reading for honors at Oxford, with symptoms which an Oxford practitioner attributed to some grave affection of the brain, and was advised to throw up his work and to leave the University. He then consulted an eminent London physician, who confirmed the former opinion given by the Oxford physician, and prescribed a period of complete brain rest, and a voyage to Australia, as the best means of obtaining it. The patient went, and when he returned he was told that "he must abandon the idea of succeeding to his father's large commercial undertakings, and that he must also abandon a marriage engagement which he had contracted prior to his break-down. In other words, his prospects in life were blighted, and his despondency was commensurate with his misfortunes." The author found it to be nothing but a case of myopia $= \frac{1}{8}$, and insufficiency of the internal recti muscles. A pair of spectacles was all that he needed. These were given him; he was allowed to marry; and he returned to the author in three weeks declaring himself to be quite well. He was also seen two years subsequently, when he stated that he had never been troubled more with the "brain disease."

The American edition of this work is by Dr. John Green, of St. Louis, Mo., who is in every way equal to the task which he has so well performed. The book is replete with valuable information, and but few practitioners would fail to procure it could they once glance at its pages. J. L. T.

---

Transactions of the Texas State Medical Association, Eighth Annual Session, 1876.

If we were called upon for the most substantial evidence we could give of progress in the American medical profession, we should unhesitatingly point to such volumes as the one before us emanating from our various state medical societies. This is one which reflects honor upon the state from which it proceeds, not only as a literary and scientific performance but as a triumph of typography. Its mechanical execution is admirable, showing that the useful arts are keeping pace with medical improvement in our remote settlements.

The president's (Dr. Brown) address was carefully prepared, and contains important statements. He says the profession of medicine is growing in the confidence and esteem of the people of Texas, which is the natural result of its manifest advancement in skill and intelligence. He bears hard on the medical schools that resort to "the artifices of trade" to secure students, and make "the manufacture of doctors so disgustingly easy." We doubt the advantage of popularizing medical knowledge, and of educating the people in the principles of medicine, as he proposes; for it is our observation that the readiest dupes and most active abettors of quackery are the persons who have a smattering of medical science, which is all that the masses can possibly acquire. Nor have we any hope of his obtaining help from the legislature, "wrestle" with it as he may, in behalf of the regular profession. Texas will hold on, as older states have done, to the principle of showing no preference by law to any school of medicine. The spirit of Dr. Brown's address is excellent, and its effect upon the profession and the people of his giant young commonwealth will be healthful. In style it would bear toning down decidedly; and the sensible author, when he comes to review his discourse, will see that its force would not have been impaired if he had spoken in simpler language and a calmer tone. Plain words, rather than the pomp of oratory or high-flown language, befit medical subjects.

The eucalyptus globulus is treated of elaborately in a prize essay by Dr. Richard Bibb, but without giving any of the author's experience or deductions respecting the new remedy.

Dr. John H. Pope has a carefully prepared report on the progress of medicine, confining his review to the former year, and giving a list of remedies lately introduced into the pharmacopœia. He alludes to the direction which medicine in our day, much more decidedly than ever before, is taking toward the prevention of epidemic diseases, over which when they break out we seem to have very little control. Nothing could exhibit our profession in a light more truly noble than this devotion to preventive medicine. In so far as we succeed in our endeavors, we diminish our professional income; but such a thought, so far from influencing the labors of physicians, has hardly entered their minds. The fact is one which challenges the admiration of mankind.

The report on gynecology, by Dr. Thomas D. Wooten, is founded on his individual observation and experience, and has the advantage of presenting independent views on all the questions of practice to which he refers. The report will be read with great interest by practitioners.

Not much of novelty or interest is brought out by Dr. W. J. Burt, in his short report on the anatomical and physiological differences between the white and negro races.

The reports of Dr. J. R. Taylor and Dr. J. T. Norris, on climatology and epidemics, are too brief to afford much information. That by Dr. A. H. Kilpatrick on indigenous medical resources, is more substantial. From the account given of cockle-bur (*Xanthium strumarium*), that familiar plant would appear to have decided therapeutic powers. According to Dr. Kilpatrick, it is a vesicant, an antidote for snake-bite, a styptic, and is good "in all affections of the kidneys or bladder." A doubt of its efficacy is apt to start up in the mind when any remedy is so much extolled. But let this be tried as a diuretic in strangury, scalding urine, and other urinary troubles, as proposed in this report.

Five cases of diphtheria are reported by Dr. T. J. Heard; and his history is followed by a paper on dislocations of the shoulder, by Dr. Greensville Dowell, illustrated by several good wood-cuts. A case of lithotomy is reported by Dr. W. H. Park; and Dr. Eads reports miscellaneous cases, which are of value as increasing the statistics of medicine and surgery. Drs. Murphy and Long relate a case of cystitis, in which they used injections of nitrate of silver with success; and a case of sessile polypus of the meatus urinarius in a female, removed by the bromide of potassium and tannin, is reported by Dr. T. J. Heard. Cases are related briefly by Dr. G. W. Holcom and Dr. T. D. Manning, and three interesting cases of imperforate hymen are reported by Dr. S. R. Burroughs. Dr. Kilpatrick gives two remarkable cases of retention of the fetus after death, to which Dr. A. E. Ford adds one of a similar character; in none of them did the health of the mother suffer. A case of double vagina is reported by Dr. J. W. Fennell, in which, before labor could be accomplished, he was obliged to divide a septum between the passages, which he did with a curved, probe-pointed bistoury, and the child was safely de-

livered by the natural efforts. Meteorological tables conclude this vólume of transactions, of which we take leave with the remark that it shows the medical profession of Texas to be capable of great things. Forty years ago, when that territory became free, there was hardly a medical society in the United States that could boast of a volume of transactions in every way so creditable as this.
L. P. Y.

---

Cyclopædia of the Practice of Medicine. Edited by Dr. H. VON ZIEMSSEN. Volume VI, Diseases of the Circulatory System; and Volume XI, Diseases of the Peripheral Cerebro-Spinal Nerves.

The portly volumes of this great work continue to appear at short intervals, and fully sustain its reputation. Eight authors were engaged on the sixth volume, which contains upward of a thousand pages, including an ample index. Six of these are professors in as many German universities— Rosenstein, Schrœtter, Lebert, Quincke, Vogel and Wagner; the other two are Dr. Bauer and Dr. Steffen. The eleventh volume was written by Professor Erb, of Heidelberg.

As this work has been in progress, the question has often been asked—Why, when we have so many able works in our own tongue on Practice, should we go to Germany for another? There is this manifest advantage in it, that it enables our physicians to view therapeutics from a foreign stand-point; it shows them the opinions of men abroad, admitted to be as learned, as thoughtful, as laborious as any in the world. And then, divided as the labor has been, the work is far more thorough than it could possibly have been made by a single author. It will form in itself, when completed, a library on the subject; and while it will not supersede the treatises of American and English authors on the practice of medicine, it will be studied with reference to points relating to medical science, which are necessarily discussed in them with less fullness. It undoubtedly makes one of the most valuable of all the contributions made in latter years to the literature of our profession.

**The Medical Men of the Revolution** An Address before the Alumni Association of Jefferson Medical College. By J. M. Toner, M. D. Philadelphia, 1876.

Dr. Toner is placing his professional brethren under great obligations to him by his generous efforts to rescue from oblivion the names and services of the early physicians of America. Some years ago he favored the profession with biographical notices of the medical men who flourished before our war of independence; in the address before us, forming a volume of one hundred and forty pages, he gives us an account of those who were concerned in our revolutionary struggle. In both he has brought to light many incidents in the medical history of our country which will be read with interest by all physicians. The extent of the services rendered by the members of the profession to their country, outside of their profession, is, we believe, not generally understood even by physicians themselves. It is not generally known that "there was scarcely an office, civil or military, that at some time a physician did not fill," as is made to appear by the author of this address.

The address is not a eulogy, but a calm, historical record of names, dates and facts in biography, showing a patience and industry of research of which few physicians in our country are capable. It gives the names of twelve hundred physicians who participated, directly or indirectly, in the war, and of thirty-six who held official rank in the army. Of these the most illustrious fell at Bunker Hill; but there were others who, living longer, rendered greater services to the cause than Warren. It was a physician—Dr. Ephraim Brevard—who drew up, at Charlotte, in North Carolina, the famous declaration of independence, which preceded by a year that of Mr. Jefferson. But we must refer our readers to the address itself for other instances.

We acknowledge our obligations to Dr. Toner for this charming little book, and we thank him especially for introducing into it the following letter from Washington to one of his generals: "A few days ago I received a very polite letter from Dr. Boyes, surgeon of the fifteenth regiment (British), requesting me to return him some valuable medical manuscripts taken in the brig Symmetry. He says they are packed in a neat kind of portable *library*, and consist of Dr. Cullen's Lectures on the Practice of Medicine, thirty-nine or forty volumes; Cullen's Lectures on the Institutes of Medicine, eighteen volumes; Anatomical Lectures, eight volumes; and Dr. Black on Chemistry, nine volumes, the whole in octavo. If they can be found I beg that they may be sent up to me, that I may return them to the Doctor. I have no other view in doing this than that of showing our enemies that *we do not war against the sciences.*" L. P. Y.

## Salicylic Acid—The Experience of Maine Physicians in its Use.
Reported by HENRY GERRISH, M. D., of Portland.

In a pamphlet of fifteen pages, reprinted from the Transactions of the Maine Medical Association, the following diseases have been treated with this comparatively new remedy: Acute rheumatism has been cured by doses of seven to ten grains every hour or two, the fever and swelling usually subsiding within forty-eight hours. One case of chronic articular rheumatism treated successfully by doses of the acid from one to two drachms daily; also several cases of subacute rheumatism entirely relieved by doses of seven to ten grains every two hours. Rheumatic neuralgia yielded readily to its use; but lumbago and sciatica would not. One case of chronic diarrhœa apparently cured by its use. Locally it has been used with more or less success in diphtheria, pharyngitis, gangrene, cystitis, etc. It causes no serious derangement of the stomach, but has an effect somewhat similar to quinia in causing a ringing of the ears. It is usually given in wafers, but also in water, with borate of soda to facilitate the solution.

A Practical Treatise on the Diseases, Injuries, and Malformations of the Urinary Bladder, the Prostate Gland, and the Urethra. By SAMUEL D. GROSS, M. D., LL. D., D. C. L., Oxon, etc.

This is the third edition of this work, by the veteran Professor of Surgery in the Jefferson Medical College, and appears revised and edited by Dr. Samuel W. Gross, the son of the learned author, who, with the industry of the father, has rewritten much of the work, and brought it fully up to the knowledge extant on the subject. It has been so long before the profession that no extended review of it would be admissible; and it has been so well received that it needs no recommendation to the medical profession. Every surgeon in the country will deem it necessary to his library, and every physician who has a troublesome case of urinary disease will consult it with advantage. On whatever subject Dr. Gross writes it is well understood that he is exhaustive, so that the reader may expect to find in this treatise all of value that is known to the profession touching the affections considered in its pages.

---

Yellow Fever and Malarial Diseases, Etc. By GREENSVILLE DOWELL, M. D., Professor of Surgery in Texas Medical College, etc.

Dr. Dowell has written from experience in this monograph, having, as he informs us in his introduction, treated in hospitals and in private practice over two thousand cases of yellow fever. He believes that the disease can be treated successfully, and has written on the subject for the instruction of the people as well as the profession. His work is illustrated by two chromos, exhibiting the appearance of the skin, liver and intestines in the worst cases. The author accounts for want of system in his treatise by explaining that it was written and published at different times; and in collecting the several memoirs together, he deemed it unadvisable to change them. It will be looked into with interest by all physicians who are likely to encounter yellow fever.

# Clinic of the Month.

---

TREATMENT OF ACUTE RHEUMATISM BY SALICIN.—Dr. T. Maclagan, in the Lancet of October 28th, speaks as follows of the treatment of acute rheumatism by salicin:

In my original paper on the subject,* the following conclusions were given as the result of my then experience of the remedy: First, we have in salicin a valuable remedy in the treatment of acute rheumatism; second, the more acute the case, the more marked the benefit produced; third, in acute cases, its beneficial action is generally apparent within twenty-four, always within forty-eight, hours of its administration in sufficient dose; fourth, given thus at the commencement of the attack, it seems to arrest the course of the malady as effectually as quinia cures an ague, or ipecacuanha a dysentery; fifth, the relief of pain is always one of the earliest effects produced; sixth, in acute cases, relief of pain and a fall of temperature generally occur simultaneously; seventh, in subacute cases, the pain is sometimes decidedly relieved before the temperature begins to fall; this is especially the case when, as is frequently observed in those of nervous temperament, the pain is proportionally greater than the abnormal rise of temperature; eighth, in chronic rheumatism, salicin sometimes does good where other remedies fail; but it also sometimes fails where others do good.

A further experience of the remedy has confirmed me in the accuracy of these conclusions. In not one case of acute rheumatism have I found salicin fail to produce a speedy cure of the disease. I have, therefore, nothing to add to, nothing

* Lancet, March 4th and 11th, 1876.

to detract from, the conclusion, "that, given in sufficient dose at the commencement of the attack, salicin seems to arrest the course of acute rheumatism as effectually as quinia cures an ague, or ipecacuanha a dysentery. "

The point to which, in this communication, I would direct special attention, is the dose which should be given:

*Dose.*—What I said on this point in my former paper was as follows: "The dose of salicin is from ten to thirty grains every two, three or four hours, according to the severity of the case. Fifteen grains every three hours is a medium dose for an acute case. It is very possible that less might suffice; for I have not tried to find the minimum dose. It is very certain that a much larger dose may be given without producing discomfort."

Further experience has led me to the conclusion that it is well to give the larger dose; and that the best way to get the full and speedy benefit of the remedy is to saturate the system with it as quickly as possible. The more speedily this is done, the more speedily are the fever and pains subdued. I now, therefore, give the salicin to adults in a dose of twenty to thirty grains every two hours; in very acute cases I give that quantity every hour till pain is relieved. With relief of pain, sleep returns, and the hourly dose can not be adhered to. But it is well to give twenty grains, at least, every two hours during the day, till the temperature is down to the normal. For a week afterwards the same dose should be given four times a day. Salicin is an excellent bitter tonic; in my experience as good as quinia, and not apt to disagree as the latter is. I have always found cases of acute rheumatism treated by it convalesce very rapidly; treated in the old way, convalescence from that disease is a slow and tedious process.

I am specially anxious to call attention to the necessity for giving salicin in large and frequently repeated doses, because, in some of the cases which have been reported in the journals since my original paper was published, the dose given was too small to produce benefit. To give "from thirty to sixty grains per day " is to do justice neither to the patient nor the remedy; and to report a case in which such a dose was given as one indicating the "inability of salicin to arrest the disease," is to draw an inference which is unwarranted by the facts, and which tends to throw unmerited discredit on a remedy whose ability to arrest the progress of acute rheumatism has already been demonstrated in numerous cases. A case of acute rheumatism which gets from thirty to sixty grains in twenty-four hours— *i. e.*, an average of less than two grains in the hour—receives practically no treatment, and is of no value as evidence either for or against salicin.

The conclusions to which I have come with reference to the action of salicin on the cardiac complications of acute rheumatism are :

First. That given sufficiently early and in sufficient dose, salicin prevents these complications.

Second. That its free administration is the best means of staying their progress after they have occurred.

Third. That such general treatment does not exclude the usual local measures—leeching, poulticing, etc.

Fourth. That the beneficial action of the salicin on the heart ceases when the temperature falls to the normal.

Fifth. That salicin is powerless to remove the effusion which remains after the fever has ceased. To touch the gums with mercury, slightly but quickly, I regard as the most hopeful means of attaining this end.

It is right that I should add that my experience of salicylic acid leads me to regard it as having much the same action as salicin, as an antipyretic and antirheumatic. All that I have said of the alkaloid I believe to be equally applicable to the acid. The advantage of the former is that it is an excellent bitter tonic, and never causes troublesome symptoms ; except in some rare cases such tinnitus aurium as results from a two or three grain dose of quinia. The disadvantage of the latter is, that it generally causes irritation of the throat, and frequently induces sickness ; in one case I found it give rise to troublesome irritation of the bowels.

TREATMENT OF SPASMODIC STRICTURE OF THE ŒSOPHAGUS. — Dr. Morell Mackenzie, London Medical Times and Gazette, October 21, gives the following :

Whenever the cause, whether of constitutional or local origin, can be discovered, it should be removed. All reflex sources of irritation—-especially those connected with the gastro-intestinal and uterine systems—should be most carefully sought out, and, if possible, got rid of. The nervous system must be braced up by moral, as well as by hygienic and medicinal agencies. It must not be forgotten that the hysterical disposition prevails in by far the largest number of cases. The mind should, if possible, be kept employed by regular and interesting occupation, or by change of scene and travel. Certain nervine tonics are specially valuable, such as the valerianate of zinc. I generally give it in combination with assafœtida, but it acts very well alone.

The dietary in these cases is of the greatest importance. If the spasm is very severe, thickened liquids should be given ; and it is well to bear in mind that warm drinks are much less apt to bring on spasm than cold ones, and in nine cases out of ten if the drink is sweetened it is better borne. Many patients discover these circumstances without medical advice. Gradually the food may be thickened, and panada* may be allowed. If the case progresses favorably, the patient will be able to return by degrees to ordinary diet. Stimulants should not as a rule be allowed, and all *piquant* food should be prohibited. It is the greatest mistake to force these patients to take solid food. They may sometimes be tricked out of their malady when it is slight and recent, but rough measures always fail.

As regards local treatment, much can be done with the continuous current. The electrode should be introduced into the

---

* Panada is generally made of chicken or some white meat, but mutton and beef may be employed. The essence of the meat should first be extracted, and the residue reduced to the finest pulp. The whole should then be mixed together and passed through a fine sieve. It should then be heated, and in the case of invalids should be served with fresh gravy.

œsophagus at least once a day, and kept in position as long as the patient can bear it. I generally use a ten or twelve-celled battery. The application should be made soon after a meal, so that a considerable time may elapse between the treatment and the next time of deglutition. The muscles should also be galvanized externally. This treatment generally requires to be continued for some weeks or months. Sometimes great benefit, and indeed a complete cure, may be obtained by passing bougies. It is best to use an instrument with a metallic or ivory knob, and, if possible, to keep the extremity of the instrument opposite the seat of spasm. This treatment affords relief in the same way that passing a sound sometimes relieves irritability of the neck of the bladder. I have never obtained any satisfactory results from the application of stimulating or astringent solutions to the œsophageal mucous membrane. It has already been pointed out how easily those cases dependent on flatulent dyspepsia can be cured. It must not, however, be forgotten that in a large number of instances the dysphagia is a mere fancy, there being, in fact, no spasm. By passing a bougie and assuring the patient that there is no obstruction, such persons may sometimes become aware of the groundlessness of their sensations, but they are often more difficult to cure than true spasm.

ON AN AUSCULTATORY SOUND. — Dr. Ralph W. Leftwich, Lancet, October 14th, has the following:

The application of mediate auscultation to the detection of stone, though not new, has hitherto, I believe, been confined to the somewhat awkward expedient of placing a stethoscope upon the hypogastrium while the sound is rotated in the bladder. The "auscultatory sound," here described, is in many respects an improvement upon this. It consists essentially of an india-rubber tube, one end of which is provided with an ear-piece and the other stretched over the handle of a sound. The tube should be about twenty-five inches in length, and of a quarter of an inch bore. It must be composed of extremely soft and moderately thick india-rubber. The sound itself should be of solid steel ; and, although the ordinary form answers very well, it is a decided advantage to have the extremity of the handle cylindrical or conical, so as to preserve the lumen of the tube. The ear-piece, made of vulcanite, is similar to that of a Grüber's otoscope or a Stern's stethoscope; it is intended to be inserted into the meatus, and maintains its position there best if bent to an obtuse angle.

Thus constructed, the instrument will be found to conduct sonorous vibrations with remarkable intensity and delicacy; indeed, the lightest rub on a polished surface can be heard with ease. In using it, it is necessary that the ear-piece be inserted into the meatus with sufficient firmness to retain its position there without being held. The sound should be held lightly between the finger and thumb and manipulated in the usual way; the grating noise, however, is so distinct that the tapping movement occupies a secondary place, and is of most use in refining the diagnosis and in distinguishing between a calculus and a deposit on the walls of the bladder. The value of the instrument in the simple detection of calculus is tolerably evident, but there can be little doubt that, with practice, its sphere of usefulness will be much extended.

CASE OF TRANSVERSE FRACTURE OF THE PATELLA TREATED BY A NEW METHOD.—W. T. Grant, M. B., of the Royal Infirmary of Edinburgh, (Edinburgh Medical Journal, October,) shows the principle of this new method by relating the following case :

J. R., aged fifty-six years, laborer, was admitted to the surgical wards, Royal Infirmary, August 7, 1876, suffering from transverse fracture of the patella, the result of indirect violence, there being also bruising of the knee on which he had fallen at the time of the accident. After an interval of two days to let the swelling subside a little, under Mr. Bell's sanction the limb was put up in the following manner: The leg was packed on an inclined splint, extending from the heel to near the gluteal fold; the lower fragment was then firmly fixed in position and steadied by a strap of plaster passing right round the leg; a semilunar splint of Hyde's poroplastic material was now carefully modelled to the thigh, just above the margin of the upper fragment, and this held in position by two stout pieces of strapping, the whole being surrounded by a few turns of a convergent spica bandage.

After allowing the splint to "set," I now took two steel hooks (about the size of those used by Malgaigne) and fixed them firmly into the splint, one on each side of the patella, the hooks being connected with a steel chain about three feet long; this was attached to the ordinary pulley-extension apparatus with a weight of nearly four pounds. On allowing this to act, the upper fragment was at once felt to be drawn closely down, while the lower remained in position, and after twenty-four hours the approximation had so gone on that only with difficulty could the line of separation be felt; now it is just recognizable by a line of thickening running across the bone. The patient suffered no discomfort, except at first a sense of dragging, which soon passed off. This method seems to me to present the advantage of being comparatively painless, while exact apposition of the fragments may be obtained by the use of a moderately applied force, which is not so great as to inconvenience the patient by pressure on the joint or by limiting movements conducive to comfort in bed.

Since using the above, I am glad to see in the August number of the Dublin Journal that Dr. Hornbrook, in America, has been using the same principle of continuous extension by means of straight strips of plaster passing above the patella, with which he has got excellent results, bony union being obtained in all his three cases.

CALLOUS FORMATION IN THE NOSTRIL.—Dr. C. Ritter, of Bremervörde, in the Memorabilien, August 24, 1876, relates the following case:

A man sixty years old presented himself to me, who wished to be relieved of an obstruction of the left nostril. For about sixteen years he had not been able to breathe through the left nostril. There flowed from it continually a clear, badly smelling fluid, and upon pressure a thick, offensive mass of a purulent appearance emptied itself from the nose in various quantities. The interior part of the nostril was entirely filled with this thick, offensive, coherent, purulent matter. After this it was not likely that one would expect to find a polypus; a bony formation was found, from which small pieces were removed with the forceps before the whole mass could be extracted. These pieces combined, presented the imprint of the nasal cavity. The open cavity to which the flat-formed excrescence had been attached was entirely filled with this purulent matter. The extent of the plate in length and breadth was one and a half centimeters, and the thickness nearly a centimeter. I believed now that the specimen was a necrosed nasal bone, incrusted with a chalky substance. After remaining some time in muriatic acid the outer surface of a foreign body was visible, resembling the incrusted mucus itself. Every time muriatic acid was applied there was evolution of carbonic acid from the pieces of the yellowish mass. The microscopical appearance showed a similarity to the mucous discharge. In about a week the last slimy flakes were dissolved, and on the inner portion of the foreign body I found a reddish colored cherry-stone, easy to cut, and within it was found the true kernel. Every part of the cherry-stone was permeated with that same abominable odor of the nasal discharge.

CAUSTIC PROPERTIES OF BROMIDE OF POTASSIUM.—M. Perrant states—*Archives Générales*, October—that he has obtained excellent results from the bromide of potassium, either in powder or in concentrated solution, in certain ulcerating tumors of the maxillary bones. Repeated cauterizations have destroyed the pathological tissues without causing pain in the adjacent parts.

# 𝔑otes and 𝔔ueries.

An Old Medical Thesis.—Many a medical student, who intends to be a candidate for graduation next spring, is just now vexing his mind with thoughts as to his thesis, and with work upon its preparation. The Christmas holidays will bring him little recreation, for all leisure time must be given to this labor, which he thinks so important. Lo! the hundreds of reams of paper that have been the receptacle of the crude thoughts of medical students, or of the carefully culled extracts from standard authors in medicine, and the thousands of bolts of ribbon, that have been consecrated upon the venerable altar of theses! Alas, if the anxious workers should know what fate awaited these best productions of their brain or pen, in all probability never entirely read—possibly not even glanced at—by any one but themselves, how quickly many an ambitious hope would perish. In our old medical colleges there are hundreds or thousands of these forgotten relics, time sprinkling dust upon their pages, eating away their once fair characters, and remorseless moths devouring their faded ribbons, or irreverent mice chipping silks and paper for beds of parturition and nurseries—masses measured by bushels, by boxes, by piles only fit to "be cast as rubbish to the void." And what has been will be. As are now the theses of past years, so will be those of 1877.

A few of our medical colleges have wisely abolished the rule requiring these exercises of the medical student's knowledge, or of his transcription, but most of them run in the old ruts, and uphold a "custom more honored in the breach than in the observance." And, therefore, the mass of our American medical students must pass into the state of doctorhood bearing the cross of a thesis as a mark of fitness.

But suppose their productions were required in Latin, how the anxiety we have alluded to would be turned into dire consternation. It is not probable that fifty per cent. of our medical students have ever studied Latin at all, and of that number not ten per cent. could claim to have been well instructed in Latin composition. It might be a comfort for those incompetent to endure this severe test, to think that possibly some of their teachers were not themselves latinists; indeed if the truth must be told, the doctor is to be envied who has not more than once found a professor in a medical college who was not even a respectable English scholar, who could neither speak nor write his mother tongue correctly, and who would be promptly rejected as a teacher in a common school. Medical schools now and then prove to be uncommon schools in one respect, at least.

We have been led into this train of thought by having before us a Latin thesis written in 1771, by Jonathan Elmer, M. B. Dr. Elmer was one of the few who, in Philadelphia, June 15, 1771, received the degree of M. D., Professors Morgan, Shippen, Kuhn and Rush, being members of the faculty. With only four theses a thorough perusal was highly probable, and with such a corps of teachers absolutely inevitable. The thesis being in Latin, *dissertatio medica inauguralis*, was no concealment to men of the classical learning these men had; some of them, indeed, having themselves testified that learning in Latin theses when graduated at the University of Edinburgh.

Dr. Elmer dedicated his dissertation to Benjamin Franklin, *viro perillustri*, and to his son, William Franklin, 'the Governor of New Jersey. He was then twenty-six years of age, but had already made some mark as a writer by a criticism, in 1767, of Dr. William Shippen's theory of the choroid being the immediate seat of vision; by an essay the same year on the motion of the heart; and by another on the different constitutions of the air and the diseases connected therewith, in 1769, for the American Philosophical Society, of which society he became a member in 1772, Dr. Franklin being the President. Knowing these facts in his history, we look with increased interest at this printed pamphlet of twenty odd pages of well-written Latin, in its production antedating five years the Declaration of Independence.

The subject of the dissertation, putting it in plain English, is the Causes and Remedies of Thirst in Fevers.

The author could draw not only from Hippocrates, Celsus, Boërhaave, Hoffman, Whytt, Sanctorius, Von Swieten, and Mead, but did not disdain Quintillian, Cicero, and Lucan.

We do not care to have our readers follow him through his ingenious reasoning as to the causes of thirst in fevers; the acrimony of the blood, and the increased irritability of the nervous system, playing an important part. When he comes to discuss treatment he observes: *Tolle causan, cessabit effectus,* in philosophia aphorismus est celeberrimus et argumento nostro aptissimus. Of course, therefore, remove the fever and the thirst will cease. But where this can not be done, or while it is being done, relieve the thirst.

First in his list of remedies he places pure water, and quoting from Baron Von Swieten's Commentaries a case of the successful use of this agent cold, gives a half-way endorsement of cold drinks in fevers—a wonderful admission and advance for 1771. Then follow as remedies acidulated drinks, acescent liquors, ripe fruits, neutral salts, anodynes, anti-spasmodics, and the list is concluded with *epithemata* and *enemata*.

Dr. Elmer returned to his Jersey home, and entered upon the hard life of a country practitioner, making his rounds on horseback. He became eminent in his profession. Dr. Rush remarked of him, that in "medical erudition he was exceeded by no one in the United States." He bore an honorable part in the Revolutionary struggle, and after a while, in consequence of feeble health, abandoned practice, and worthily filled important positions, both legislative and judicial—the former not only being state but national. Some of his descendants are now worthy successors to his medical honors and labors, living almost in the daily view of his grave, and working in the same field where he lived his useful life.

The earliest recollections of our own childhood are identified with the scenes where Dr. Elmer's professional labors had been performed; and in the dim distance of forty years the sluggish creek, the slow vessels following its wearisome windings, loitering, lingering in its seaward journey as if loth to leave its muddy banks, with their ragged edges black and shining with the tide's ooze; the level marsh, the sandy soil over or through which wheels noiselessly move; the peaceful calm and stillness; a few miles off the small, sleepy village of Greenwich, that in its infancy long ago was expected to be a formidable rival to Philadelphia, and that ought to be as memorable for the burning of obnoxious tea in 1774 as Boston for casting it into the water, and that is memorable as the birthplace of one of the most illustrious of physicians, Dr. George B. Wood—all seem more like a vision from "Dreamthorpe" than a page from memory. But we are wandering where our readers can not accompany us.

Have we any regrets that the Latin theses have ceased? Nay, let the English, too, become a thing of the past. But let us by no means discourage classical culture on the part of medical students. Greek and Latin they ought to have, not in full college measure, but only half, giving the rest of the time that ordinarily is devoted to these studies to German and French, and instead of the higher mathematics let them learn to use the pencil and the brush. When will wiser views of education take possession of teachers, and needed reforms be made? All grades of learning should be but stepping-stones in the individual's pathway—equipments for his special work in life. Those who are looking forward to the different learned professions, should have their educational paths diverge much sooner than they do. Life is short, and preparation for its special and highest duties should be commenced much earlier than it is. When the reform indicated is accomplished, we will have better preachers, better lawyers, and better doctors, even though the last may not be able to write inaugural dissertations in Latin.

INDIANA, ILLINOIS AND KENTUCKY TRI-STATE MEDICAL SOCIETY.—This society held its second annual meeting in the court-house in Vincennes, Ind., on the 21st, 22d and 23d of November. The attendance was good, and the papers read, and the discussions elicited by them, were very interesting.

Dr. Smith, of Illinois, read a paper on Ergot. This remedy, he stated, is becoming one of the most popular medicines in use; and that in 1807 he believed its use was as well understood as an excitant to uterine fibers, by many eminent practitioners, as it is at the present time. The writer gave his own and others' experience of ergot, in hastening tardy labor, preventing ante-partum and post-partum hemorrhage and abortion. After mentioning a number of diseases in which ergot is used, he said: "There is one other malady in which ergot has been given with results that would almost warrant me in ascribing to it specific powers. The malady I refer to is morning sickness of females. Some twelve years ago I ascertained that ergot would put a stop to this vomiting at any time from the first month to the end of pregnancy, and I have given it in every case I have had, and have not been disappointed in its use, nor have I ever seen labor induced when given for this trouble. The fluid extract is given in ten to fifteen drop doses three times a day."

An animated discussion arose at the conclusion of this paper as to how the remedy could both produce and prevent abortion, and as to its physiological action in arresting vomiting. The explanation was that ergot wisely given contracts bleeding vessels, thus removing the cause of abortion; when given in larger doses it induces contraction of the uterine fibers, and thus the expulsive overcomes the retentive force of the uterus. Its modus operandi in allaying vomiting was explained by its action upon the uterine fibers, contracting them and lessening the caliber of the vessels, relieving any irritation, and thus arresting the sympathetic symptom. An inquiry was made as to when one should cease administering ergot in a case of threatened abortion, so as to produce contraction of the vessels and not the expulsive efforts of the uterus.

The only rational answer given was to administer cautiously, see the patient frequently and watch carefully.

Dr. J. W. Compton, of Evansville, Ind., read a paper entitled "Solution and Absorption of Medicines: a plea for Digestible Medicines." It was asserted that many medicines have always been, and still continue to be, administered in indigestible forms, and that the gastric and intestinal juices are unable to dissolve them so that they may be absorbed and produce their intended therapeutical effect. This view was maintained by citing cases. One patient vomited twenty-four recently made quinia pills, which had remained in the stomach from one to five days; another passed pills from the bowels which had remained in the alimentary tract the same length of time. The conclusion was, that loss of time and loss of life must necessarily result on account of the administration of insoluble medicines.

Following this paper was one by Dr. Ireland, of Louisville, Ky., giving a thorough resumé of gynecology and obstetrics, out of which grew quite a discussion as to whether chloroform is applicable in all cases of labor, and also whether anæsthesia should be complete. Drs. Smith of Vincennes, Compton of Evansville, Mitchell of Terre Haute, and Professor Byford of Chicago, participated in the discussion. Drs. Smith and Compton, having met with frequent cases of alarming hemorrhage following the relaxation produced by this remedy, do not, as a rule, administer it unless requested by their patient. Dr. Mitchell had never seen hemorrhage follow the use of chloroform during labor. He had used it, until within the last few years, in almost every case occurring in his practice since 1849. He favored complete anæsthesia. Prof. Byford thought there was no danger when the agent was properly administered. His method was to give the patient a handkerchief saturated with chloroform, and allow her to hold it and inhale the vapor till her hand fell, thus giving it in a small quantity, not desiring to produce complete anæsthesia unless in the last stage of labor, or in a primipara, under which circumstances it did not usually decrease the expulsive force.

· In operations during labor it is necessary to produce complete anæsthesia. He had seen no bad effects follow the use of this agent, and in cases where the indications are that hemorrhage will occur, give ergot conjointly with the chloroform. Ether, if used, will have to be administered in larger quantity and for a longer time.

Dr. B. Tauber, Lecturer on Laryngoscopy, Rhinoscopy, and Diseases of the Throat, etc., in the Miami Medical College, Cincinnati, Ohio, read a paper "On the Local Treatment of the Larynx." He exhibited to the society the laryngoscopic case, devised by him, containing the instruments necessary to make topical applications to the larynx. It contains a three inch concave reflector, with Kræmer's head-band, six laryngoscopical mirrors, an insufflator, with Schrœtter curve, a brush for the larynx, and also one for the pharynx, a laryngeal cauterizer and sound, a tongue depressor, two powder-boxes, two bottles for solutions, and a crucible. Price, twenty-five dollars.

Dr. Byford delivered a most useful and interesting address upon the deleterious influences operating upon girls in the second decade of their lives. He first spoke of the importance of this period in life, of the differences, physical and mental, between man and woman, and of the peculiar responsibilities and sufferings belonging to the latter. Are the requirements which society makes of girls, as to education and as to social life, calculated to secure to them healthy womanhood? The girl at about ten years, needing abundant exercise in the open air, is kept in the house, arrayed in fine clothes, sent to school in a crowded room, overworked mentally, too great lessons are assigned, and she is admonished not to "loiter" on the way on her return home at the close of school. Physical development is thus arrested. At the age of fifteen she is sent to boarding-school to complete her education; fifty per cent. are more or less injured by the discipline inflicted, and often return home invalids. They are subjected to physical restraint; just so many hours are allowed for study, usually too many; so many for sleep, and usually too few; so many for walking, for singing, for praying, for attending church, but no time for unrestrained frolic and fun; their enjoyment is of a kind suitable for the aged, tending to curb the spirit of youth, and not to develop it. Who is to be blamed? Not the proprietors of boarding-schools; society demands it; the more rigid, the more popular the school.

The dress and toilet of the fashionable young girl are unnatural and unhealthy. She must be corseted, corded, bustled, pulled-back, padded, etc.; twenty-five per cent. of breathing-room is encroached upon; three-fourths of all the muscles are cramped. Society demands it; society is everybody. Does a healthy woman exist? Unless there is a reform in the hygienic conditions relating to woman, she will soon become "traditional," a thing of the past.

The accomplishments which society demands of a young lady are a smattering of French and Italian, music, dancing, etc.; all soon forgotten after marriage. Does it pay to compromise health for these attainments, if they be so classed? What is gained? Husbands. Young men allow their fancy to control them, and later regard woman as an expensive luxury. Give girls a sound education, and a change will take place in these matters. The men of this country work harder than those of any other country. With woman the reverse is true. Useful labor is the only source of true happiness. Reform the training of our youth; the laws of health should be made known to the masses. This knowledge must be disseminated by the medical man; he must remove these great evils, if it is ever done. As we value our services to our fellow-men, so we must expose the damaging habits of our fellow-men. We need a hygienic "Moody," one who, by his voice and pen, can arouse the masses to a sense of their duty, and bring them back to their original state of health and consequent happiness. Until we accomplish this, the medical profession can not claim that its mission is fulfilled.

The address of Dr. J. W. Thompson, of Paducah, Ky., the President of the Society, was chiefly historical, and was remarkable not merely for the learning displayed, but also for the philosophic spirit which informed it. He made a brilliant contrast between the fame of two of the most eminent of Kentuckians, the sage of Ashland and the surgeon of Danville—Henry Clay and Ephraim McDowell; that of the former gradually lessening with the lapse of years, from the fact that it was identified with policies and issues that were transitory in character; while that of the latter increases with the progress of medicine. McDowell, by devising and executing ovariotomy, has added three thousand years of active life to woman. We shall not attempt a synopsis of the address, which delighted all who heard it, and reflected so much honor upon the author and his state.

Dr. J. O. Stillson, Jr., of Bedford, Ind., read a paper on European Medical Education as compared with American. After a few introductory remarks, the following question was propounded: ''What, then, are our universities and their graduates in comparison with those of other countries? what is the standard of merit, the actual worth, the dignity of the practitioner in the United States, when compared with those of Germany or France?'' In order to answer this question it will be proper to consider the following points: First, the European student of medicine, when he enters and when he leaves lectures; second, the methods of teaching and the time required; third, the position of the doctor of medicine in society; fourth, is their example worthy of imitation, and have we a right to claim help from legislation in favor of whatever endeavors may be made? On the continent the learned professions stand on the same level, and are open only to students who pass rigid examinations in Latin, Greek, Mathematics, Chemistry and Natural Philosophy. The learned bodies are of one accord in insisting on thorough preparation before entering medical lectures. Professors Von Jaëger and Billroth have expressed themselves of this opinion, for the following reasons: ''By compelling the student to make preparation for the sake of admission as a matriculant, he acquires the methods and means of research in the ever-inexhaustible fields of science; he acquires the respectable habits of thinking and study, so neces-

sary to him as a student. Medicine thereby becomes attractive, and offers itself only to those who really have a talent and
a capacity for its pursuit. This advance having been made,
his progress in lectures is so much the more rapid that the
usual term of five years might be very much shortened, and
thereby be real economy in the end." There are those who
shrug the shoulders and shake the head at the thought of a
physician needing a liberal or classical education; and argue
that the medicine of the educated man will of itself fail, let it
do its best, when the grim specter of the hour-glass and scythe
crosses the threshold, and when the angels come for little
Johnnie; and that all the Latin of Celsus, or the Greek of
Hippocrates, will not throw off a diphtheritic membrane or
restore a too long neglected enteritis.

The requirements upon the continent are not so much those
of time nor age, but actual merit and ability to undertake
and prosecute the study of medicine. They are not averse to
the admission of ladies when they pass the same tests upon
the same terms as gentlemen. Ladies are seen as students
of medicine at Zürich, Berne, Göttingen, Vienna and Paris.
During the session just closed, there were twelve young lady
students at the Ecolé de Médecine in Paris, and one young
lady from America was interne at the Pitié.

The Doctor then enumerated the various examinations for
each year of the five years' course, and the laws which govern the practice of medicine in Europe; and stated that reform
in the teaching and practice of medicine in our own country
was necessary, for the scores of doctors graduated were far in
excess of the demand; and many were practicing within the
borders of Indiana who had never attended a medical lecture;
men who can not describe the simplest chemical reaction or
the most essential physiological law, whose knowledge of
therapeutics goes no farther than a half-dozen formulæ gotten
from some antiquated volume of Domestic Medicine, whose
libraries consist of a few volumes, and who rarely see a medical periodical. Medicine has to do with the dearest interests
of man, with the sorrows and joys of individuals and of house-

holds, with life and death. Let us, therefore, pray for reform in our colleges, reform in the profession, and for help from our law-makers, that candidates from all schools of medicine be required to obtain license to practice after having been subjected to trial before proper examining and licensing boards. The laws and principles of justice and humanity demand it; and the weal and woe of the many is of far more importance than that of the few.

Dr. William Dickinson, of St. Louis, Mo., a specialist in that city in ophthalmology for about twenty years, was present, and by invitation read a paper upon "The Functions and Affections of the Third Cranial Nerve." These were well illustrated by the narrative of a most interesting case, presenting all the chief manifestations of lesion of this nerve, viz., ptosis (paresis of the levator); strabismus divergens (paresis of the internal rectus); inability to rotate the globe upward (paresis of the superior rectus), or to rotate downward (paresis of inferior rectus); mydriasis (paresis of ciliary nerves, enervating the circular fibers of the iris); and loss of power of accommodation (paresis of ciliary nerves, enervating the ciliary muscle). The hearing of the patient, a man of about thirty years, was greatly impaired, and observably during the last year. The faculty of vision was not impaired, for when tested by means of a perforated card, he could read even the smallest print. The senses of taste and smell were unaffected, nor was the sensibility of the fifth cranial nerve, nor its motor functions, in any degree impaired. All the cranial nerves on the right side retained their normal exercise. He never had suffered from injury to the head, but had syphilis ten years since, and was then believed to have been cured; at least he has suffered from no subsequent symptoms. A brother, much his senior, died of apoplexy at about the age of fifty years.

The present affections supervened suddenly upon awakening one morning, after having contracted a severe cold; the ptosis first, and the others in immediate succession. Since all the subdivisions of the third nerve, including the inferior

oblique, were affected, and these divisions taking place immediately upon the escape of the nerve into the orbit, the lesion
most palpably resides in the sphenoidal fissure, or at some
point in its course between its origin in front of the pons
varolii and the sphenoidal fissure, or at its origin, probably in
the corpora striata. Of all the cranial nerves the third is more
liable to paresis or paralysis than any other, except the ab-
ducens (sixth); and of the former the superior branch anima-
ting the superior rectus is the one most frequently met with.
Rheumatism is the most fruitful cause of paralysis of the latter,
and is the most amenable to treatment by a brisk cathartic
and the ordinary antidotes of the general disease. The most
frequent of intracranial causes is pressure, from tumors of
great variety, especially those of syphilitic origin. Serous or
sanguineous effusions are also common causes; and if the
trunk be affected all its distributions must consequently suffer.
Among other causes may be enumerated effusion into the
ventricles, concussion of the brain, basilar meningitis, certain
narcotics, tubercular deposits, syphilitic nodes at the base of
the brain.

Peripheral disease from the last cause is the most common,
and there is generally orbital periostitis as well. Von Gräfe
thinks that about one-third of the cases of paralysis of the third
cranial nerve are due to this cause. Having made the diagnosis that pressure was the cause of the symptoms presented,
the treatment has been chiefly pot. iod. in full doses; hydg.
bichlo., hydg. prot. iod., and the use of galvanism, after the
manner employed by M. Benedikt, of Vienna. The continued
current is by him preferred, and must not be prolonged usually
beyond one-half minute at each sitting. He says: ''In most
cases a curative action was only produced when the excitement was relatively weak, and when no trace of muscular contraction was produced. The proper measure of the strength
of the current is always furnished by the sensitiveness of the
fifth pair, yet the intensity of it must be such as to produce
a slight sensation in the parts affected.''

In mydriasis the copper pole should be placed on the closed

eyelid, and the zinc pole over the neighborhood of the cheek-bone. In ptosis the copper pole may be either on the fore-head or may be applied by means of a short catheter-like rheophore to the mucous membrane of the cheek; while the zinc pole is drawn over the lid. And to act upon the internal rectus or superior oblique, the zinc pole must be drawn over the skin of the side of the nose, near the inner angle of the eye, while the upper is on the forehead or in contact with the mucous membrane of the cheek. Under this treatment, perseveringly pursued, the patient has nearly recovered from all the affections enumerated.

Dr. George W. Burton, of Mitchell, Ind., read a paper on Puerperal Peritonitis, taking the position that there was no such disease as a "specific puerperal fever;" that the doctrine of "epidemics" can not be sustained; that the disease so called may arise from a number of different causes, auto-genetic and hetero-genetic.

Interesting papers were read by Dr. Ezra Read (an abstract of which will be found in this number), also by Dr. J. B. Arm-strong, of Terre Haute, and by other members, a synopsis of which we were unable to get, except that of Dr. Read.

Resolutions were passed concerning the death of Dr. Hitt, of Vincennes, Ind. ; also a paper was read on the life and char-acter of Dr. Hitt, by Professor Byford. There were seventy-one members in attendance. The next meeting will be held at Evansville, Ind., commencing on the third Tuesday in Oc-tober, 1877.

The following officers were elected for the ensuing year: President, Dr. W. H. Byford, Chicago, Ill. ; first Vice Presi-dent, Dr. J. L. Dismuke, Mayfield, Ky. ; second Vice Presi-dent, Dr. G. G. Barton, Washington, Ind. ; third Vice Presi-dent, Dr. H. H. Deming, Peoria, Ill. ; Recording Secretary, Dr. G. W. Burton, Mitchell, Ind. ; Corresponding Secretary, Dr. F. W. Beard, Vincennes, Ind. ; Treasurer, Dr. A. Patten, Vincennes, Ind.

The society is emphatically a working body; and if this meeting is a criterion of what may be expected in the future, their meetings will be anticipated by the profession with much pleasure and practical interest. We are indebted to Dr. T. C. Donnell for the interesting report given of this meeting.

To Subscribers.—We want to say a few earnest words to you in this final number of the American Practitioner of the year 1876, words which we hope you will carefully read, faithfully remember, and promptly act upon. Some of you have followed the fortunes of our journal, first and fast friends, from its origin in 1866 as the Cincinnati Journal of Medicine. Others more recent in accession, we can not doubt are equally faithful.

More than thirty thousand dollars has been expended upon the journal in the eleven years of its existence. We wish we could say that subscribers and advertisers had paid all this. But we know, to our sorrow, this can not be said.

Shall not the journal, in its twelfth year, be freed from all pecuniary embarrassments? Few medical journals in the United States have a larger circulation, the most not near so large. But we are sure this circulation can be much increased. Not a single subscriber but can add one or more to the list. Will you not, in this month of December, make the hearts of Editors and Publishers happy by promptly remitting your own, and the subscription of some friend, for 1877? Do this, and the monthly issue of the American Practitioner, instead of being fifteen hundred or two thousand, as in·1876, will be twice that in 1877.

If any subscriber has become delinquent through negligence, let him repent and remit.

In attention to subscriptions, we trust contributions will not be forgotten. Every one meets with cases in practice that will interest and instruct the great body of the profession, and let him bring them forward for such interest and instruction.

We confidently appeal to subscribers thus to help us, and to help us now, and we promise in return our best gratitude, and the best work in your behalf we are capable of doing.

HARVEY AND CESALPINUS.—HISTORICAL FRAGMENT BY DR. SAMPSON GAMGEE.—"Who discovered the circulation of the blood?" is a question to which the majority of well-informed persons would answer, "William Harvey." Nor would the reply of professed physiologists, in this country at least, be different. Professor Ceradini, of Genoa, has recently* published an elaborate monograph advocating the prior claims of Cesalpinus, and, after honoring him with a monument in Rome, it is proposed to insert a tablet to his honor on the portals of the University of Pisa, in which he taught for some years before he took up his residence near the Vatican, as physician to Pope Clement VIII. This plea on behalf of Cesalpinus is only a revival. Moreri,† so early as 1732, urged on his behalf, that "it would be robbing him of a very precious glory not to mention that he had known the history of the circulation of the blood."

A few dates are here essential. Cesalpinus was born at Arezzo in Tuscany in 1519, and died in Rome in 1603, his chief works having been published from 1569 to 1593. William Harvey was born in 1578, went to Padua in 1598, returned to England in 1602, was appointed lecturer on anatomy and surgery to the College of Physicians in 1615, published his "Exercitatio Anatomica de Cordis et Sanguinis Motu" in 1628, and died in 1657. Thus Cesalpinus's work was accomplished before Harvey's had begun.

Cesalpinus knew the pulmonary circulation, as Servetus and Realdus Columbus had done before him, though independently. Cesalpinus first employed the word "circulation," and certainly went far, by experimenting and reasoning, to demonstrate the greater, or systemic, as well as the lesser or pulmonary circulation. Considering, as the Italians claim, that their illustrious countryman had proved and knew the whole doctrine, the question remains, Did the world learn it from him? or did the great truth, so far as he was concerned, lay dormant in his folios until exhumed by the learned of succeeding gen-

* Lancet, November 4, 1876, p. 663.

† Le Grand Dictionnaire Historique; nouvelle et dernière édition, en 10 vols. Paris, 1732. Art. Cesalpinus. Vol. II, p. 675.

erations? That Harvey's essay is a model of clear and concise reasoning has never been questioned, and Buckle's* claim is incontestably a valid one—that the discovery of the circulation of the blood was first made *perfectly intelligible* by Harvey.

Cesalpinus was a great naturalist, who spent his long life as a student.† Harvey toiled through a busy, restless life, and fought his way, winning renown for himself and his doctrines by energy of resolve and eloquence of pleading. If he was not by his contemporaries reputed to be the author of the doctrine of the circulation, how was it that, after he left Padua, the great theme of discussion was "De Paradoxo Harvejano?" Why did John Rolan, the learned professor of the University of Paris, specially confute him? Why did Leichner in 1646 entitle his essay "De Motu Sanguinis, Exercitatio Anti-Harveiana?" Why did Zacharia Sylvius, in 1648, say, in the preface to his edition of Harvey's work, "*Novam* quandam et *inauditam* de motu cordis et circulatione sanguinis sententiam?"

It seems to me unanswerable that, by the verdict of his contemporaries and immediate successors, Harvey was the reputed discoverer of the circulation; they, the world, learned the new doctrine from him.

If this be conceded, the question is still open, Did Harvey discover all the doctrine he taught? He gives credit to Galen, to Realdus Columbus, and a few others, but makes no mention of Cesalpinus; but there is no proof that he knew his works. Certain it is that great works were published in Italy at that time, which obtained very little circulation and remained comparatively unknown, to-wit, Ruini's "Anatomia del Cavallo," which contains a most extraordinary sketch of the circulation of the blood. This marvelous passage, so far as I know, never attracted attention until my friend Professor Ercolani, of Bologna, set it forth with justifiable national pride.

* Miscellaneous and Posthumous Works, Vol. II, p. 203. London, 1872.

† "La vie du botaniste d'Arezzo s'est écoulée toute entière dans le silence du cabinet." (Nouvelle Biographie Universelle. Paris: Firmin Didot, 1854. Vol. IX, p. 439.)

That Harvey was, however, under greater obligation to his predecessors than he had the candor to acknowledge, there is some reason for believing. In the first paragraph of his intro duction he says: "As we are about to discuss the motion, action, and use of the heart and arteries, it is imperative on our part to state what has been thougbt of these things' by others in their writings, and what has been held by the vulgar and by tradition, in order that what is true may be confirmed, and what is false set right by dissection, multiplied experience, and accurate observation." In this admirable spirit of intended candor did Harvey begin his work; he concluded it in a very different disposition, if we are to judge from the last para- graph in his dedicatory letter to his very dear friend, Dr. Ar- gent, the excellent and accomplished President of the Royal College of Physicians. "I had no purpose to swell this trea- tise into a large volume by quoting the names and writings of anatomists, or to make a parade of the strength of my mem- ory, the extent of my reading, and the amount of my pains; because I profess both to learn and to teach anatomy, not from books but from dissections; not from the positions of philosophers, but from the fabric of nature; and then because I do not think it right or proper to strive to take from the ancients any honor that is their due, nor yet to dispute with the moderns, and enter into controversy with those who have excelled in anatomy, and been my teachers."

I submit, with much deference, it was not a question of de- tracting or disputing, but of doing justice. To his president Harvey disavows the study of literature; in his introduction, he as clearly tells us that he purposes devoting himself to working up the literature of his subject. International jeal- ousy apart, it would be most interesting to follow up the steps of the great discovery—one of the most gradual of any of the great discoveries of truth. The present fragment is only put forth as a suggestive contribution, but not without hope that some leisure may allow of its development, if it should be deemed worthy of it. (Lancet.)

DESCRIPTION OF AN ENLARGED CLITORIS.—Scultetus, in his Armamentarium Chirurgicum, 1666, refers to enlargement of the clitoris in the following strong language: Enorme, inutile, molestum et damnificum generi fœmino clitoridis incremen-tum. As we read this passage, after having stopped to ad-mire "damnificum" in such connection, we could not help thinking of Virgil's description of the Cyclops, Æneid, book third—

Monstrum horrendum, informe, ingens, cui lumen ademptum—

and we wondered if Scultetus had not this description in his mind, when he was accumulating such vigorous adjectives for clitoral hypertrophy.

MEDICAL EDUCATION.—Dr. McCall Anderson, in an address on this subject, published in the Lancet, November 11, 1876, says: Since the days of my student life great changes have taken place in the prescribed curriculum and in the subjects of examination; and although I am far from thinking that these are in every way to be commended, I am free to admit that, in two respects at all events, they are on the side of progress, namely, as regards the institution of a preliminary examination, and the giving of greater prominence to the practical departments. That a preliminary examination was urgently called for few can doubt, but if proof is required, it may be found in the answers given to the following questions submitted to candidates by one of the examining boards:

Question—What is meant by the antiquity of man? An-swer—The wickedness of men.

Q.—The "Letters of Junius?" A.—Letters written in the month of June.

Q.—The Crusades? A.—A war against the Roman Catho-lics during the last century.

Q.—The first meridian? A.—The first hour of the day.

Q.—To speak ironically? A.—To speak about iron.

Q.—A Gordian knot? A.—The arms of the Gordon family.

Q.—The Star Chamber? A.—Place for viewing the stars.

Q.—To sit on the Woolsack? A.—To be seated on a sack of wool.

Q—A solecism? A.—A book on the sun.

Q.—The year of jubilee? A.—Leap-year.

We could have appreciated this last answer more heartily had it emanated from one of the female medical students.

CPSIA information can be obtained
at www.ICGtesting.com
Printed in the USA
BVHW082056201118
533619BV00011B/1587/P